Progress in Drug Research
Fortschritte der Arzneimittelforschung
Progrès des recherches pharmaceutiques
Vol. 44

Progress in Drug Research
Fortschritte der Arzneimittelforschung
Progrès des recherches pharmaceutiques
Vol. 44

Edited by / Herausgegeben von / Rédigé par
Ernst Jucker, Basel

Authors / Autoren/ Auteurs
George deStevens · V. Zingel, C. Leschke and W. Schunack
Paul D. Hoeprich · Richard M. Schultz · P.K. Mehrotra, Sanjay Batra and
A.P. Bhaduri · Anil K. Saxena and Mridula Saxena.

1995   Birkhäuser Verlag
            Basel · Boston · Berlin

Editor:

Dr. E. Jucker
Steinweg 28
CH-4107 Ettingen
Switzerland

© 1995 Birkhäuser Verlag, P.O. Box 133, CH-4010 Basel, Switzerland
Softcover reprint of the hardcover 1st edition 1995
Printed on acid-free paper produced from chlorine-free pulp

ISBN-13:978-3-0348-7163-1   e-ISBN-13:978-3-0348-7161-7
DOI: 10.1007/978-3-0348-7161-7

Contents · Inhalt · Sommaire

Foreword

Volume 44 of "Progress in Drug Research" contains six reviews and the various indexes which facilitate its use and establish the connection with the previous volumes. The articles in this volume deal with problems of drug discovery during "The golden age of drug research", with histamine H_1-receptor agonists; with antifungal therapy; with antifolates in cancer therapy; with menses-regulating agents and with developments in anticonvulsants.

In the 36 years that PDR has existed, the Editor has enjoyed the valuable help and advice of many colleagues. Readers, the authors of the reviews, and last but not least, the reviewers have all contributed greatly to the success of this series. Although the comments received so far have generally been favorable, it is nevertheless necessary to analyze and to reassess the current position and the future direction of such a review series.

So far, it has been the Editor's intention to help disseminate information on the vast domain of drug research, and to provide the reader with a tool with which to keep abreast of the latest developments and trends. The reviews in PDR are useful to the non-specialist, who can obtain an overview of a particular field of drug research in a relatively short time.

The specialist readers of PDR will appreciate the reviews' comprehensive bibliographies, and, in addition, they may even get fresh impulses for their own research. Finally, the readers can use the 44 volumes of PDR as an encyclopedic source of information.

It gives me great pleasure to present this new volume to our readers. At the same time I would like to express my gratitude to the authors who willingly accepted the task of preparing extensive reviews. My sincere thanks also go to Birkhäuser Verlag, and, in particular to Mrs. L. Koechlin and Mssrs. H.-P. Thür, E. Mazenauer and G. Messmer. Without their personal committment and assistance, editing PDR would be a nearly impossible task.

Basel, May 1995   DR. E. JUCKER

Vorwort

Der vorliegende 44. Band der Reihe «Fortschritte der Arzneimittelfor-schung» enthält sechs Beiträge sowie die verschiedenen Register, welche das Arbeiten mit diesem Band erleichtern und den Zugriff auf die vorher-gehenden Bände ermöglichen.

Die Artikel des 44. Bandes behandeln wiederum verschiedene aktuelle Themen dieses komplexen Forschungsgebietes, wobei jedoch der erste Beitrag einen interessanten Rückblick auf die Arzneimittelforschung des «goldenen Zeitalters» vermittelt. Die übrigen Beiträge befassen sich mit Histamin H_1 Rezeptoren, mit Pilzerkrankungen und ihrer Therapie, mit einigen Entwicklungen im Gebiet der Krebserkrankungen, mit neueren Möglichkeiten der Empfängnisverhütung und schliesslich mit Problemen der neueren Antikonvulsiva.

Seit der Gründung der Reihe sind 36 Jahre vergangen. In dieser langen Zeitspanne konnte der Herausgeber immer auf den Rat der Fachkollegen, der Leser und der Autoren zählen. Manche Anregung empfing ich auch von den Rezensenten. Obwohl die grosse Mehrzahl der Besprechungen positiv war, stellt sich doch immer wieder die Frage nach dem Sinn und Zweck der «Fortschritte».

Nach wie vor ist es unser Ziel, neueste Forschungen in Form von Übersich-ten darzustellen und dem Leser auf diese Weise zu ermöglichen, sich verhältnismässig rasch und mühelos über bestimmte aktuelle Richtungen der Arzneimittelforschung zu informieren. Er erhält damit die Möglichkeit, sich in diesem komplexen und rasant sich entwickelnden Fachgebiet auf dem laufenden zu halten. Dem Spezialisten hingegen, bieten die «Fort-schritte» eine wertvolle Quelle der Originalliteratur dar, erlauben ihm Vergleichsmöglichkeiten, und sie können u.U. seine eigenen Untersuchun-gen befruchten. Für alle Leser stellen die «Fortschritte» mit ihren umfang-reichen Registern eine nützliche Quelle von enzyklopädischem Wissen dar, so dass das gesamte Werk auch als Nachschlagewerk dienen kann.

Zum Gedeihen dieser Reihe haben vor allem die Autoren beigetragen; ihnen allen sei hier gedankt. Dank gebührt auch dem Birkhäuser Verlag, insbe-sondere Frau L. Koechlin und den Herren H.-P. Thür, E. Mazenauer und G. Messmer.

Basel, Mai 1995   DR. E. JUCKER

Progress in Drug Research, Vol. 44 (E. Jucker, Ed.)
© 1995 Birkhäuser Verlag, Basel (Switzerland)

Heterocyclic diversity: The road to biological activity

By George deStevens[1]

The Charles A. Dana Research Institute, Drew University, Madison, New Jersey, USA

---

[1] This scientific autobiography is dedicated to my wife Ruby, who for 45 years has been a staunch supporter of all my endeavors.

1   Prologue

In a previous review [1] written for this series I presented an account of some of my experiences during my 25-year tenure with CIBA and then CIBA-Geigy. These reflections emphasized primarily my role in management, especially as it related to my responsibilities as Executive Vice President and Director of Research, and the background related to decisions concerning the research and development process and the decision-making which led to bringing certain medicinal products into the physician's armamentarium. Several cogent factors associated with organizational matters and operational principles were also stressed. These and other thoughts were presented in a retrospective account and served to summarize my career as a manager of large multi-faceted research and development programs. On reflection, what experiences prepared me for this role?

On discussing this question with the Editor of this series, we agreed that a review describing my own personal scientific research programs from their conception through execution, with emphasis on the ideas, motivations and circumstances associated with this search for molecules with potential biological activity might offer some insight to the resolution of the above query.

Obviously each generation of chemists uses the tools and methods available at the time to achieve his/her goal. In this review, I would like to show how certain chemistry evolved in my laboratory, the problems that surfaced, how they were solved and which potential and actual new drugs were discovered, keeping in mind that at the time there were no computers, MS and NMR were in their infancy, combinatorial chemistry libraries were unimaginable, molecular biology was not yet an established discipline and consequently, the cloning and expression of receptors and the use of recombinant DNA for the synthesis of enzymes and other important proteins were not available. My generation used intuition, imagination and great experimental skill to synthesize *grams* of material for biological testing. These thoughts will be elaborated in more detail in the pages to follow. Thus, let us embark on this road to biological activity by starting at the beginning.

Having survived 10 months of intensive combat in Europe (1944–1945) with the 42nd Rainbow Division (7th Army), I returned to civilian life in April 1946 to continue my education at the leading bastion of Jesuit education in the U.S., Fordham University. Eventually, I did my doctoral research with Professor F.F. Nord, who had been a staff member of the Kaiser Wilhelm Institut at Berlin-Dahlem until the Nazi Laws for the

Restitution of the Civil Service forced him to leave Germany. My work involved the enzymatic isolation of native lignin from bagasse (sugar cane fiber) followed by structural studies. Nord's research programs strongly emphasized biochemical approaches to organic chemistry problems. Consequently, my training was firmly grounded in learning the fundamentals of not only organic chemistry, but also of biochemistry, enzymology and microbiology. These principles were incorporated in the laboratory. Thus, sterilized bagasse preparations were inoculated under microbiological conditions with a brown rot fungus, *Lentinus lepideus*. Over a period of time, depletion of the cellulose content caused liberation of chemically unaltered lignin. Structural studies on this native lignin gave much information on the molecular composition of the natural polymeric substance. This work led to the publication of 15 peer reviewed papers [2]. However, the work was filled with a certain amount of frustration since lignin is a high molecular weight amorphous material and consequently, sharply defined crystalline materials were difficult to come by.

Thus, on completion of my thesis research, I was quite convinced that my next scientific endeavor would be directed toward the synthesis of small crystalline molecules. In February of 1953, I joined the Photo Records Division of the Remington Rand Corporation. Therein I became involved in the synthesis of heterocyclic compounds to be used in the preparation of cyanine dyes, which are essential in sensitizing silver chloride in emulsions used in the photographic process.

Cyanine dyes are prepared by the reaction of a 2-methyl-N-quaternarized heterocycle with the appropriate condensation agent. These dyes contain at least two auxochromic nitrogen atoms, the one ternary and the other quaternary, the one nitrogen lying in one heterocyclic nucleus and the other lying in the other heterocyclic nucleus, the two nitrogens being connected by a conjugated carbon chain. This resonating system acts as a chromophore and the intensity of color which these substances elicit (as measured in wave lengths in the ultraviolet and the visible) is a consequence of the degree of unsaturation in the molecule and the nature of the two heterocyclic nuclei.

Thus, the synthesis of new heterocycles is the source of new and potentially more useful cyanine dyes. This was the initial impetus for my lifelong interest in heterocyclic chemistry. Some of the heterocycles I prepared were 2-methyl-5,6-dihydro-4-cyclopentathiazole [3], 2,7-dimethyl-4-isopropyl-4,5,6,7-tetrahydrobenzothiazole [4], 2-methyl spiro (4,5)decano (6,7d)thiazole [5], 2-methyl-4,5-dihydro-3-naphthothiazole [6], 2-methyl-5,6,7,8-

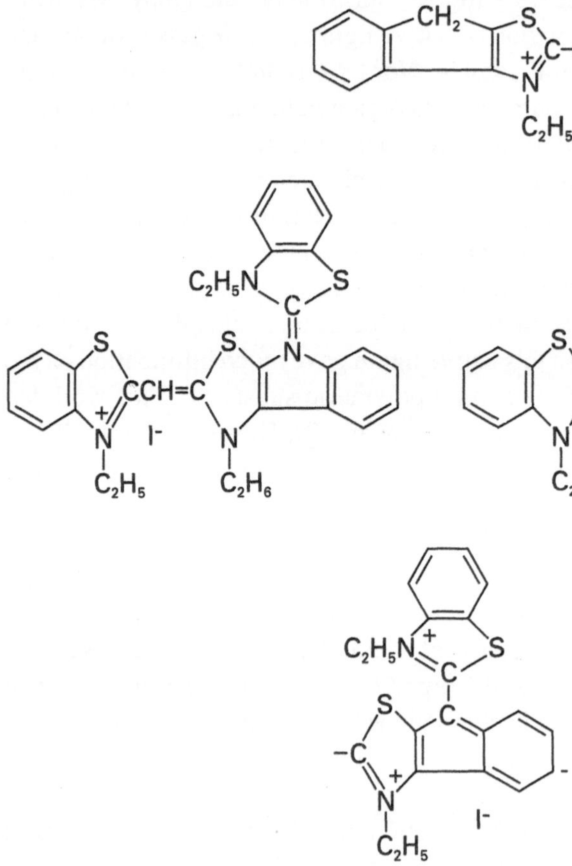

Fig. 1
Cyanine dye containing indenothiazole moiety

tetrahydro-4-cycloheptathiazole [7], 2-methyl spiro (4,4)nonano (1,2d)thia-
zole [8], 2-methyl-4,5,6,7-tetrahydro benzoxazole [9] and 2-methyl -
(2,1d)indenothiazole [10]. The indenothiazole [11] was unique in that it
gave cyanine dyes in which two modes of resonance were operating, one
through the normal cyanine type structure and the other through the chromophore resulting from condensation at the activated methylene group of
the indeno moiety. The unusual property of these dyes was that they
exhibited two absorption maxima because of the double chromophore as
shown in Figure 1. This type of phenomena had not been noted heretofore
in cyanine dyes.

Although this was intriguing research, it was apparent to me that I was very much more interested in pursuing a career in the life sciences. By the Spring of 1955, a number of important discoveries had come from the laboratories of the pharmaceutical industry; prednisone, aureomycin, streptomycin, the sulfa drugs, antihistamines, chlorpromazine and reserpine. Such outstanding contributions to medicine fired the imagination of this young researcher to seek to become a part of this exciting endeavor. Consequently, I called Professor Nord and told him of my plans. He immediately suggested that I write to Dr. Emil Schlittler, formerly of CIBA, Basel, and recently appointed Director of Chemical Research of CIBA Pharmaceutical Company in Summit, New Jersey. My interview with Schlittler went well and so in the Summer of 1955, I became a member of the newly formed organic synthesis group in Summit. According to Schlittler, my mission was straight-forward. *Do excellent chemistry and do my best to try to discover biologically active substances.*

In those days the biologists had set up general screens in animals (rodents, dogs) for evaluating certain potential therapeutic effects; e.g., CNS (stimulation, depression, anxiety), hypertension, diuresis, analgesia, antiparasitics, antivirals, etc.). The biologists also committed a considerable amount of their time to develop new animal models simulating a human disease. Since these were all *in vivo* general screens, it was necessary to submit 2 to 3 grams of test compound for a complete primary evaluation. If activity of note was discovered, then additional quantities were required and, as a rule, the structure activity relationship (SAR) study followed.

I point this out since today the focus of drug discovery is on biochemical targets. Mechanism-based testing initially involves *in vitro* methods which measure enzyme inhibition, receptor agonism or antagonism and ion channel modulation. Under these circumstances *only milligram* quantities of substance are required for testing and to facilitate matters mixtures can be tested from which the active agent can be identified, all of which would not be realizable in an intact animal.

Be that as it may, let us return to the golden age of drug discovery.

2   Analgetics

The first project I was assigned to was the search for a non-narcotic analgetic. Little did I realize the enormity of the challenge. The question was, where to begin? A study of the literature at the time indicated that the pyrazolones, aminopyrine and phenylbutazone, represented a class of compounds which exhibited analgesia without causing addiction. Their shortcoming was their propensity for causing agranulocytosis. It occurred to me that other heterocyclic systems might share the analgetic effect without causing the deadly side effect. To maintain the structural logic of my approach, I decided that the best chance for finding analgetic activity was to construct a heterocycle in which a carbonyl was juxtaposed between a nitrogen and another hetero atom in a 5-membered ring system.

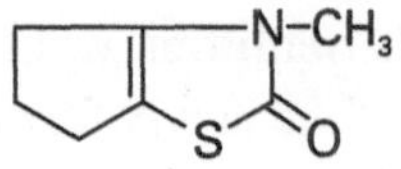

Fig. 2
Su-4027

One of the first compounds I submitted for testing was Su-4027 (Figure 2). This substance proved to be very effective in all animal analgetic tests, but exhibited a narrow therapeutic ratio. Nevertheless, it served to confirm my hypothesis of the structural requirements. Various synthetic pathways lead-

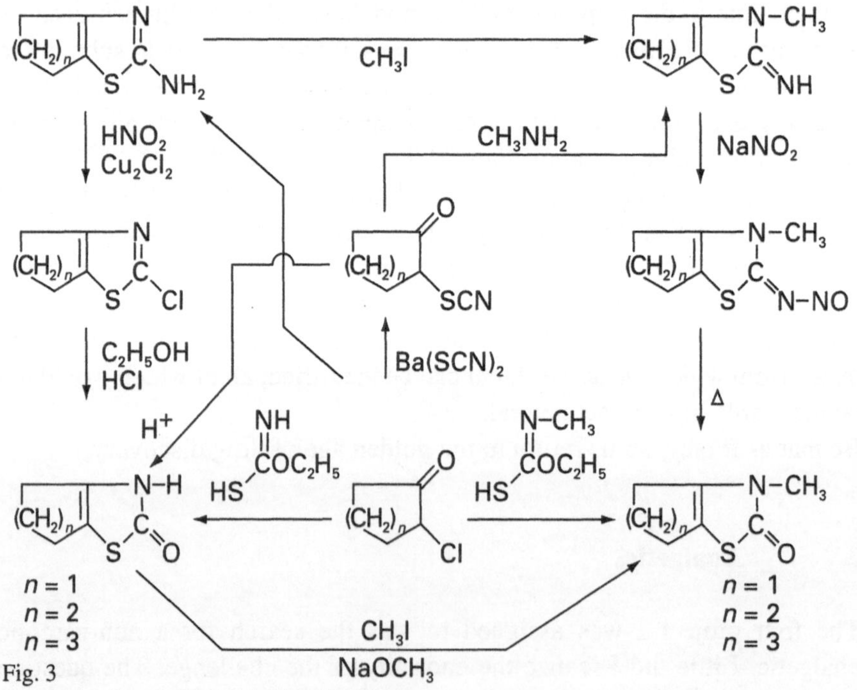

Fig. 3
Synthesis of cycloalkeno-d-thiazoline-2-ones

ing to various cycloalkenothiazoline-2-ones [12] are shown in Figure 3. An extensive SAR program revealed the following:

1. Fusion of the cycloalkeno group to the thiazoline-2-one was necessary. The 6-membered ring compounds were more active than the 5- or 7-membered compounds. Aromatic (benzothiazolin-2-one) or 4,5-disubstituted compounds were inactive.
2. Substitution on nitrogen other than methyl increased toxicity.
3. Replacement of a methylene group in the cycloalkane portion with oxygen (pyran), sulfur (thiopyran) or nitrogen (piperidine) reduced activity.

The above-described thiazoline-2-one derivatives also appeared to be lipophilic. Thus, a variety of basic derivatives was synthesized to increase water solubility and thus increase absorption and possibly expand the therapeutic ratio (Figure 4).

Su-4432 [13] was synthesized as shown in Figure 5. This substance was found to be almost as potent as morphine in experimental animals and was devoid of addiction potential. In addition, it had a wide therapeutic ratio. It was submitted for evaluation in humans, and at doses of 100 mg per day in 100 patients for 6 months, it proved to be equivalent to codeine in reducing

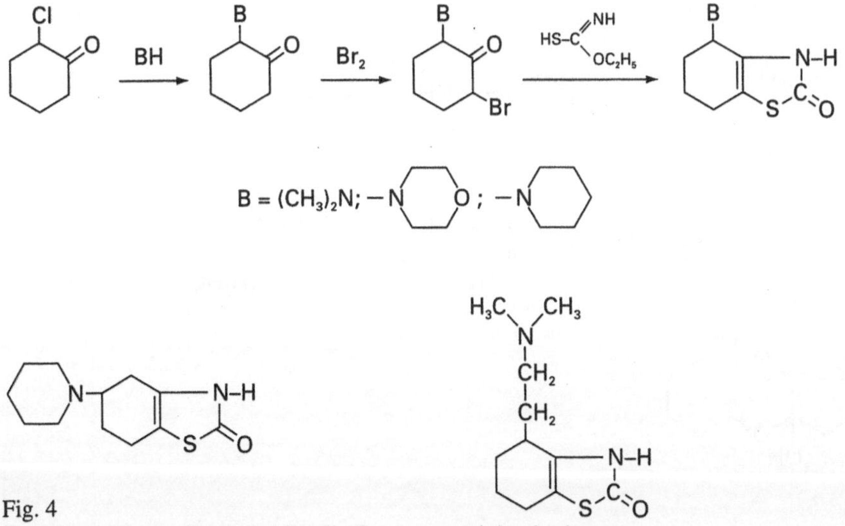

Fig. 4
Synthesis of cycloalkeno-d-thiazolin-2-ones containing basic groups

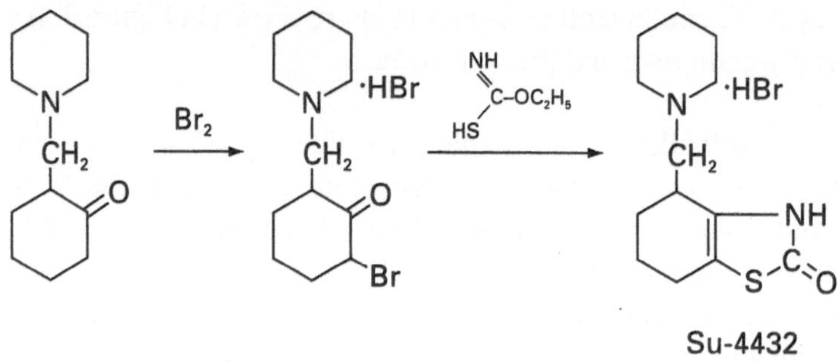

Fig. 5
Synthesis of Su-4432

pain. As plans were being finalized to expand clinical trials to Phase III, a report came in indicating that over a period of time in a small number of patients Su-4432 caused inflammation of the optic nerve, a side effect which was not noted in animal toxicity studies. Fortunately, this effect was reversible. Su-4432 was removed from further clinical trials and for obvious reasons this series was no longer pursued.

Ongoing at the time was the synthesis of other heterocycles containing structural features similar to 4,5,6,7-tetrahydrobenzothiazoline-2-one. As shown in Figure 6, the synthesis of 4,5,6,7-tetrahydrobenzimidazole-2-one and 4,5,6,7-tetrahydrobenzoxazoline-2-one was straight-forward, although surprisingly the reaction of ethyl carbamate with the dimer of α-hydroxy

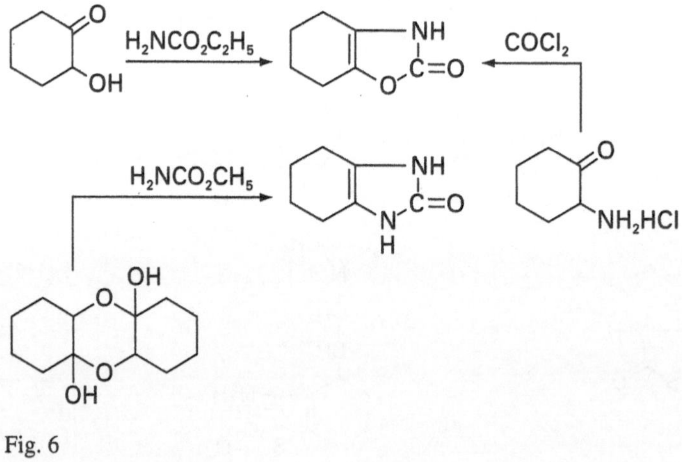

Fig. 6
Synthesis of tetrahydrobenzoxazole-2-one and tetrahydrobenzimidazolone

cyclohexanone gave a 90% yield of the imidazolone [14]. These substances had analgetic activity in animals comparable to the prototype, but were quite toxic. Thus, replacement of sulfur with nitrogen or oxygen was not advantageous.

A further variation of the prototype thiazoline-2-one was the thiazin-2-one [15]. The corresponding compounds were prepared through the condensation of the appropriate α-halocyclic ketone with thioglycolamide (see Figure 7). However, these substances were completely devoid of activity, thus re-enforcing the original hypothesis that the carbonyl group should be between a nitrogen and another hetero atom within the cyclic system.

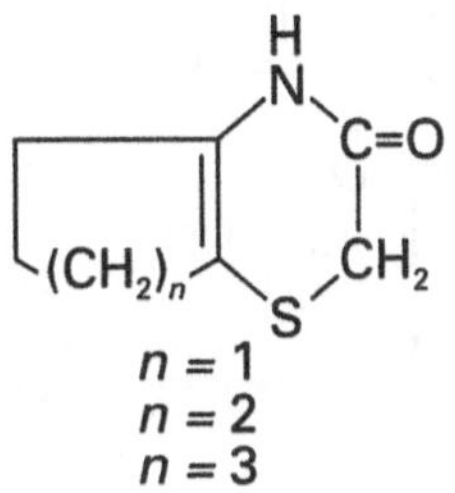

$n = 1$
$n = 2$
$n = 3$

Fig. 7
Cycloalkenothiazinones

Finally, it was of interest to prepare some 5,6,7,8-tetrahydroquinazolines and 6,7-dihydro-5-cyclopentapyrimidines [16] (See Figure 8 for the latter series). None of the substances prepared within this class exhibited analgetic properties. However, a surprising chemical transformation was noted. The 1-methylmercapto-quinazoline (5,6-bicyclic) derivative was transformed to the 5,5-bicyclo compound, 5,6-dihydro-4-cyclopentaindazalone. The mechanistic rationale for this transformation is shown in Figure 9. Strong infrared absorption bands at 2700–2200 cm^{-1} in addition to several chemical transformations in which the 3a position of the heterocycle and the basic N_1-position were selectively substituted supported the assignment of the dipolar or zwitterion form to this type of compound [17].

At this point, I wish to acknowledge the significant input and contribution of Louis Dorfman, at the time (1950–1980) Director of Analytical and Spectral Research at CIBA, in this and other discussions in this review relating to the assignment of structure based on the spectral properties of the molecules under study.

Another approach in the search for a non-narcotic analgetic was to seek to improve upon the properties of propoxyphene (Figure 10); that is, increase potency, reduce toxicity and minimize the addiction potential. Initially,

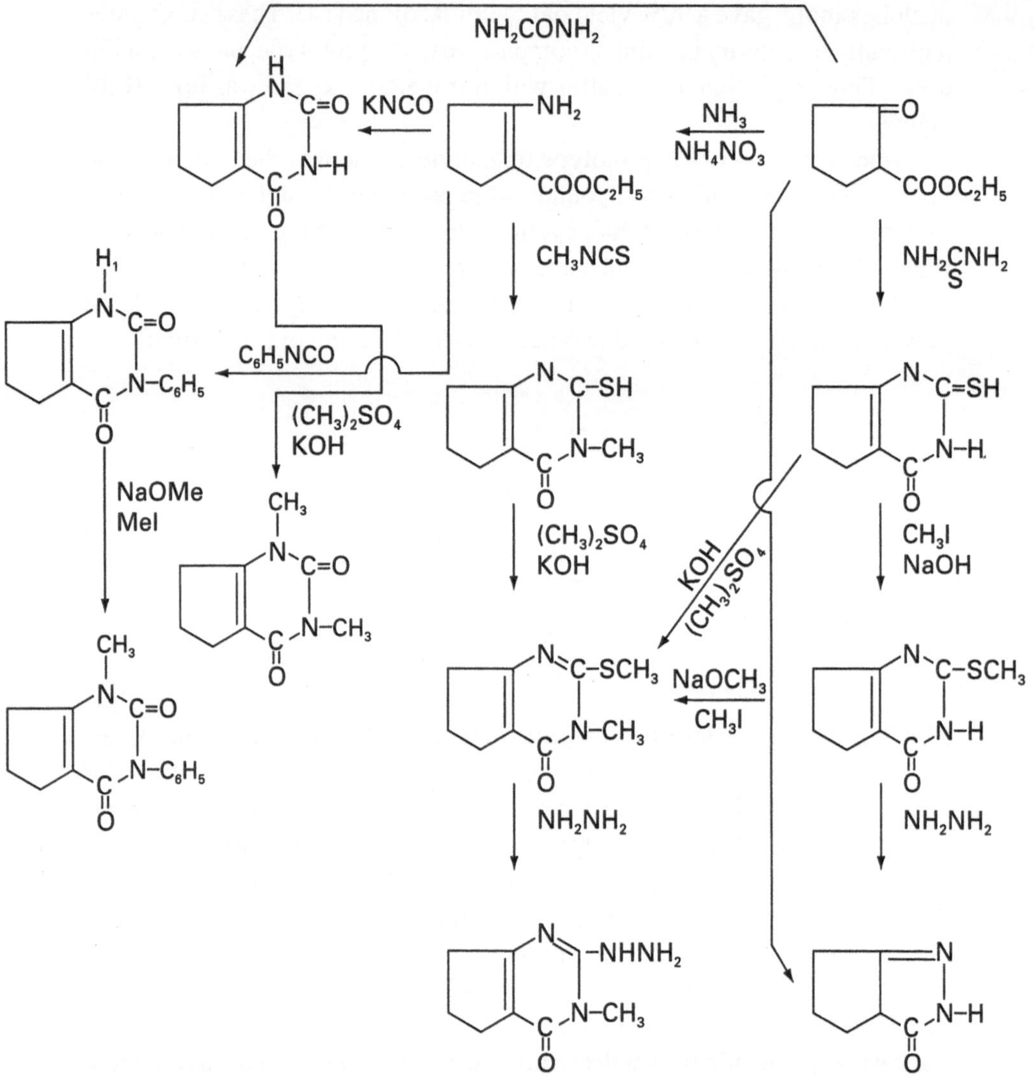

NH_2CONH_2

KNCO

$-NH_2$

$COOC_2H_5$

NH_3
NH_4NO_3

$COOC_2H_5$

CH_3NCS

C_6H_5NCO

$(CH_3)_2SO_4$
KOH

NH_2CNH_2
S

$N-C_6H_5$

NaOMe
MeI

CH_3

CH_3

CH_3

$N-C_6H_5$

$(CH_3)_2SO_4$
KOH

KOH
$(CH_3)_2SO_4$

$N=C-SCH_3$ NaOCH$_3$
CH$_3$I

$N-CH_3$

$N=C-SCH_3$

$N-H$

NH_2NH_2

CH$_3$I
NaOH

NH_2NH_2

$-NHNH_2$

$N-CH_3$

Fig. 8
Synthesis of various cyclopentapyrimidines

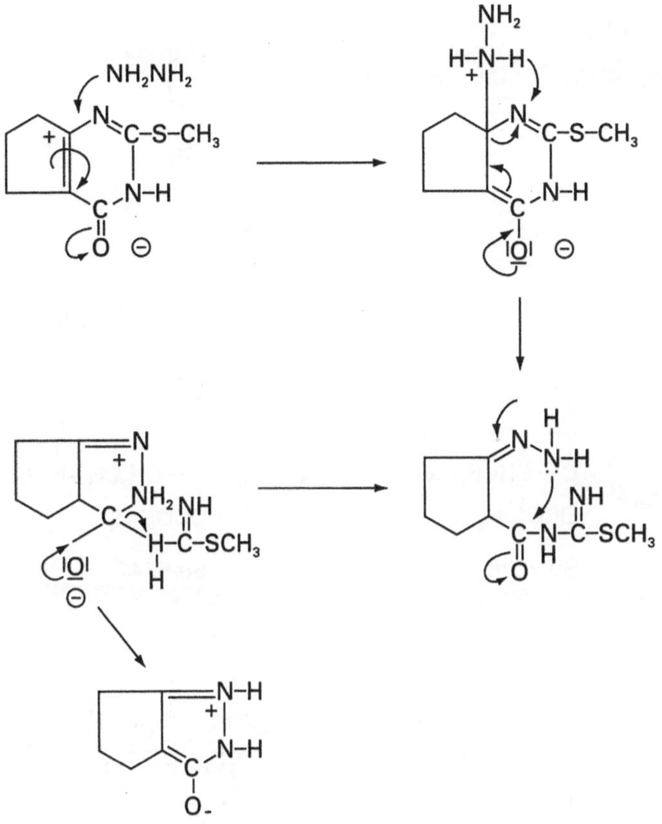

Fig. 9
Mechanism for formation of cycloindazalone

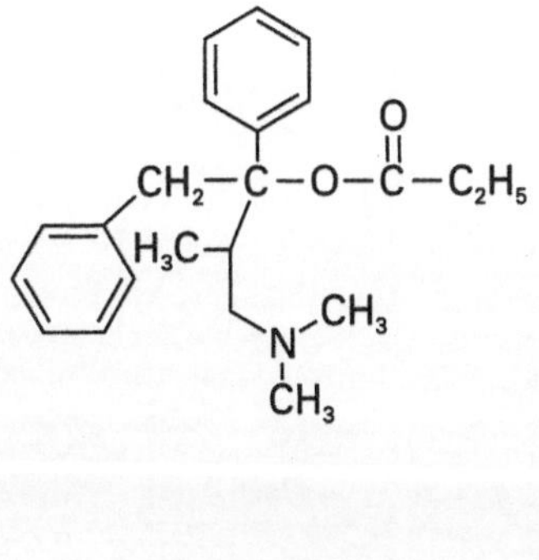

Fig. 10
Propoxyphene

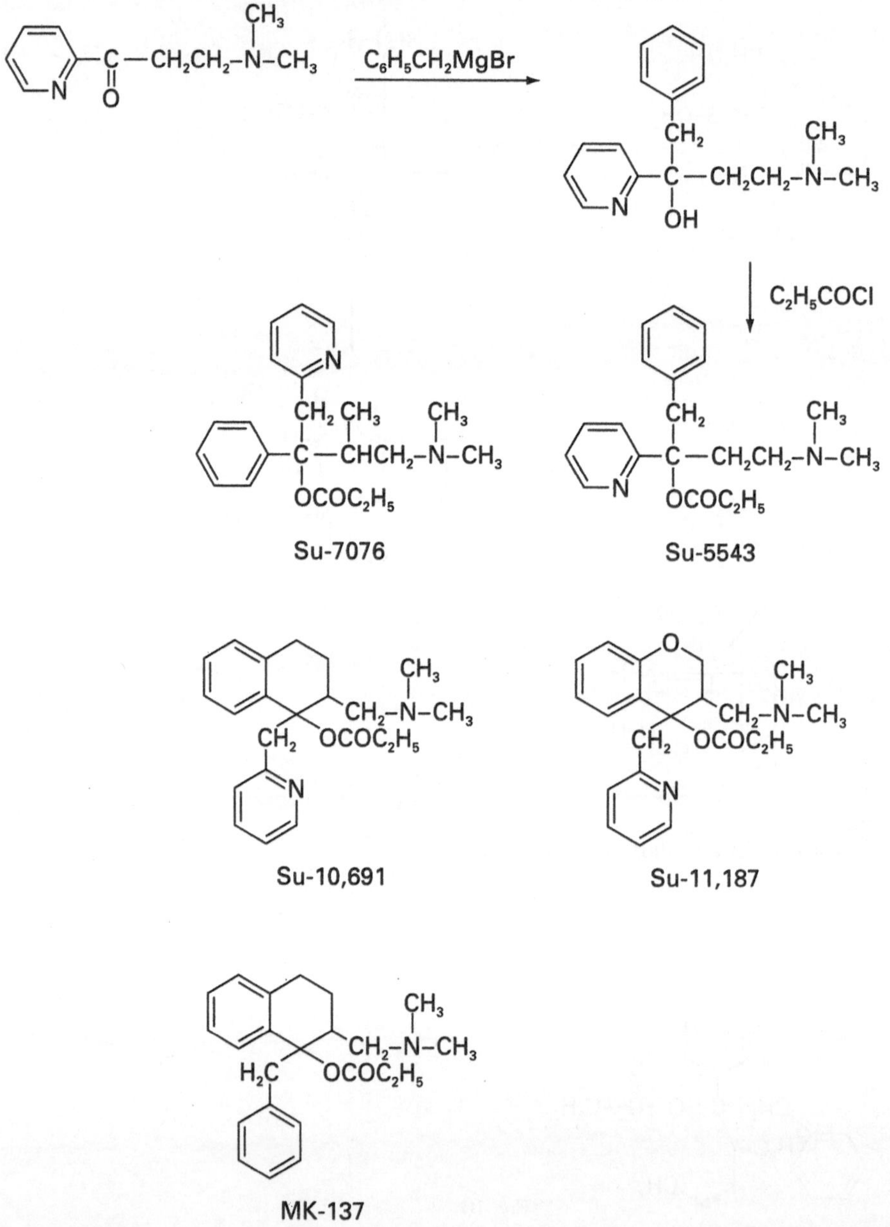

Fig. 11
Modifications of propoxyphene

Dr. Charles Huebner and I decided to prepare a pyridine analog of pro-poxyphene. Much to our surprise, Su-5543 was completely devoid of analgetic effects (Figure 11). However, the reversal of the aromatic group, giving rise to the 2-picolyl derivative (Su-7076), yielded an analgetic twice as potent as propoxyphene. The ameliorating effect on analgetic activity due to the incorporation of a 2-picolyl group in the molecule had not heretofore been reported. This unexpected finding then prompted us to prepare substances with restricted conformation, thus enabling the molecule to fit more exactly on the receptor. We synthesized a large number of tetralin, chromane and thiachromane analogs of Su-7076. The most effective of these cyclic analogs were Su-10,691 and Su-11,187, the former was five times more potent than morphine, whereas the latter was approximately equal to morphine when tested in experimented animals [18].

Concomitant with our findings, Patchett [19] of Merck, Sharp and Dohme reported the analgetic potency of MK-137 to be about one-half that of morphine.

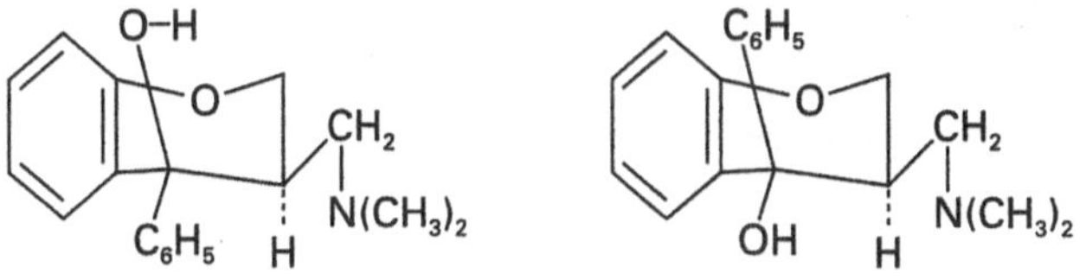

Fig. 12
Stereochemistry of chromane alcohol racemates

In the chromane series, we were able to demonstrate unequivocally that of the two diasterioisomeric alcohols shown in Figure 12, on reaction with propionyl chloride, the isomer in which the hydroxyl and the adjacent hydrogen are in the transdiaxial conformation yielded exclusively the dehydration product ($\Delta^{3,4}$ chromane) whereas the other isomer gave rise in 95% yield to the analgetically active compound. The other active substances were conformationally related to the chromane series through chemical and spectral (NMR) comparisons.

In spite of the high potency and rapid onset of action of these cyclic substances, unfortunately they also were antagonized by nalorphine, eliciting high addiction liability and tolerance. For this reason, further development was terminated.

These two major programs in analgetics taught me how difficult medicinal research really is. It was certainly exciting and fulfilling to find through experiment that one's hypothesis in planning the design of compounds for a particular biological effect indeed was realized and did give rise to the desired action in animals. However, to then translate this to a medicinal product was quite another matter.

Suffice it to point out that several years later, some of these ideas were incorporated in a joint project with Dr. Neville Ford and Dr. Richard Carney. Our objective was to synthesize a rapidly acting phenylpropionic acid. It was reasoned that the pharmacokinetic properties of the prototype sub-stance could be markedly improved by incorporating an amino group in the molecule to simulate an amino acid and thereby increase water solubility and thus enhance oral absorption. Our rationale was eventually realized with the NDA approval of pirprofen [20] (Figure 13) by the FDA and its introduction in several countries in Europe and Japan as an effective analgetic with a rapid onset of action.

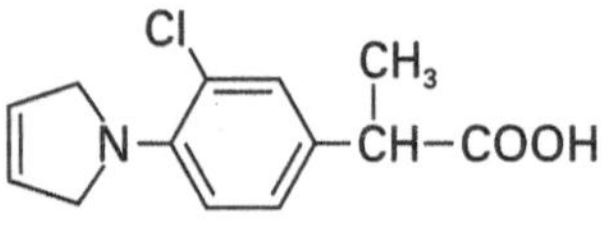

Fig. 13
Pirprofen

3   Diuretics

As my research on cycloalkeno-d-thiazolin-2-ones was coming to a close, Emil Schlittler called me into his office and told me that, although I should continue to pursue my work on analgetics, he also felt that I should start to think about cardiovascular problems. I had already been doing some ex-ploratory work on sulfonylureas as hypoglycemic agents. He said he was more concerned with the importance of CIBA staying at the forefront in the antihypertensive field. His discovery of reserpine and its complete pharma-cological evaluation by Professor Hugo Bein of CIBA, Basel, had been responsible for the company's strong position in cardiovascular medicine. In the ensuing days I reflected on our conversation and particularly about the recent report (1957) by Novello and Sprague [21] of Merck, Sharp and Dohme on the synthesis of disulfonamides and especially chlorothiazide. Chlorothiazide was important since it was the first non-mercurial orally active diuretic drug not dependent for its activity on carbonic anhydrase inhibition, such as acetazolamide. Its potential as an antihypertensive agent was generally recognized, although its high dose (250–500 mg twice daily) and some tendency at high doses for eliciting carbonic anhydrase inhibition were considered limiting factors at that time.

My initial approach was to synthesize a disulfonamide structurally related to saccharin (Figure 14). Thus, mchlorotoluene disulfonamide was oxidized to the corresponding saccharin derivative, which was then catalytically reduced to the fully saturated cyclic system. These showed some degree of diuretic activity, but clearly were not comparable to chlorothiazide. However, it did not escape my attention that the fully saturated compound still had diuretic effects.

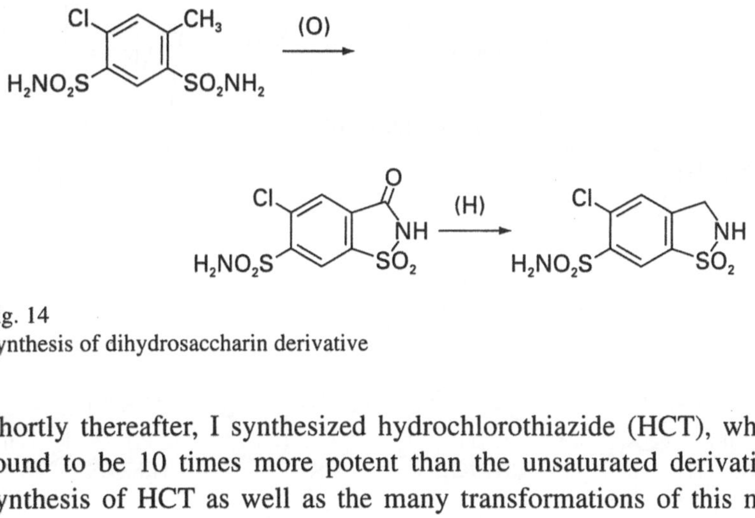

Fig. 14
Synthesis of dihydrosaccharin derivative

Shortly thereafter, I synthesized hydrochlorothiazide (HCT), which was found to be 10 times more potent than the unsaturated derivative. The synthesis of HCT as well as the many transformations of this molecule through methylation and acetylation at the 2,4 and 7 positions, as well as the oxidative transformation of these derivatives to the corresponding chlorothiazide derivatives are outlined in Figure 15. Also, a wide variety of derivatives was prepared by reaction of 5-chloro-2,4-disulfamyl aniline with different aldehydes. Working with my collaborator, Dr. Lincoln Werner, and two assistants, Sal Ricca and Angelina Halamandaris [22–24], over a period of 3 years, we prepared over 400 derivatives of this class from which a number of significant factors evolved (Figure 16).

1.   Whereas in the chlorothiazide series, only the prototype showed any significant activity, in the hydrochlorothiazide series substitution in the 2- or 3-position of the benzothiadiazine 1,1-dioxide gave rise to

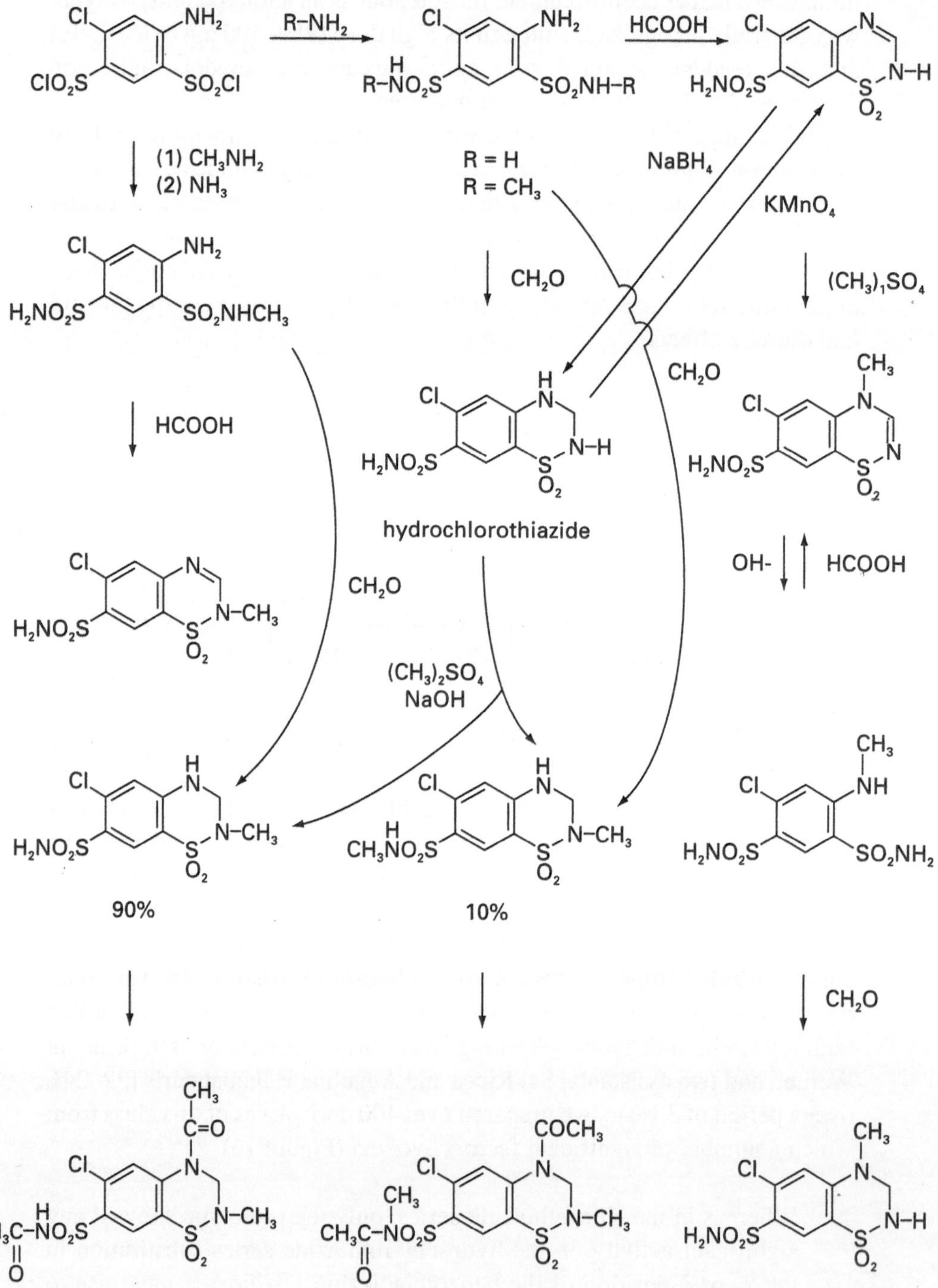

R–NH₂ → R-NH2 reaction scheme

(1) CH₃NH₂
(2) NH₃

R = H
R = CH₃

HCOOH

NaBH₄

KMnO₄

CH₂O

(CH₃)₁SO₄

HCOOH

CH₂O

hydrochlorothiazide

CH₂O

OH-   HCOOH

(CH₃)₂SO₄
NaOH

90%

10%

CH₂O

Fig. 15
Hydrochlorothiazide synthesis and transformations

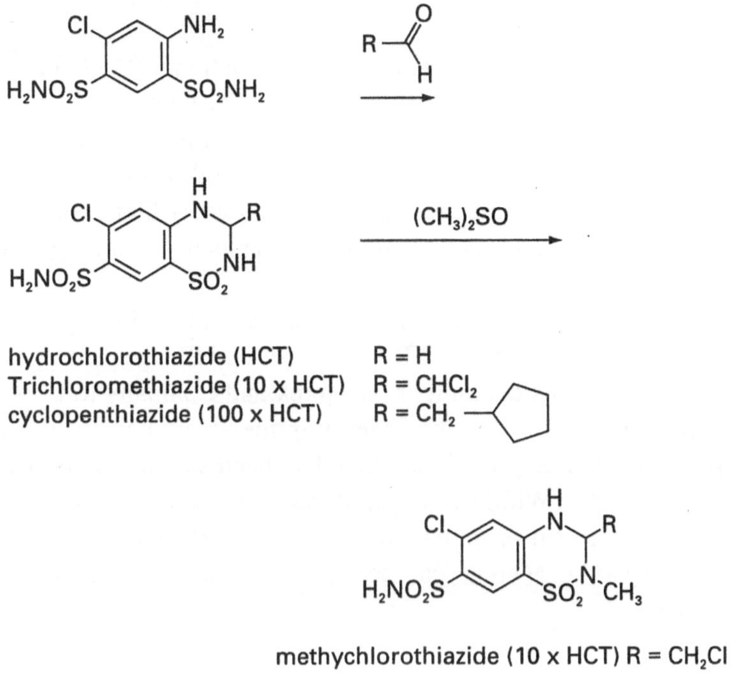

hydrochlorothiazide (HCT)   R = H
Trichloromethiazide (10 x HCT)   R = CHCl₂
cyclopenthiazide (100 x HCT)   R = CH₂ —

methychlorothiazide (10 x HCT) R = CH₂Cl

Fig. 16
Synthesis of potent hydrochlorothiazide derivatives

representative derivatives with equivalent or greater potency than hydrochlorothiazide.

2. The members of the hydrochlorothiazide series showed greater chloride excretion and lesser carbonic anhydrase inhibition than chlorothiazide.

3. A lipophilic substituent at position 3 gave very potent compounds. Cyclopenthiazide is 100 times more potent than hydrochlorothiazide and appeared to be longer acting (up to 18 hours).

In any event, hydrochlorothiazide was introduced into medical practice in February 1959 and within a short time became the drug of choice in the treatment of mild hypertension. And today, some 37 years after its discovery, it is still widely prescribed as first step therapy for mild hypertension. In addition, it is used in fixed combination with all the other antihypertensive drugs. The other thiazide modifications, most of which are covered in the CIBA patent [24], have also been used. However, none has achieved the status of standard therapy in cardiovascular medicine such as hydrochlorothiazide has.

Anecdotally, in the Fall of 1958, I attended the International Biochemistry Conference in Vienna. At the reception, Dr. Max Tishler, President of Merck, Sharp and Dohme Laboratories commented to Emil Schlittler that he had heard that CIBA had synthesized hydrochlorothiazide. Schlittler confirmed this and called me over and introduced me to Tishler, who said, "Well done. I am sorry you are not on my team." Thus began a long-term friendship.

An interesting vignette associated with hydrochlorothiazide involved our legal department. On the morning CIBA received its NDA approval, our corporate counsel called his counterpart at Merck and Company to inform him of the approval. On learning this, Merck immediately began to push FDA for approval of their application, which had been submitted almost 6 months later than CIBA's. Within 10 days, Merck also received approval of their NDA and CIBA lost its competitive advantage. When asked why he called his counterpart at Merck, our corporate executive said, "It was professional courtesy."

4   Modified natural products

4.1   Polycyclic indoles

During the 1950's and 1960's CIBA was well known for its strong research programs in alkaloids and steroids. In such an environment, it was inevitable that discussions amongst chemists from the natural products and the synthetic groups often could be quite animated and gave rise to a plethora of ideas. In studying the structures of these natural substances, it was my perception that straight-forward group modifications of the molecule in question would not really lead to a drug of real value. For example, many variations of reserpine were prepared, but none offered any advantage over the original substance. I was more intrigued in synthesizing from basic starting materials heterocycles which would bear some skeletal resemblance to the natural substance, but with unique and unusual features. In so doing, it was hoped that the resulting new compounds would have potentially useful biological properties.

Our initial efforts were directed towards synthetic analogs of the indole alkaloid Rutecarpine (Figure 17) about which very little was reported in the

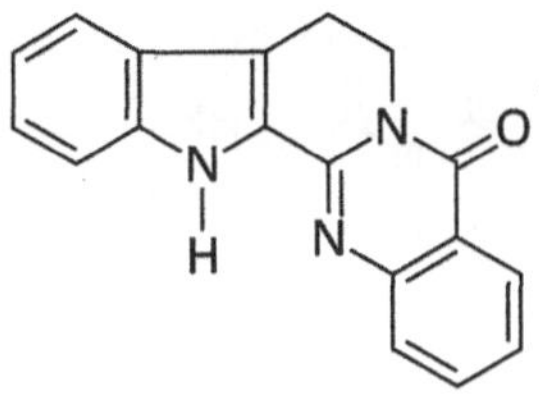

Rutecarpine 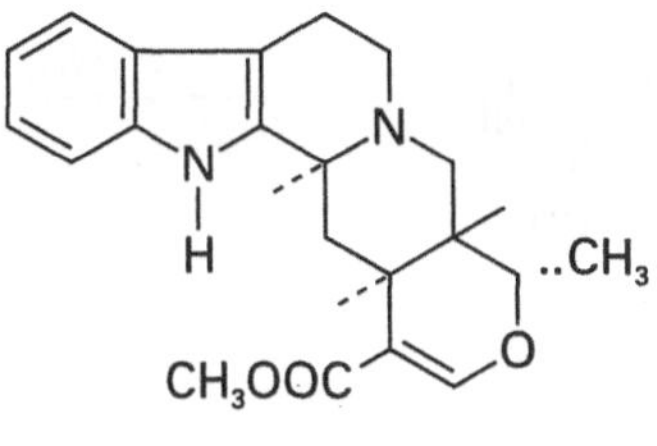   Ajmalicine

Fig. 17
Structure of Rutecarpine and Ajmalicine

literature in 1961. It was the goal of this phase of our research to prepare tetracyclic indoles [25] with a hetero atom in ring D other than N_b. In Figure 18 are shown the transformations which were carried out to prepare the 3-methylaza and the 3-oxaindolo [2,3a] quinolizine derivatives. In each case, substitution at position 4 in ring D was controlled by the aldehyde used in this intramolecular Mannich reaction.

Further modifications of ring D of these tetracyclic indoles were concerned with compounds containing a hetero atom at position 2 of indole [2,3a] quinolizine. In Figure 19 is shown the series of reactions which gave rise to the ring D piperazine and D morpholine analogs [26]. Of these substances, only the piperazine derivative showed a good antihypertensive effect in the renal hypertensive rat. However, this effect was of short duration. Substitutions at the 2-aza-position with various substituents did not result in compounds with sustained blood pressure lowering effects.

Now it appeared that an obvious extension of this work would be to prepare pentacyclic indoles containing heteroatoms in ring E. Ajmalicine (see Figure 17), containing oxygen in ring E, served as a model. Representative examples of some new pentacyclic indoles are shown in Figure 20.

The pentacyclic compound in which ring E contains the pyrimidine ring system had a marked calming effect on experimental animals. In some respects it was pharmacologically similar to reserpine. However, its site of action appeared to be supraspinally, primarily in the brain stem. Unfortunately, on repeated dosing this substance caused severe sedation. An extensive structure-activity study was not successful in separating the two effects. The stereochemistry of these polycyclic indoles is straight-forward, as shown in Figure 21. Since we have in a majority of the compounds only one asymmetric center (i.e., C_{12b} in the tetracyclic series and C_{13b} in the

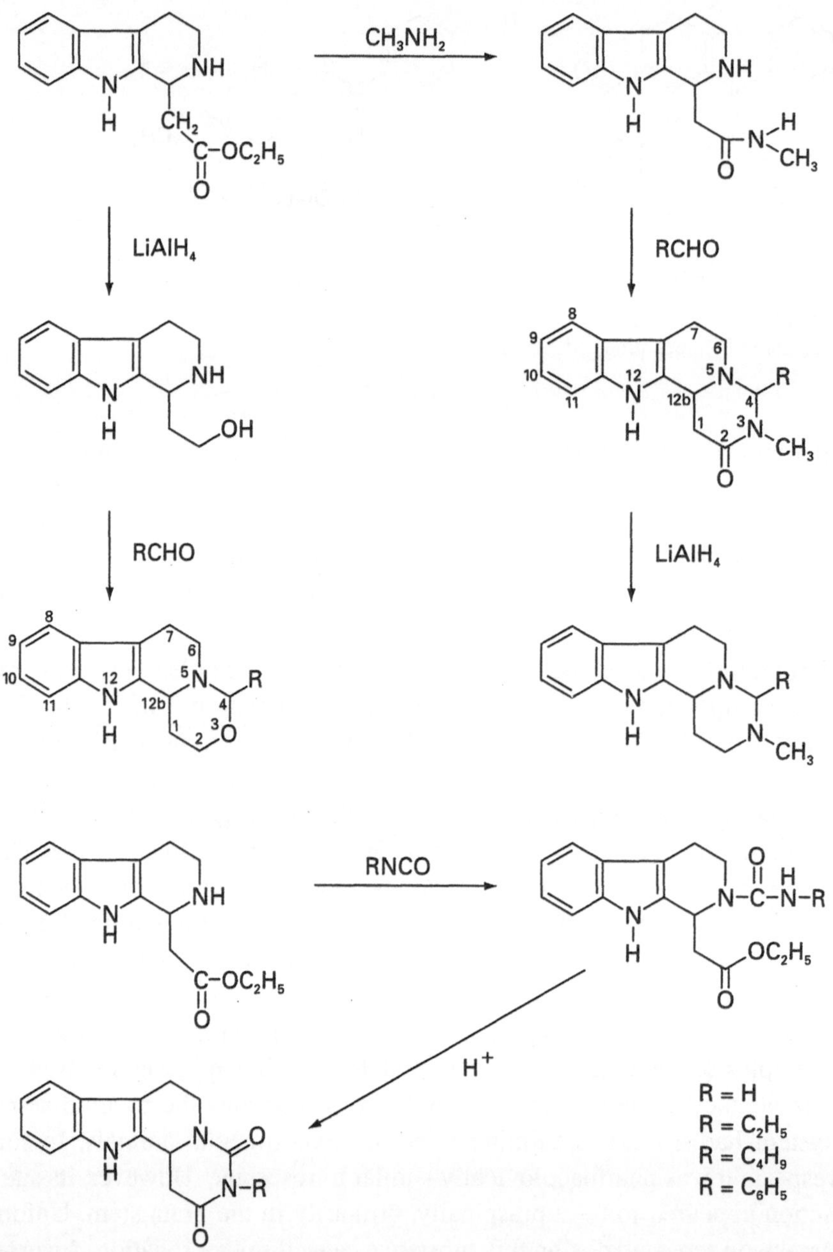

Fig. 18
Synthesis of tetracyclic indolo [2,3-a]-quinolizines

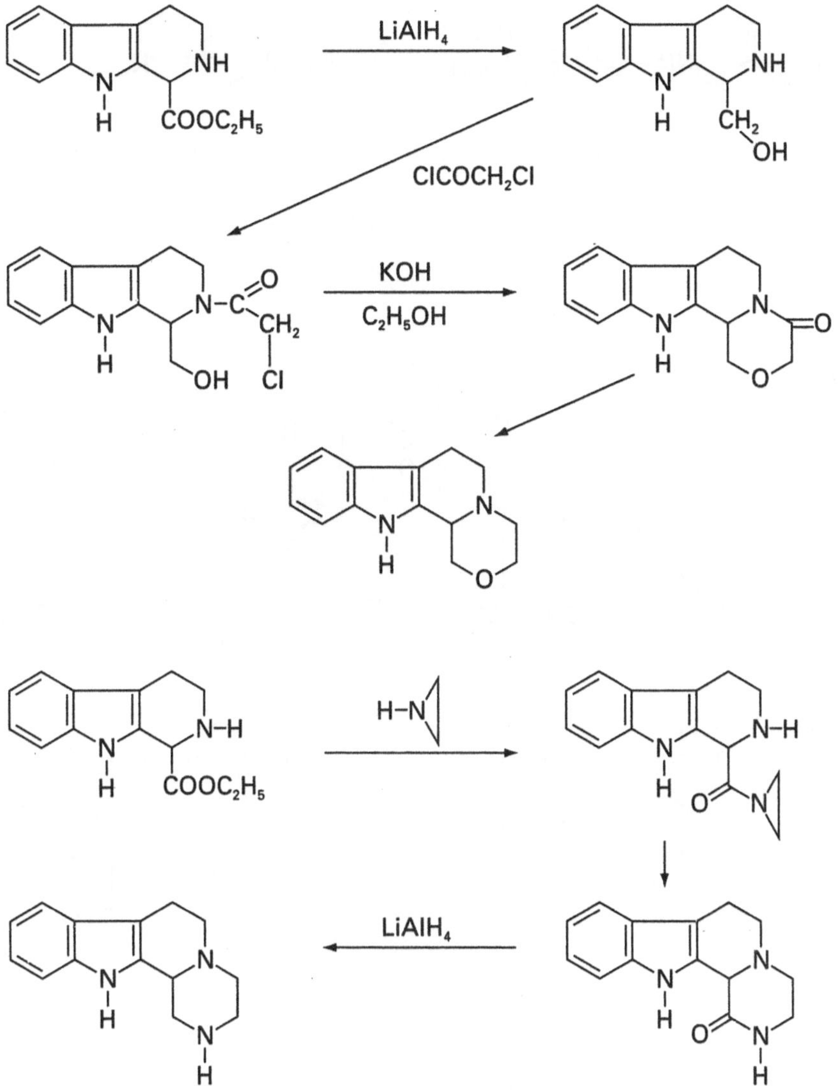

Fig. 19
Synthesis of tetracyclic indolo [2,3-a]-quinolizines

pentacyclic group), the hydrogen at this carbon is either in the axial or equatorial conformation.

The AA' conformers are thermodynamically more stable than B and to substantiate the axial conformation of the hydrogen at the asymmetric center infrared absorption spectroscopy was used with advantage. The

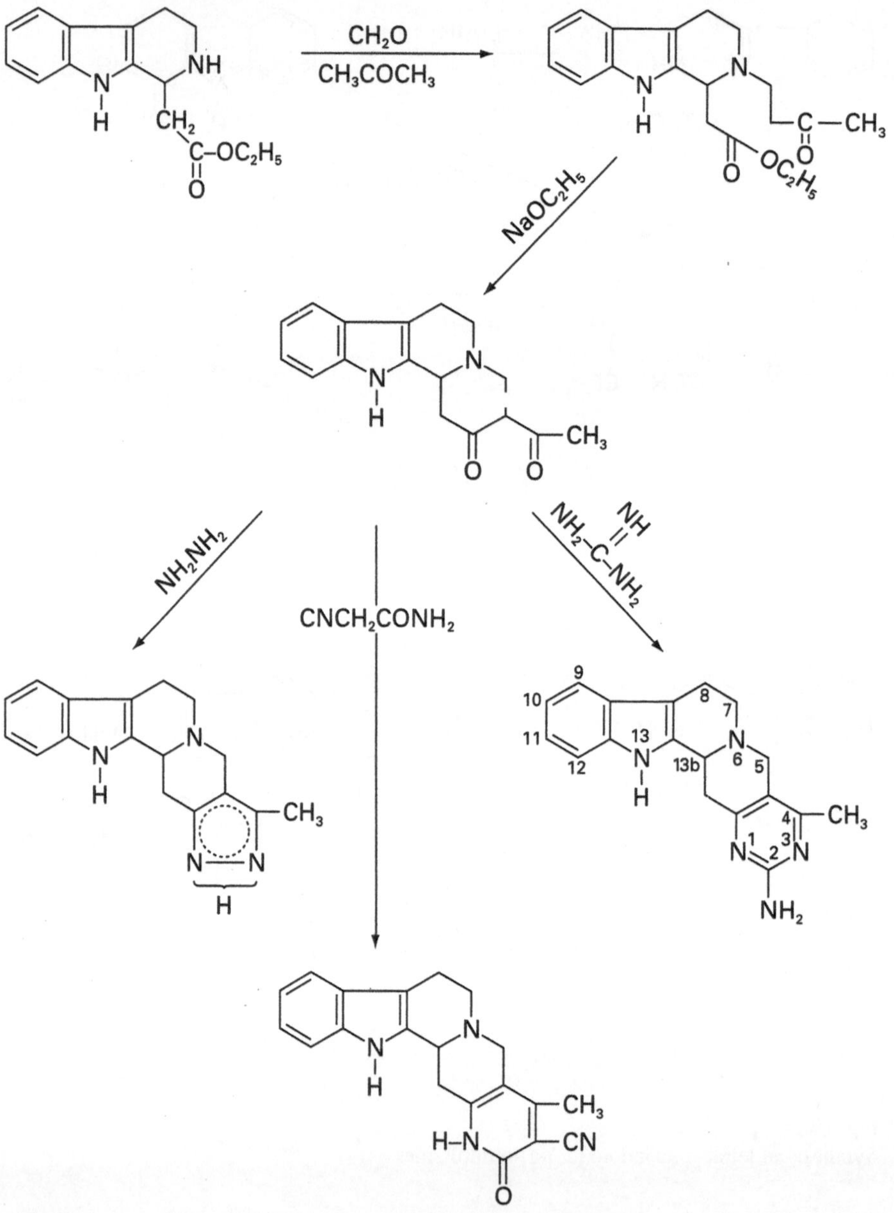

Fig. 20
Synthesis of pentacyclic indolo [2,3-a]-quinolizines

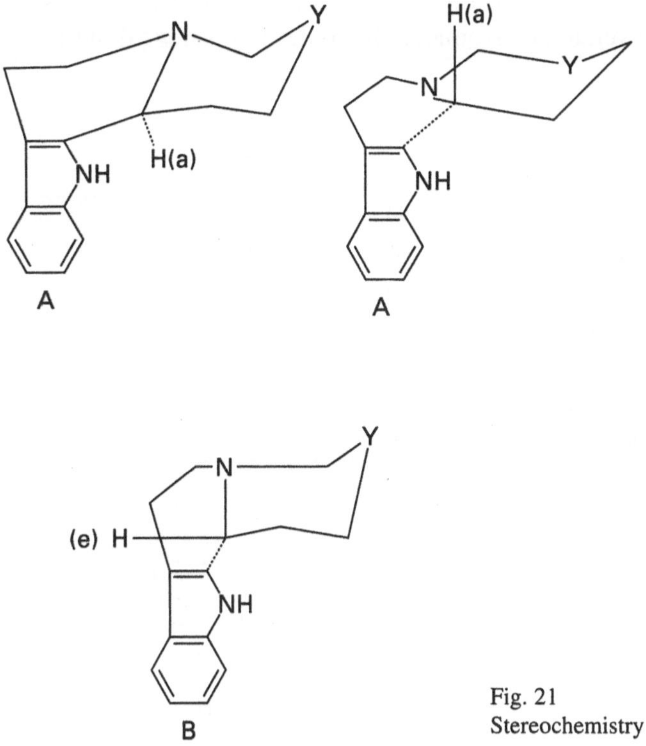

Fig. 21
Stereochemistry of polycyclic indoles

above-described compounds exhibit at least one and in many cases three absorption bands or plateaus in the 2700 cm^{-1}–2800 cm^{-1} region of the infrared. Bohlmann [27] had demonstrated that in the quinolizidines the presence of absorption bands in this region is associated with an axial hydrogen at the bridgehead carbon adjacent to the basic nitrogen. The spectral data thus confirmed the assigned axial conformation.

Finally, we had decided to round out our polycyclic indole research by preparing some compounds with alkyl substituents in ring C alpha to N_b. Dr. Herbert Blatter, following well-trodden paths, carried out the condensation of indole-3-carboxaldehyde with various nitro alkanes in refluxing glacial acetic acid containing $(NH_4)_3PO_4$. Although the corresponding α-alkyl tryptamine derivatives were obtained, it was noted that a marked reduction in yield in the intermediate resulted in going from nitroethane to nitropropane. In working up the reaction mixture Blatter was able to isolate a by-product which had a strong band in the infrared at 2238 cm$_{-1}$, the region characteristic for the nitrile group absorption. To make a long story short, this chance observation turned out to be a *new one-step general method* for the conversion of aromatic aldehydes to nitriles (Table I).

Table I.
Percent yield of aromatic nitriles from aldehydes

Nitrile	%
3-Cyanoindole	60
5-Bromo-3-cyanoindole	41
3-Cyano-7-azaindole	40
p-Dimethylaminobenzonitrile	77
p-Chlorobenzonitrile	50
3,4,5-Trimethoxybenzonitrile	74
p-Isopropylbenzonitrile	30

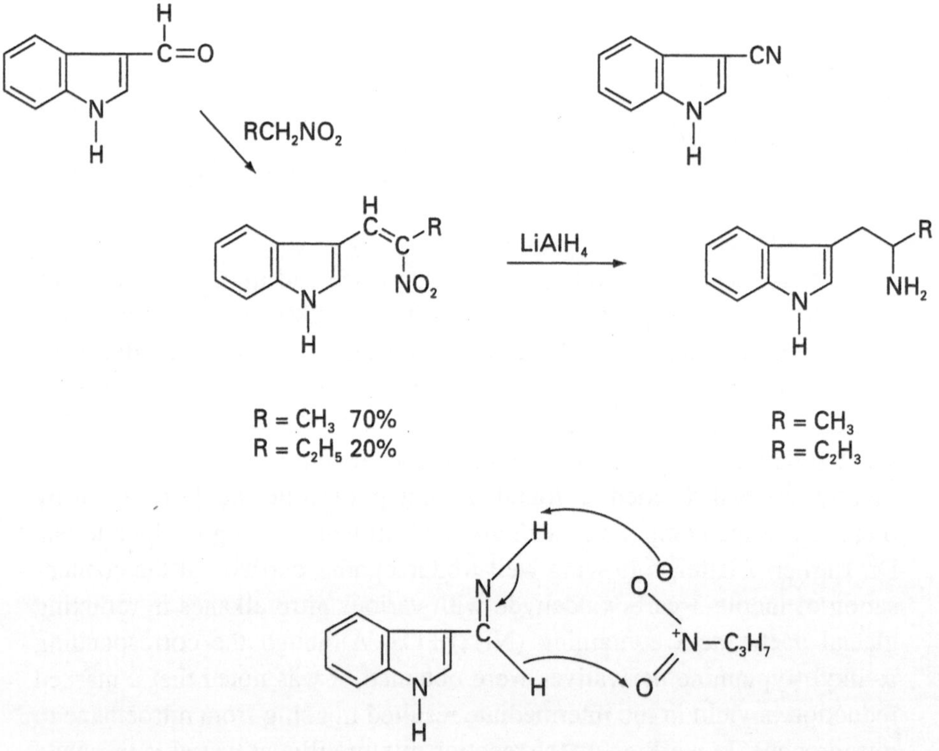
RCH₂NO₂
LiAlH₄
CN
NO₂
NH₂
R = CH₃ 70%
R = C₂H₅ 20%
R = CH₃
R = C₂H₃
N–C₃H₇

Fig. 22
Mechanism for formation of aromatic nitriles from aldehydes

A reasonable mechanism for this reaction consists in a concerted transition state complex whereby the 1-nitropropane engages in an attack on the intermediate imine (formed from the ammonium salt) with concomitant hydride shift [28] (Figure 22).

4.2   Steroids

Our excursion into steroids was brief, but theoretically satisfying. The steroid research at CIBA, Basel had led to the introduction of the androgen

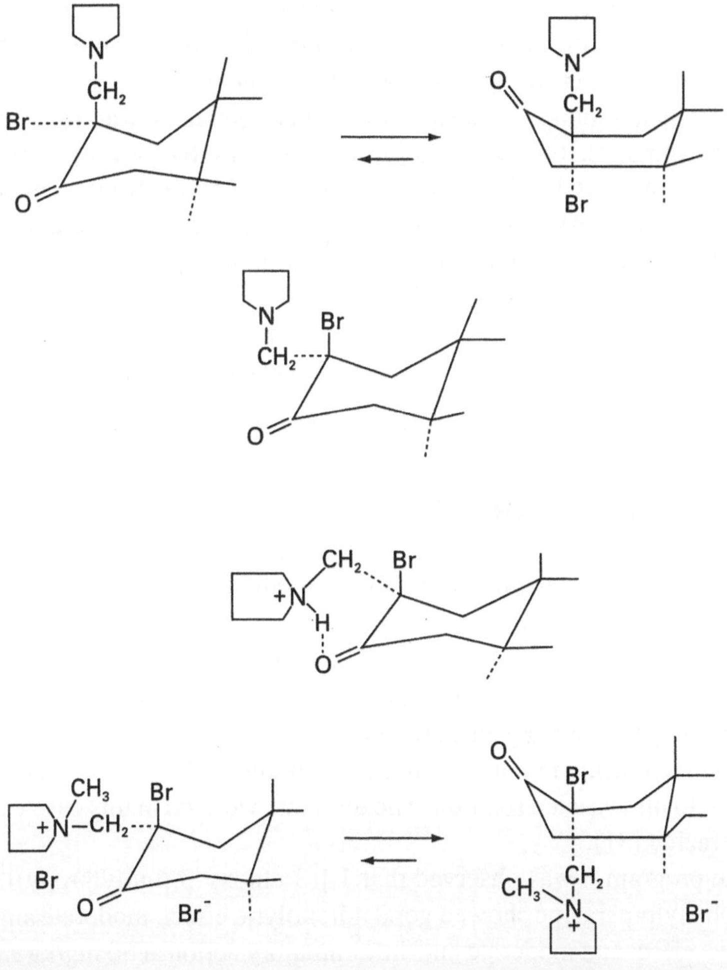

Fig. 23
Stereochemistry of 2-bromo derivatives of androstane-3-one Mannich bases

methandrostenolone. The application of the Mannich reaction to steroids up until 1959 had been limited to a report by Julian on the preparation of 16-dimethylamino dehydroisoandrosterone. With my highly capable associate Angelina Halamandaris, we began to explore the synthesis of 2-substituted Mannich bases of 17-β-hydroxy-5α-androstane-3-one [29]. The Mannich bases so formed were devoid of hormonal activity. However, it was of theoretical interest to study their brominations under kinetically controlled conditions [30]. Due to unfavorable 1,3-diaxial interaction, it was anticipated that the boat form would prevail (Figure 23). Under those circumstances the axial halo ketone rule would give rise to a negative Cotton effect. In fact, a *positive* Cotton effect was realized. Thus, the axial bromo ketone of the chair confirmation was the product. It is conceivable that the hydrogen bonding effect of the proton and the carbonyl aids significantly in the A ring maintaining the chair form. This constraint was removed through the formation of the methobromide salt of the Mannich base (carbonyl absorption at 1710 cm_{-1}). Bromination of this substance under kinetic control gave rise to the 2-bromo derivative whose infrared carbonyl absorption band was displaced to 1730 cm^{-1}. Although axial bromination did occur, in the absence of hydrogen bonding effects plus the strong diaxial 1,3-bromine-methyl interaction resulted in the conformation "flip" to the more stable boat form with equatorial bromine. That the 4-bromo derivative was not formed was shown by alternative synthesis.

5   Piperazine derivatives

It should be emphasized that up until we began this work in 1962, the only drugs on the market containing the piperazine ring system were generally described as tranquilizers and antihistamines. Our research on indole [2,3a] quinolizines suggested that the piperazine moiety could be useful in the design of antihypertensive agents. However, it was decided to break away from the fixed conformation of the tetracyclic indole system and to prepare molecules with unrestricted rotation. The template we used in this case was phenylpiperazine [31].

Early in the program it was observed that 1-[(3-ethoxy-3-p-tolylpropy)]3-methyl-4-phenylpiperazine showed good adrenolytic effect, moderate antihypertensive effect and moderate anti-inflammatory action at 50 mg/kg s.c. in the granuloma pouch test in rats. Figure 24 illustrates the general mode of synthesis of these compounds. At this point, Dr. Robert Mull joined the

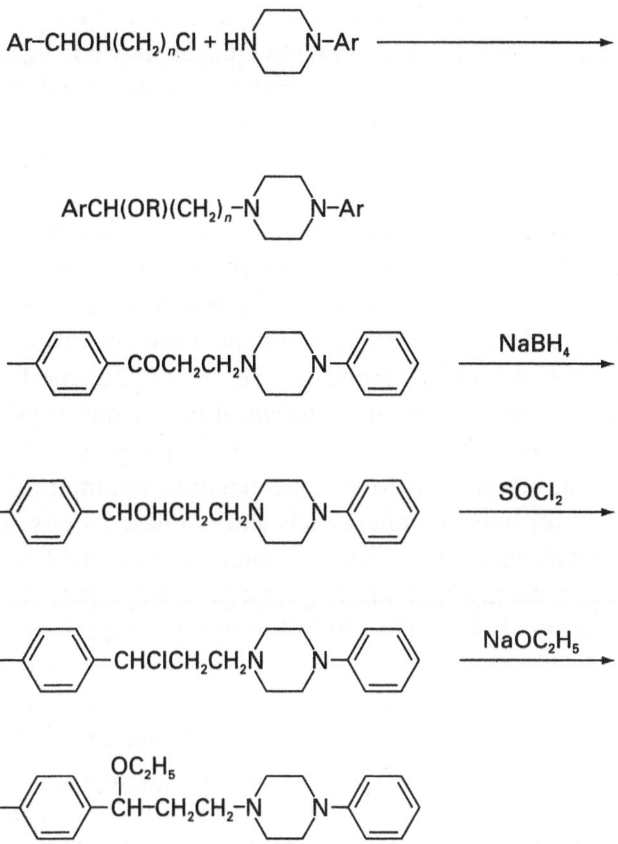
Ar–CHOH(CH2)nCl + HN N–Ar
ArCH(OR)(CH2)n–N N–Ar
COCH2CH2N N
NaBH4
CHOHCH2CH2N N
SOCl2
CHClCH2CH2N N
NaOC2H5
OC2H5
CH–CH2CH2–N N

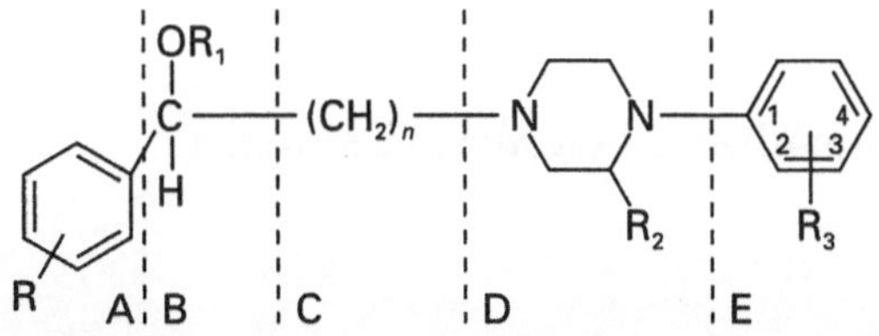
OR1
C
H
(CH2)n
N N
R2
R3
R
A
B
C
D
E

Fig. 24
Synthesis of phenylpiperizine derivatives

program to study this class in depth, determining the effect on activity with appropriate changes from A to E in the general structure as shown in Figure 24. Each parameter was varied selectively so that a minimum number of compounds would be prepared before choosing the compound which displayed maximum antihypertensive effect without any adrenolytic or anti-inflammatory properties.

Well over 50 compounds were synthesized and tested. The substance in which R = H, $R_1 = C_2H_5$, $R_2 = H_1$ and $R_3 = 4\text{-}CH_3$ was found to have excellent antihypertensive effects when tested orally at 4 mg/kg in unanesthetized dogs for 12 days. Most interestingly and unexpectedly, this compound (Su-9896) at a dose of 6 mg/kg administered orally to 12 unanesthetized dogs caused a pronounced diuretic and saluretic effect. To our surprise, this was the only member of the class to show a diuretic action. It was not anti-inflammatory and its adrenolytic effect appeared to be minimal.

Su-9896 was submitted for human clinical trials and in Phase I study was found to be well tolerated. Phase II studies corroborated the animal pharmacology in that doses of 50 mg b.i.d. orally gave a good antihypertensive effect and a modest diuretic action. The clinical trials were expanded and for a while we thought this substance would go all the way. But as more patients were brought into the trial, it was observed that some suffered syncope with sudden loss of consciousness. This was believed to be due to an excessive postural hypotensive effect. Lowering dosage and less frequent administration did not appreciably reduce this adverse reaction. Clinical feedback to the biology laboratory indicated that Su-9896 was probably acting centrally. At the time the identity of the α_2-receptor and its role as an autoreceptor in the brain in controlling sympathetic flow had not been elucidated. In retrospect, it is more than likely that Su-9896 was acting in part as a potent α_2-antagonist.

6   Seven- and eight-membered heterocyclic systems

6.1   Benzazepines

In 1963, in the course of some broad clinical testing of the CIBA antihistamine, Antistine®, it was noted that this drug also exhibited rather good antiarrhythmic effects, although heavy sedation was observed at therapeutic doses. A joining of the two aromatic rings of this drug forms a morphanthridine derivative (Su-11,636) which showed some structural similarities

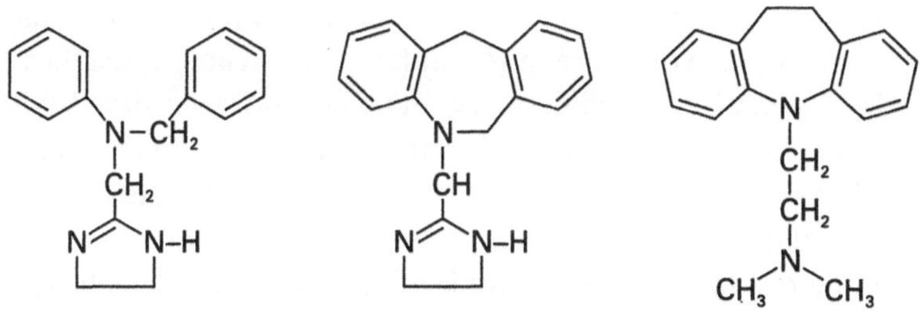

Antistine   Su-11636   Imipramine

Fig. 25
Antistine and related compounds

to imipramine (Figure 25). Su-11,636 did show good antiarrhythmic action in humans, but also displayed disturbing central effects. This prompted us to consider that the molecule was too closely related to the tricyclics and thus to look at it from a different perspective.

That is to say, if one envisions the dissociation of one of the benzene rings (as noted by the heavy arrow in Figure 26) from the morphanthridine ring system and then connects the same by a single bond to the 7-membered ring, the result is a 3-phenyl-2,3,4,5-tetrahydro-1-benzazepine, and indeed this heterocycle could readily be synthesized from 2-phenyl-1-tetralone derivatives by a Schmidt ring expansion reaction followed by reduction [32, 33].

Su-13,197 was found to be several times more potent than Antistine as an antiarrhythmic in experimental animals. In fact, the mode of action was quite different from quinidine and procainamide. The clinical trials also confirmed the activity in man and without causing sedation or other central effects. CIBA carried out extensive clinical trials with this substance over a period of two years and it certainly was of great help to the patients. However, individuals with compromised cardiac conditions suffering arrhythmic epi-

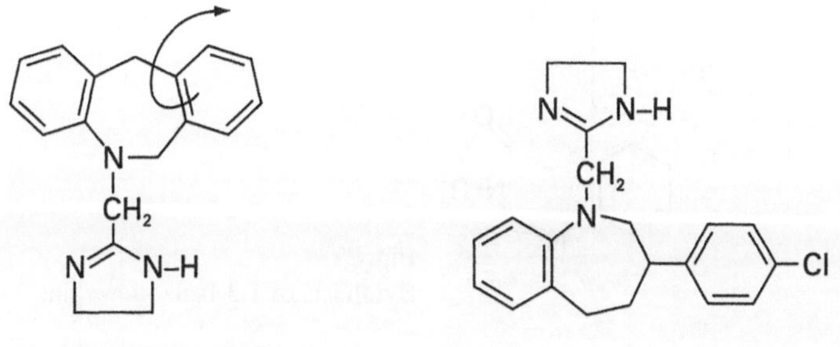

Fig. 26
Su-13,197

sodes are high risk patients under any circumstance. As a result during the trials, a small number (3 out of 127) expired, although it did not appear these deaths were drug related. Nevertheless, the FDA in 1967 considered this percentage unacceptable and thus put all trials on hold, our protestations notwithstanding. Su-13,197 was eventually terminated and because of the FDA attitude, we also closed out our antiarrhythmic research program. In passing, it is of interest to note that the imidazoline derivative of 1-phenyl-3-benzazapine was devoid of antihistaminic or antiarrhythmic effects.

6.2   Benzodiazepines

As often happens in medicinal research, when a drug of novel structure and biological activity is introduced into medical practice it is followed by a flurry of activity by scientists seeking to improve its biological and toxicological profile. Such was the case with the 1,4-benzodiazepines, chlordiazepoxide and diazepam, discovered by Dr. Leo Sternbach of Roche.
Our interest in 7-membered heterocycles was surely stimulated by the Sternbach discovery; however, as the saying goes: "Why go fishing in the same lake with everyone else?" In surveying the field, it immediately became evident that research on 1,3 and 2,4-benzodiazepines was surprisingly unexplored. Thus, our objective was *not* to search for another anxiolytic agent, but to synthesize some representative examples of these unknown benzodiazepines as part of a lead discovery program.
In our initial efforts, the internal condensation of the *o*-amino-N-acyl

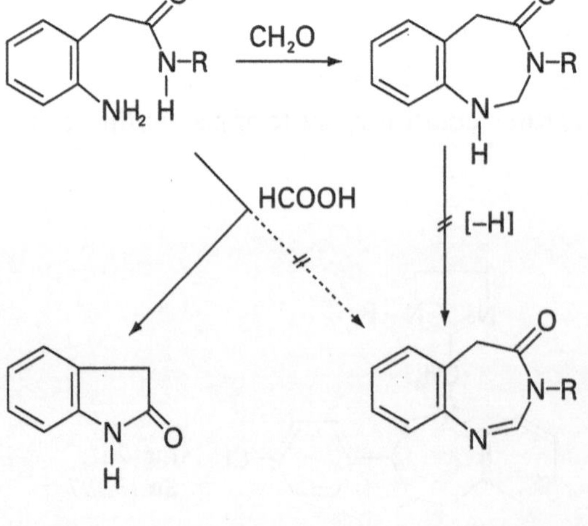

Fig. 27
Synthesis of 1,3-benzodiazepine

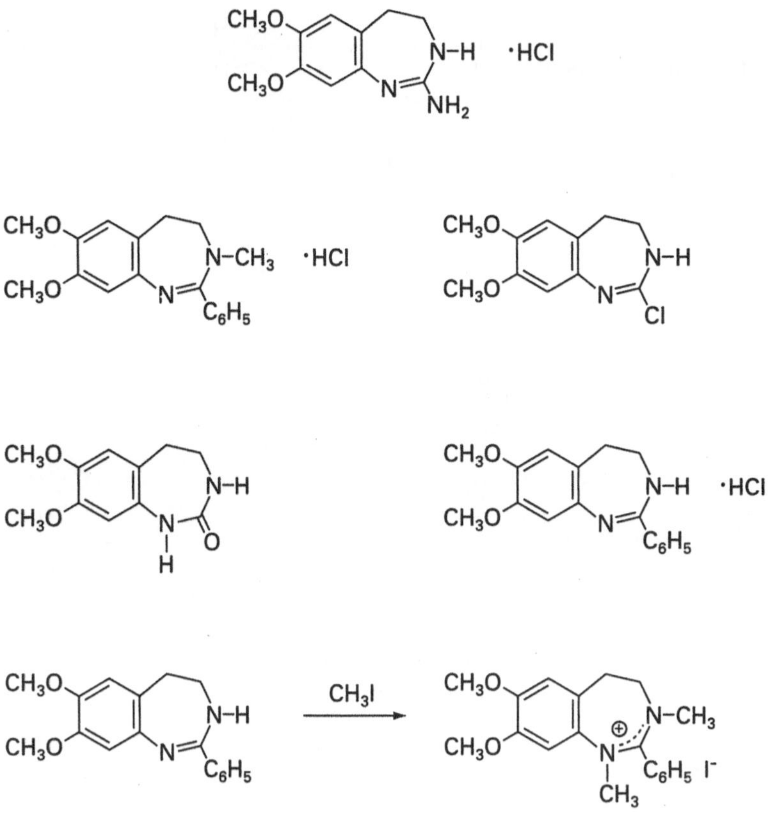

Fig. 28
Derivatives of 1,3-benzodiazepines

phenylethylamino derivative with formaldehyde gave rise to the desired 1,3-benzodiazepines[31] and their subsequent reduction formed the completely saturated system [34] (Figure 27). However, all attempts to synthesize the unsaturated system with formic acid resulted in the formation of oxindole or oxindole polymer. At about this time, Dr. Herman Rodriguez, a new Ph.D. from Professor Sharma's group at Penn State, joined our team and the problem was turned over to him. In a series of studies, he solved some of the problems of stability of intermediates and introduced new synthetic approaches. In Figures 28 and 29 are listed a group of representative 1,3- and 2,4-benzodiazepines, which were submitted for biological evaluation [33, 35]. The 3-amino and 3-dimethyl-amino-2,4-benzodiazepines elicited significant antihypertensive activity. The latter sub-

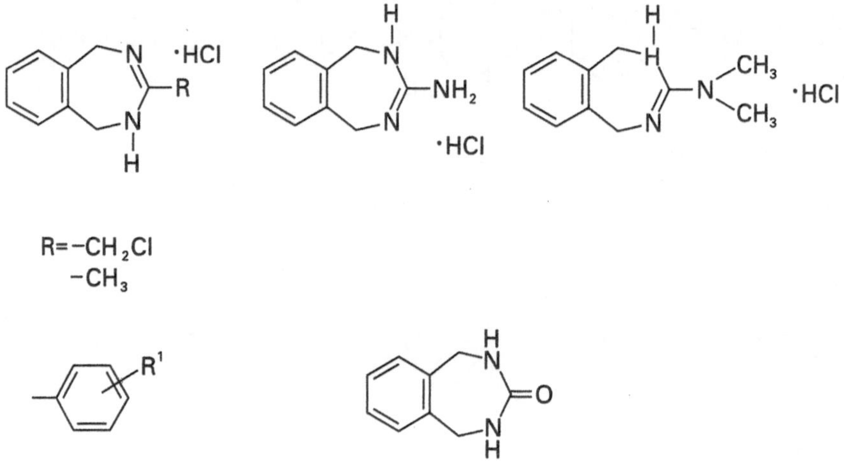

R=−CH₂Cl
  −CH₃

Fig. 29
Derivatives of 2,4-benzodiazepines

stance was prepared for evaluation in humans. However, 90 days toxicity studies in rats precluded further study of this series.

6.3   Octazocines

Our initial entry into eight-membered ring chemistry goes back indirectly to 1955 when Dr. Paul Schmidt of CIBA, Basel, spent a six-month sabbatical in our laboratories in Summit. Schmidt, at the time, was very much interested in microbiological problems and in the process, prepared a series of amidoximes, which were found to be trypanocidal. In the Fall of 1955, Schmidt returned to Basel to a most successful career in which he eventually became Stellvertretender Director of the Synthetic Team of CIBA and then CIBA-Geigy. He and his colleagues in Basel were responsible for the discovery of several important drugs; oxprenelol, niridazine, sulfaphenazone and maprotoline.

In any case, the amidoxime problem was taken over by Robert Mull, who expanded it considerably and drove it in a different direction when he synthesized Su-4029, which was found to elicit potent antihypertensive effects in experimental animals [Figure 30]. This substance went into clinical trials and, in the able hands of Dr. Irvine Page of the Cleveland Clinic, was found to be antihypertensive in humans, but it also caused fever.

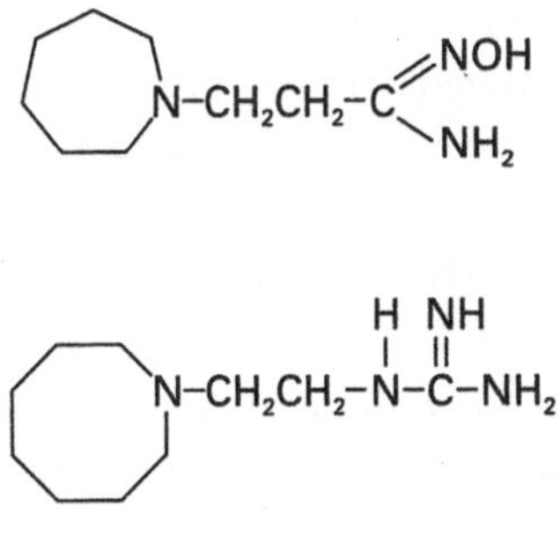

Fig. 30
Su-4029 and guanethidine

After an extensive structure-activity study, Mull [36] prepared guanethidine, which became and still is the most effective antihypertensive drug in patients with severe high blood pressure.

As an extension of the benzodiazepine research, Mull and I began to explore

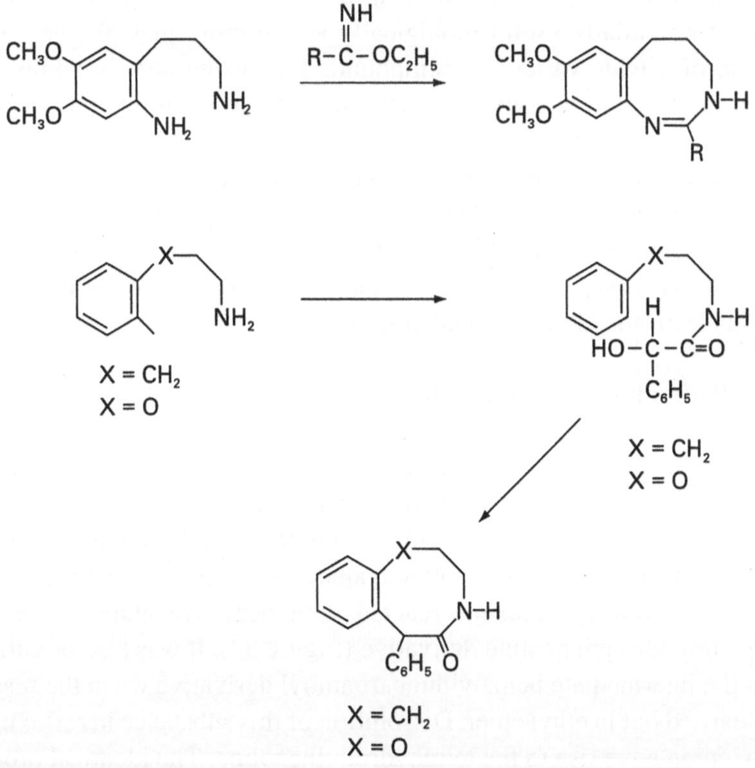

Fig. 31
Synthesis of 1,3 benzodiazocines, benzazocines and benzoxazocines

the synthesis of the unknown benzazocines [33] (Figure 31). When 2-amino-4,5-dimethoxyphenylpropylamine was allowed to react with various imidates the 2-substituted 1,3-benzodiazocines were formed. Yields in excess of 50% were achieved only when highly dilute solutions were employed. The benzazocin-2-one and the benzoxazocin-5-one were also obtained in good yields by running the cyclization reaction of the glycol-amide intermediate under high dilution conditions. Although we learned much about the synthesis and chemistry of these substances and their derivatives, none displayed biological activity worthy of further pursuit.

7   Unusual chemistry searching for biological activity

It had always been my contention that the potential of a synthetic medicinal chemistry program depended a great deal on the flexibility of the interme-diates used. In other words, the diverse use of the intermediates in the synthesis of potentially useful biologically active molecules allowed the preparation of a wide variety of compounds for testing and, in addition, facilitated the structure-activity relationship study in permitting the prepa-ration of selective derivatives leading to the most active clinical candidate in a series within the shortest period of time. Parenthetically, in the 1960s, this was suggestive of a cerebral combinatorial chemistry library approach to drug discovery. Very limited indeed, but at the same time empowered by *intuition, observation for the unexpected and experience*, and not by com-puters and electronically automated systems.

7.1   Pyrimidines and quinazolines

The preparation of the novel N-substituted pyrimidines and quinazolines came about by the unexpected chance observation of the formation in quantitative yield of a thiopyrimidine from the condensation of ethyl β-anilinocrotonate with benzoylisothiocyanate [32] (Figure 32). Similarly, the enamine, anilinocyclohexene reacted with benzoylisothiocyanate to yield the tetrahydroquinazoline derivative (Figure 33). It was also possible to obtain the intermediate benzoylthiocarbamoyl derivative when the reac-tion was carried out in ethyl ether. Dissolution of this substance in refluxing tetrahydrofuran gave rise to the tetrahydroquinazoline. The identical prod-uct could be obtained through the condensation of N-phenylbenzimidoyl isothiocyanate with morpholinocyclohexene [38, 39].

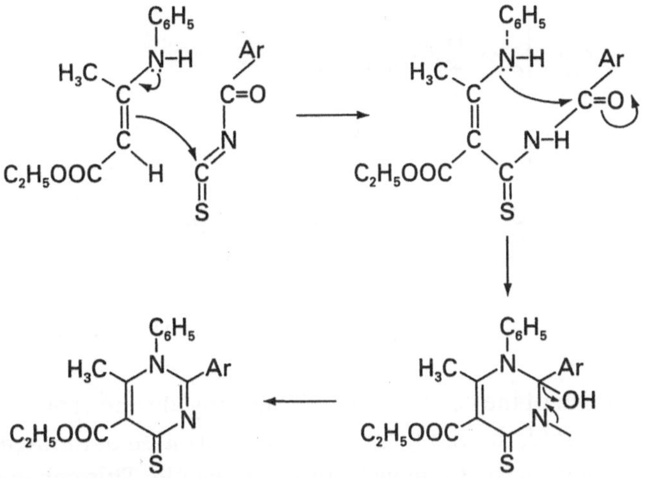

Fig. 32
Synthesis of 1,2-disubstituted pyrimidinethiones

The N-phenylbenzimidoyl isothiocyanate intermediate was found to be most versatile in that it readily underwent intramolecular ring closure to 2-phenyl-4(3H) quinazolinethione in refluxing benzene (Figure 34). This proved to be a unique general synthesis of these substances. The cyclization occurs regardless of the presence of electron withdrawing or electron

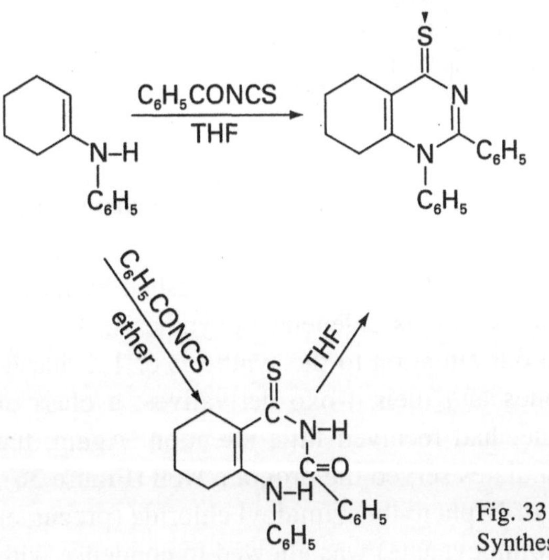

Fig. 33
Synthesis of tetrahydroquinazolinethiones

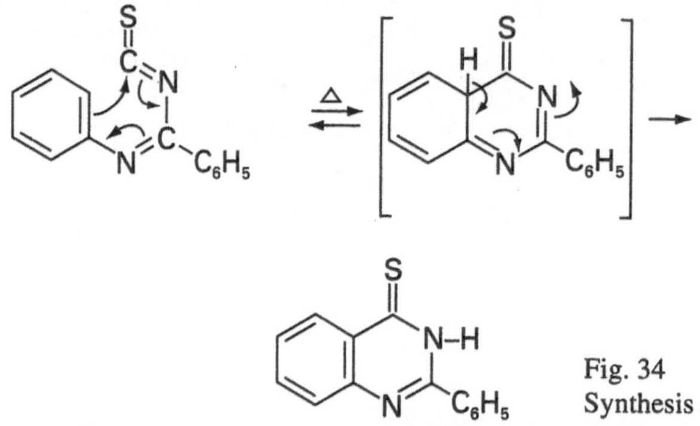

Fig. 34
Synthesis of 2-phenylquinazolinethione

releasing groups on either of the benzene rings. Thus, ring closure is brought about by a cyclic, concerted, thermally induced reorganization of the *sigma* and *pi* bond electrons within the framework of the molecule. This category of reaction has been designated a "no mechanism reaction" because of the difficulty, if not the impossibility, of describing precisely the transition state or states of such reactions. Such multicenter processes are neither ionic or radical. They are thermally induced and independent of extra molecular environment and are often insensitive to internal structural variation.

In passing, it should be noted that in most cases, a red crystalline imidoylisothiocyanate dimer could be isolated albeit in very low yield

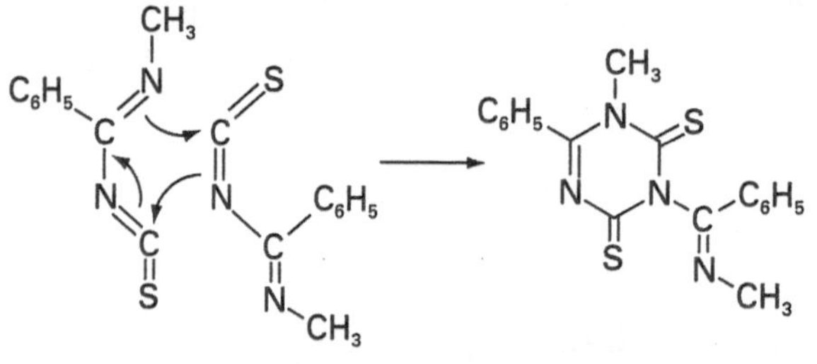

Fig. 35
Synthesis of triazinethione

(Figure 35). The triazine structure of the dimer was established by means of analytical and spectral data, as well as independent synthesis.

Finally, Blatter and I directed our attention to the synthesis of 1,2-diaryl-substituted 4-quinazolinethiones and their 4-oxo derivatives, a class of compounds which, at the time, had received little attention. Again, the availability of flexible intermediates served the program well (Figure 36). In this case, the condensation of N-phenylbenzimidoyl chloride (precursor to the previously described isothiocyanate) was allowed to condense with

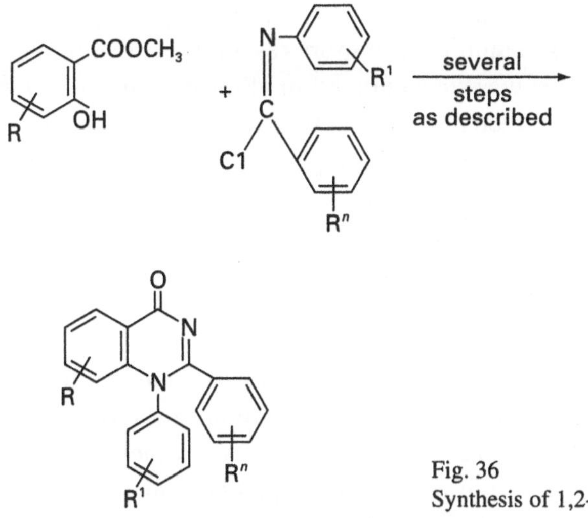

Fig. 36
Synthesis of 1,2-diphenyl-quinazolinethione

methyl salicylate and a Chapman rearrangement of the resulting product followed by saponification to the acid, conversion to the acid chloride and then amination resulted in an amide intermediate, which, when heated at 300° for a few minutes, gave almost quantitative yield of the 1,2-diphenyl quinazolone. Again, this was found to be a general synthesis of these heterocycles [40].

In 1965, I was invited to lecture at the Technion in Haifa, Israel, by Professor David Ginsburg. The presentation of these results led to a lively discussion, which continued at dinner in the restaurant adjacent to the medieval Crusader fort in Acre. One of the participants in the discussion was Dr. Elijah H. Gold, a Ginsburg doctoral candidate who eventually joined the medicinal chemistry staff of Schering-Plough, USA.

Out of the quinazoline research resulted Su-13,026 (Figure 37), a substance which exhibited analgetic effects in all experimental animal models. In addition, it was not addictive and did not elicit any of the side effects associated with narcotic-type drugs. Su-13,026, at the time of its discovery

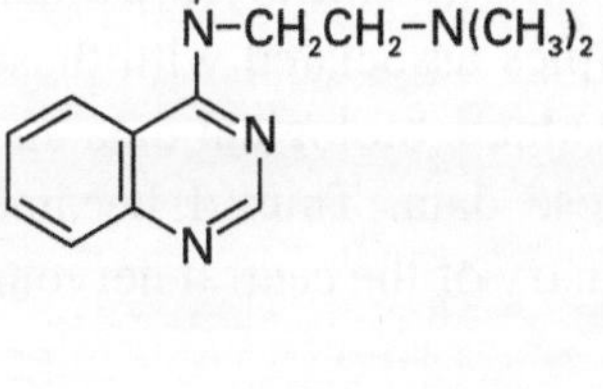

Fig. 37
Su-13,026

in 1966, did not cause ulcers in animal tests and, consequently, was not aspirin-like (cyclooxygenase inhibitor). It more resembled acetaminophen in its analgetic profile. This was substantiated in clinical trials; at 300 mg t.i.d. it was found to be an effective analgetic for mild to moderate pain. In Phase II and Phase III trials, it was clearly superior to placebo and at least comparable to and in one trial better than acetaminophen. At this point, Marketing decided it could not compete with the over-the-counter drug and, therefore, Management decided to terminate further development, in spite of the plea by Research that this was a new chemical entity with its own profile and potential in medicine.

I would only add that it is frustrating to the medicinal chemist to invest so much time and energy in a research program only to have it brought to an end by a cautious Marketing Department, the members of which in any case always think retrospectively with regard to the potential market for new products.

8   Epilogue

Herein, I have presented some of the research I personally was involved with from 1950 to 1967. In particular, I have attempted to give the rationale behind the design of certain molecules and how unexpected developments led us into new and unexplored areas of chemistry. Many biologically active molecules were discovered, but only a few became medicinal agents. Considering the unfavorable odds facing the medicinal chemist, in this regard I consider myself quite fortunate with the success I did have. Early on, I recognized the odds were overwhelming. For this reason, I set up a strategy based on *heterocyclic diversity*. Aware that many naturally occurring substances showing biological activity contain nitrogen, oxygen and sulfur within their structural framework, I intuitively surmised that the odds could be turned to one's favor if one synthesized a wide variety of new and different heterocyclic compounds for biological evaluation.

The consequence of this experience was that because of the different biological activities of the compounds I synthesized, I came in contact with biologists of different disciplines. Such interfaces allowed me to learn much about the animal tests and the biological principles associated with these tests. It also was of great value in learning to evaluate biological data and to appreciate the statistical significance of these data. Thus, I became conversant with the pharmacology and biochemistry of the central nervous system and cardiovascular renal system also learned much endocrinology, microbiology and enzymology. These interdisciplinary experiences were most useful in appreciating the demanding effort in maintaining the highest standard in the selection of a substance for further development.

As noted in this review, several substances I worked on went into clinical trials and some became drug products. My involvement in following the progress of these substances taught me much about toxicology, drug metabolism, pharmacy, process development, analytical chemistry, clinical research and last, but not least, dealing with the FDA.

Thus, to return to the question posited at the beginning of this review, the answer at first glance is not obvious. The end result certainly was not planned. However, as my research programs and experiences expanded and took on many different directions, I learned continuously what is required to turn a lead compound into a clinical candidate and finally into a drug. Most importantly, I learned that this was a group effort which required the concerted, committed effort of many scientists of different disciplines working in harmony toward a common goal. Maybe for all of the above, in 1967, I was placed in charge of the research and development operations of CIBA and then later CIBA-Geigy in the United States. The accomplishment of that period (1967–1979) has been duly recorded on the occasion of the American Chemical Society naming me in 1991 to be the first recipient of the E. B. Hershberg Award for Important Discoveries in Medicinally Active Substances [41].

References

1   G. deStevens: Progress in Drug Research 29, 97 (1985).
2   F. F. Nord and G. deStevens: Handbuch der Pflanzenphysiologie (Lignins and Ligni-
     fication) X, 390–441 (1958).
3   G. deStevens: U.S. Patent 2,882,160, April 14, 1959.
4   G. deStevens: U.S. Patent 2,892,835, June 30, 1959.
5   G. deStevens: U.S. Patent 2,892,836, June 30, 1959.
6   G. deStevens: U.S. Patent 2,905,666, September 22, 1959.
7   G. deStevens: U.S. Patent 2,916,487, December 8, 1959.
8   G. deStevens: U.S. Patent 2,916,488, December 8, 1959.
9   G. deStevens: U.S. Patent 2,892,937, June 30, 1959.
10   G. deStevens and R. H. Sprague: U.S. Patent 2,912,434, November 10, 1959.
11   R. H. Sprague and G. deStevens: J. Am. Chem. Soc. 81, 3095 (1959).
12   G. deStevens, A. Frutchey, A. Halamanda alamandaris Luts: J. Am. Chem. Soc. 79,
     5263 (1957).

13   G. deStevens, A. F. Hopkinson, M. A. Connelly, P. Oke and D. C. Schroeder: J. Am. Chem. Soc. *80*, 2201 (1958).

14   G. deStevens: J. Org. Chem. *23*, 1572 (1958).

15   G. deStevens, A. Halamandaris and L. Dorfman: J. Am. Chem. Soc. *80*, 5198 (1958).

16   G. deStevens, A. Halamandaris, P. Wenk, R. A. Mull and E. Schlittler: Arch. Biochem. Biophys. *83* (1), 141 (1959).

17   G. deStevens, A. Halamandaris, P. Wenk and L. Dorfman: J. Am. Chem. Soc. *81*, 6292 (1959).

18   G. deStevens, A. Halamandaris, P. Strachan, E. Donoghue, L. Dorfman and C. F. Huebner: J. Med. Chem. *6*, 357 (1963).

19   A. Patchett and P. Giarruso: J. Med. Pharm. Chem. *4*, 403 (1961).

20   R. W. J. Carney and G. deStevens: U.S. Patent 3,766,260, October 16, 1973.

21   F. C. Novello and J. M. Sprague: J. Am. Chem. Soc. *79*, 2028 (1957).

22   G. deStevens, L. H. Werner, A. Halamandaris and S. Ricca, Jr.: Experientia XIV *12*, 463 (1958).

23   L. H. Werner, A. Halamandaris, S. Ricca, Jr., L. Dorfman and G. deStevens: J. Am. Chem. Soc. *82*, 1161 (1960).

24   G. deStevens: *Diuretics: Chemistry and Pharmacology.* Academic Press, New York 1963. (US Patent #3,163,645 issued December 29, 1964).

25   G. deStevens, H. Lukaszewski, M. Sklar, A. Halamandaris and H. M. Blatter: J. Org. Chem. *27*, 2457 (1962).

26   G. deStevens and M. Sklar: J. Org. Chem. *28*, 3210 (1963).

27   F. Bohlmann: Angew. Chem. *69*, 641 (1957).

28   G. deStevens: Rec. Chem. Prog. *23* (2) 105 (1962).

29   G. deStevens and A. Halamandaris: J. Org. Chem. *26*, 1614 (1961).

30   G. deStevens and A. Halamandaris: Experientia *XVII* 297 (1961).

31   R. P. Mull, C. Tannenbaum, M. R. Dapero, M. Bernier, W. Jost and G. deStevens: J. Med. Chem. *8*, 332 (1965).

32   L. H. Werner, S. Ricca, A. Rossi and G. deStevens: J. Med. Chem. *10*, 575 (1967).

33   G. deStevens: In: Topics in Heterocyclic Chemistry (ed. R. N. Castle). J. Wiley and Sons, N.Y., pp. 154–177 (1969).

34   G. deStevens and M. Dughi: Trans. N.Y. Acad. of Sci. *23* (7) 568 (1961).

35   H. Rodriguez, B. Zitko and G. deStevens: J. Org. Chem. *33*, 670 (1968).

36   R. P. Mull, M. E. Egbert and M. R. Dapero: J. Med. Chem. *25*, 1533 (1960).

37   G. deStevens, B. Smolinsky and L. Dorfman: J. Org. Chem. *29*, 1115 (1964).

38   R. W. J. Carney, J. Wojtkunski and G. deStevens: J. Org. Chem. *29*, 2887 (1964).

39   H. M. Blatter, H. Lukaszewski and G. deStevens: J. Org. Chem. *30*, 1020 (1965).

40   G. deStevens, H. M. Blatter and R. W. J. Carney: Angew. Chem., Int. ed. *5*, 35–39 (1966).

41   G. deStevens: J. Med. Chem. *34*, 2665 (1991).

Progress in Drug Research, Vol. 44 (E. Jucker, Ed.)
© 1995 Birkhäuser Verlag, Basel (Switzerland)

Developments in histamine H1-receptor agonists

By V. Zingel*, C. Leschke** and W. Schunack**

* Byk Gulden Lomberg Chemische Fabrik, Byk-Gulden-Straße 2, 78467 Konstanz,
Germany, and ** Institute of Pharmacy, Free University of Berlin, Königin-Luise-Straße
2+4, 14195 Berlin, Germany

1   Introduction

The story of histamine started in the early 1900's with the fundamental investigations of Dale et al. [1–3], which recognized the remarkable physiological behavior of this biogenic amine. Scientific progress over the past decades has proved that histamine interacts with specific histamine receptors as a neurotransmitter and nearly all mammalian tissues contain detectable amounts of histamine, while the physiological role is not fully understood. According to their chronological order of discovery, three subtypes of histamine receptors are pharmacologically accepted at present: H_1-, H_2- and H_3-receptors [4–6]. The effects following direct stimulation of these histamine receptors are manifold and depend on species and tissue [7, 8]. The actions of histamine can be mimicked by selective agonists or on the contrary blocked by antagonists. Stimulation of H_1-receptors leads to effects which are predominantly pathophysiological, e.g. contraction of smooth muscles (bronchi, intestine and uterus), dilatation of small bloodvessels (arteriols, veins, capillaries), increase of permeability of capillaries and release of catecholamines from adrenal medulla. Thus the possible role of histamine in allergic and inflammatory disorders has led to the development [9] and clinical introduction [10] of the first "classical H_1-receptor antagonist". The then synthesized, more potent ethylenediamines (e.g. mepyramine), colamines (e.g. diphenhydramine), propylamines (e.g. pheniramine) and the recently developed "non sedative H_1-receptor blockers", such as *astemizole* (Hismanal[R]), *terfenadine* (Teldane[R]), *loratadine* (Lisino[R]), *ceterizine* (Zyrtec[R]) or the recently marketed *azelastine* (Allergodil[R]) have up to now been useful drugs for the treatment of allergic disorders (e.g. hay fever, urticaria, drug allergy, asthma, etc.) which are continuously increasing and also for the treatment of insect stings. In contrast to that, histamine H_1-receptor agonists are not in therapeutical use at present but they have attracted increasing attention as "pharmacological tools" during the last years. Due to the wide distribution of histamine receptors in different biological systems (e.g. in organs of mammalians or cell cultures) and the velocity of investigation of effector systems, highly potent and specific agonists for the study of the function of H_1-receptors in physiological or pharmacological experiments are urgently lacking. Since endogenous histamine and very probably H_1-receptors [11] play a specific role in seizure mechanisms, a possible field of H_1-research is emerging. There is now evidence that histamine is an endogenous anticonvulsant in CNS [12, 13]. This is supported by the fact that H_1-receptor antagonists induce [14] or exacerbate [15] seizures in some cases of epilepsy. Recent experiments with selective H$_1$-receptor agonists seem to be very promising [16]. Other fields of research for highly specific H$_1$-receptor agonists are e.g. examination of H$_1$-receptor desensitization [17–19], investigation of pathogenesis of coronary spasms [20–22] or central regulation of intestinal transit [23].

Regarding other histamine receptor subtypes, stimulation of H$_2$-receptors leads to an increase of gastric acid secretion and to an increase of frequency and contractability of the heart. Peptic ulcer therapy underwent a dramatic change after the advent of H$_2$-receptor blockers [24]. After the successful introduction of the first H$_2$-receptor antagonist *cimetidine* (Tagamet^R) [25], *ranitidine* (Sostril^R, Zantic^R), *famotidine* (Pepdul^R, Ganor^R), *nizatidine* (Nizax^R, Gastrax^R), and *roxatidine* (Roxit^R) followed in recent years and are most widely used as one of the safest classes of drugs [26]. The histamine H$_2$-receptor agonist *impromidine* [27] was successfully used in the treatment of patients with catecholamine-insensitive congestive heart failure [28, 29]. The promising arpromidine [30] and other related cardio-histaminergics are still in the beginning of the long phase of drug development.

In the last years, examinations on site of occurrence und function of histamine in brain have been enforced [31–33]. Among these extensive employments it was explored that stimulation of presynaptic H$_3$-receptors leads autoregulatively to an inhibition of histamine synthesis and release from histaminergic neurons, strengthening thereby the role of histamine as a neurotransmitter [34]. Nevertheless certain effects of H$_3$-receptors connected with H$_1$- and H$_2$-receptors remain unclear. Histaminergic neurons are e.g. involved in the control of the neuroendocrine and cardiovascular systems and also in thermoregulation, the circadian rhythm of sleep and wakefulness as well as various behaviours including feeding, drinking, learning, memory, sexual and aggressive behaviour, vestibular function, cerebral vascular regulation and analgesia [35]. Lots of these effects were elucidated after the administration of the specific and potent inhibitor of histidine decarboxylase, (*S*)α-fluoromethylhistidine, a tool which depletes histamine in pharmacological studies [36]. Outgoing from the numerous influences of the H$_3$-receptor system, two therapeutic darts might warrant special attention: Centrally acting H$_3$-receptor agonists for decrease of wakefulness (hypnotics, sedatives or anticonvulsants) while peripherally acting H$_3$-receptor agonists may be beneficial for the treatment of asthma [37, 38] and gastrointestinal disorders by reducing the cholinergic and

NANC (non adrenergic-non cholinergic) neurotransmission. Under discussion is also the application of H_3-receptor antagonists for the stimulation of arousal and vigilance, cognition enhancement and appetite suppression. It could be demonstrated that the histamine level in human brain increases during normal aging, but is decreased in Alzheimer's disease [39]. In addition, Yanai et al. [40] observed an age-related decrease in H_1-receptors measured by PET (positron emission tomography) [41].

2   Biochemical effects

The H_1-receptor (H_1r) belongs to the super family of G-protein-linked receptors. The recent genomic cloning of H_1-receptors from bovines [42], rats [43], guinea-pigs [44, 45] and humans [46] led to valuable knowledge concerning the pharmacochemistry of H_1-receptor ligands. The bovine H_1-receptor possesses 491 amino acids (M_r 55 954), the rat 486 (M_r 55 690), the guinea-pig 488 (M_r 55 619) and the human 487 amino acids, thus differing strongly from H_2-receptor sequences of e.g. canine (353' amino acids, similarity approx. 30% [47]). H_1-receptors possess a large third intracellular loop and a short carboxyl terminal, which are common characteristics among Ca^{2+}-mobilizing receptors and receptors inhibiting adenylylcyclase such as muscarine M_2-receptors [48]. This is also verified by the fact that H_1-receptor antagonists are often endowed with antimuscarinic activity but not with H_2-receptor antagonism. Homology among the different H_1-receptors in total is > 60% and > 90% in the presumed transmembrane domain regions. Putative binding sites of histamine at H_1-receptors are expected to be an aspartic acid in the third transmembrane domain and a threonine and an asparagine in the fifth transmembrane domain. Other sites which were conserved among biogenic amine receptors are also present in H_1-receptors. Such sites are Asp-73 in the second transmembrane domain, the anionic and cationic amino acid pair (Asp-124 and Arg-125) at the cytoplasmic border of the third transmembrane domain, and the ten amino acid residues (Leu-455 to Pro-464) in the seventh transmembrane domain [43].
Regarding signal transduction pathways, the amino acids of the transmembrane domains of the receptor probably form a pocket where the H_1-receptor agonist binds to induce the conformation responsible for activating the G-protein (Gp), which is coupled in the region of the second and third intracellular loop with the receptor and subsequently stimulates the con-

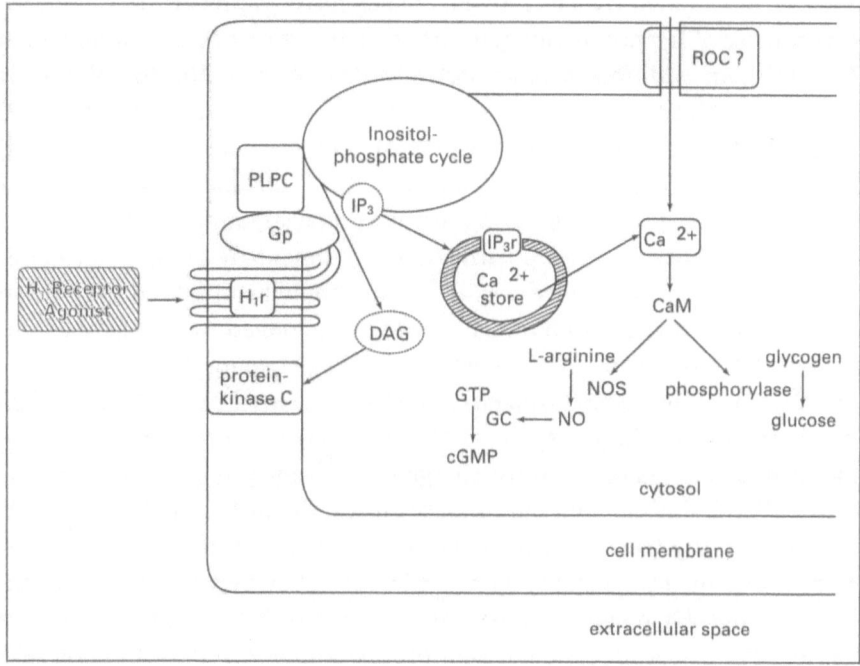

Fig. 1
Signal transduction pathways of the histamine H_1-receptor.

nected phospholipase C (PLPC) in the cytoplasmic membrane [49]. PLPC catalyzes in the inositol-phosphate-cycle the formation of inositol-1,4,5-trisphosphate (IP3) and 1,2-diacylglycerol (DAG) [50]. In the following, the ubiquitous second messenger IP3 interacts with an own receptor (IP3r) in the membrane of an intracellular calcium store, e.g. the endoplasmatic reticulum, which is responsible for Ca^{2+}-release into the cytosole under participation of ion channels [51]. After binding to calmodulin (CaM), "free Ca^{2+}-ions" stimulate the NO synthase (NOS) [52] leading to the enzymatic production of nitric oxide (EDRF) from its precursor L-arginine [53] and subsequently to the stimulation of guanylylcyclase (GC) and thus to the formation of cGMP from GTP [54]. On the other hand, Ca^{2+}-ions elicit a glycogenic response [55], which can be explained by an activation of a phosphorylase. A crucial role in signal transduction belongs to the protein-kinase C which is in fact a family of enzymes with different subspecies [56] and takes part in the enzymatic regulation of numerous functions and developments of the cell [57]. DAG and Ca^{2+} are able to stimulate protein-kinase C maximally. By a negative feedback DAG inhibits PLPC and leads to a decrease of IP$_3$ production (and also to a reduction of Ca^{2+} mobilization [58]) [59]. In addition, it is remarkable that H$_1$-receptor stimulation is connected with an influx of extracellular Ca^{2+} [60]. Possible mechanisms for this sustained effect are the opening of "voltage-dependent Ca^{2+}-channels" (VDC's) or/and "receptor-operated Ca^{2+}-channels" (ROC's). Favoured are ROC's, because during intensive investigations with the VDC-antagonist verapamil and depolarization experiments with high concentrations of K$^+$-ions no influence on Ca^{2+}-influx could be observed [61]. It can be supposed that regulation of Ca^{2+}-influx is achieved by second messengers like IP$_3$ [62, 63] or, in conjunction with its phosphorylated metabolite, inositol-1,3,4,5-tetrakisphosphate (IP$_4$) [64, 65]. However, this mechanism seems not to be obligatory in all tissues [66]. Interestingly, when the intracellular Ca^{2+}-store is fully charged, Ca^{2+}-entry is prevented, but as soon as IP$_3$ drains calcium out of these stores, the influx of Ca^{2+} switches on automatically [67]. Very recently in experiments with chinese hamster ovary cells which were stably expressed with a cDNA encoding the guinea-pig histamine H$_1$-receptor, it was also observed that histamine causes a massive release of arachidonic acid probably through the activation of a cytosolic phospholipase A$_2$ [68].

Histamine H$_2$-receptors are linked by a G-protein with an adenylylcyclase in the cytoplasmic membrane. The activation is coupled with the production of the second messenger cyclic 3',5'-adenosine monophosphate (cAMP), which is responsible for all other following effects (e.g. the activation of a H$^+$/K$^+$-ATPase in the cytosole of the parietal cell resulting in the stimulation of gastric acid secretion) [69]. Interestingly, a simultaneous stimulation together with H$_1$-receptors in the presence of Ca^{2+}-ions leads to an increase of cAMP-production [70], whereas H$_1$-receptor activation alone is inefficient [71].

The attack of histamine on H$_3$-receptors leads by a negative feedback mechanism in histaminergic neurons to a decrease of the synthesis of the biogenic amine from L-histidine (which is catalyzed by the specific histidine decarboxylase) and to an inhibition of histamine release, which can be stimulated in experiments by potassium ions. Muscarine M$_1$-receptors [72], α$_2$-adrenoceptors [73-75], and κ-opiatreceptors [76] act as heteroreceptors (presynaptically localized receptors of other neurotransmitters) on histaminergic neurons thereby inhibiting the histamine release. Details of this autoinhibition process are still unclear. Ca^{2+}-ions seem to play an important role. In examinations of the regulation of histamine release it could be demonstrated that the maximal inhibitory effect of exogenous histamine is progressively diminished when the strength of the depolarizing stimulus or the external Ca^{2+} concentration elevates [77]. Recently it was suggested that H_3-receptors are capable of inhibiting the entry of extracellular Ca^{2+} [78]. Meanwhile there is also evidence for a dependence of H_3-receptors on guanylnucleotides [79, 80], clearly showing a connection between the effector system and G-proteins [81]. In recent years, H_3-receptors could also be localized in numerous tissues of the periphery, e.g. in the guinea-pig intestine [82, 83], in human [84] or in guinea-pig lungs [85]. In these cases histamine H_3-receptors act as heteroreceptors on other neurons, influencing by this way the cholinergic, serotonergic, adrenergic, dopaminergic, and peptidergic neurotransmission.

3 In vitro screening of H_1-receptor agonists

To get an insight into structure-activity relationships scientific efforts focussed on the synthesis of compounds specifically acting on the different receptor subtypes as agonists or antagonists. After the chemical synthesis histamine receptor agonists and antagonists have to be submitted to a first "pharmacological screening". For this purpose testing models are necessary which conform with the profile of action of the original biogenic amine. These models should have a large number of the respective receptor subtypes and should allow a quantitative and reproducible evaluation of the obtained results. To gain concentration-response studies, in vitro approaches on isolated organs of animals are widely preferred. The advantage of such preparations compared with experiments on living individuals is that influences like absorption, distribution, and metabolism are negligible and that the effect of the substance to be examined only depends on the velocity (in the organ bath). Some preparations for the investigation of H_1-receptor agonists and antagonists, based on different isolated organs of the guinea-pig, are currently known. The most reliable, precise and widespread method to acquire concentration-response curves and to derive the desired pharmacological drug parameters (see later) is based on the occupation with the isolated ileum [4, 86]. All other methods have disadvantages. By examination of different H_1-receptor antagonists (e.g. mepyramine or diphenhydramine) using tracheal chain preparations [87], contractions of the trachea were observed [88]. The isolated uterus has the disadvantage that other receptors than H_1-receptors e.g. different adrenoceptors are also localized and that the procedure is sluggish (2 hours until halfmaximal relaxation [89]). Other segments of the intestine like the colon respond to an exogenous histamine stimulus with higher sensitivity which is a hint for the participation of other activators. On the tenia coli significant higher concentrations of H_1-receptor antagonists are necessary for the blockage of the stimulation effects, which can be due to additional unspecific reactions of histamine [90]. Another suitable model for H_1-receptor agonist testing is the isolated aorta [91]. Contractile responses of thoracic aorta rings can be measured in the presence of corticosteron, cimetidine, propranolol and phentolamine. H_1-receptor agonism can be verified by antagonism experiments with mepyramine.

The following text and the tables mainly contain pharmacological data from in vitro screening on five different test procedures. The H_1-receptor activity was determined on the isolated guinea-pig ileum or/and on the aorta, the H_2-receptor activity on the isolated, spontaneously beating guinea-pig right atrium [5] and the H_3-receptor activity on slices of rat cerebral cortex [6] or by using electrically stimulated longitudinal smooth muscle strips of the guinea-pig ileum [92]. These preparations are especially qualified, because the special receptor subtype is mainly responsible for the measured effect. It has to be mentioned that the interpretation of pharmacological studies using innervated muscle strips have to contend with the presence of multiple histamine receptors on muscle cells (e.g. H_1-receptors mediating Ca^{2+}-dependent contraction coexist with H_2-receptors mediating cAMP-dependent relaxation) as well as on neurons capable of releasing contractile and relaxant transmitters [93]. After recording of a complete concentration-response curve of histamine (H_1 and H_2: 10^{-8} to $10^{-5.5}$ mol/l; H_3: $0.3 \cdot 10^{-10}$ to 10^{-4} mol/l) and afterwards of the potential agonists, the subsequent evaluation follows the law of mass action and the drug-receptor-theory [94]. The pharmacological drug parameters, like intrinsic activity (i.a.), pD_2-value (for antagonists pA_2-value), pEC_{50}-values and relative activity (rel. act.) were predominantly deduced according to van Rossum [95]. As reference standard for the determination of agonistic effects histamine dihydrochloride was used (rel. act. = 100%). In the pharmacological literature the following pD_2-values of histamine are well established: 6.85 (H_1, guinea-pig ileum [95]), 6.0 (H_2, guinea-pig atrium [96]), and 7.2 (H_3, rat cerebral cortex [6]). If not indicated otherwise all tables are based on these values.

4   Histamine H$_1$-receptor agonists

4.1   Heterocyclic analogues of histamine

Histamine, the natural agonist of H$_1$-, H$_2$- and H$_3$-receptor subtypes, possesses two basic moieties: one protonable nitrogen in the imidazole ring showing a pK_a = 5.91 and the primary nitrogen of the side-chain being a significantly more basic pK_a = 9.73 [97]. At physiological pH only the primary amino group is protonated. The nitrogen atoms of the imidazole ring of histamine are indicated with N$^\pi$ and N$^\tau$ ($^\tau$ signed the N, more distanced from the side-chain), the side-chain nitrogen with N$^\alpha$ and the carbons of the side-chain with α and β [98]. The biological active form of histamine on H$_1$- and H$_2$-receptors is presumably coupled with the N$^\tau$H-tautomer of the monocation ("prototropy of histamine") [99].

The first chemical synthesis of histamine was performed by Windaus et al. [100] in the early 1900's. Afterwards numerous derivatives were synthesized, possessing the imidazole ring as a common feature. The year 1941 can be named the "year of the birth of H$_1$-receptor agonists". Walter et al. [101] synthesized a series of pyridylalkanamines and recognized that 2-(pyridin-2-yl)ethanamine (**6**) possesses (H$_1$-)histaminergic effects, whereas 4-(pyridin-2-yl)ethanamine (**10**) shows adrenergic responses. Since then, numerous heterocyclic analogues of histamine have been synthesized and screened for H$_1$-receptor activity (for an overview see [102]). From these results it was concluded that the imidazole nucleus is definitely not required for H$_1$-receptor agonist activity and the following "minimum structural requirements for an H$_1$-receptor agonist" were deduced [103, 104]: 1. The ammoniumethyl group should be in "ortho position" to a heterocyclic nitrogen atom. 2. The heterocyclic moiety needs to be able to freely rotate or at least to achieve coplanarity with the side chain.

Table 1 displays pharmacological data of some imidazole and pyridine congeners. Among the isomers of histamine only **3** ("isohistamine") is a weak selective H$_1$-receptor agonist. Among the more lipophilic imidazole derivatives (**4, 5**), recently developed in a programme of brain-penetrating histaminergic agonists, only **4** shows moderate H$_1$-receptor agonist activity. 2-(Pyridin-2-yl)ethanamine (**6**) fulfills the above-mentioned demands for an H$_1$-receptor agonist, whereas the isomers **9** and **10** only possess negligible H$_1$-receptor activity at the guinea-pig ileum. Today N$^\alpha$-methyl-2-(pyridin-2-yl)ethanamine (**7**) is the only H$_1$-receptor agonist on the market. *Betahistine* (e.g. Aequamen^R, Melopat^R) has long been used in the treat-

Table 1
H_1-, H_2- and H_3-receptor agonist activity of histamine, related imidazole derivatives and pyridine congeners.

Het–CH₂–CH₂–NR₁R₂

cpd.	Het	R₁	R₂	H₁ (guinea-pig ileum)			H₂ (guinea-pig right atrium)			H₃ (rat cerebral cortex)	
				i.a. [a]	pD₂ [b]	rel.act. [c]	i.a.	pD₂	rel.act.	rel.act.	ref.
1	imidazole (N, N–H)	H	H (histamine)	1.0	6.85	100	1.0	6.0	100	100	
2	imidazole (N–N)	H	H	0					n.d.[d]	n.d.	[109]
3	imidazole (N, NH)	H	H	0.9	4.3	0.3[e]	0			< 0.06	[106, 110]
4	imidazo-fused bicycle	H	H	0.5	pA₂[g] = 6.9	7.0	0[f]			n.d.	[112]
5	imidazo-fused bicycle	CH₃	H						n.d.	n.d.	[112]
6	pyridine	H	H			5.6	0.5		2.5	< 0.06	[105, 106]
7	pyridine	CH₃ (betahistine)	H			8.0	0.4		1.5[h]	7 · 10⁻⁶ (antagonist)	[105, 107]
8	pyridine	CH₃	CH₃	0.8		2.8			<0.13	n.d.	[112]
9	pyridine	H	H	0					[i]	n.d.	[113]
10	pyridine	H	H			< 0.001[j]			0.4[k]	n.d.	[104]

a) intrinsic activity [95], relative to histamine (max. response = 1). b) pD₂-value [95]; if not indicated otherwise values from literature are rounded up or down to 0.1. c) relative activity in percent, calculated from molar ED₅₀ ratios, relative to histamine = 100%; if not indicated otherwise values from literature are rounded up or down to 0.1. d) not determined. e) 0.1 [111]; f) inactive, negative inotropic effect observed at high doses. g) pA₂-value [95]; if not indicated otherwise values from literature are rounded up or down to 0.1. h) 10 [108]. i) pressor in cat. j) 0.01 [4]. k) 0.7 [4].

ment of Menière's disease and its triad of symptoms including vertigo, deafness and tinnitus in the form of recurrent attacks. Compound **7** is able to cross the blood-brain barrier and shows H_3-receptor antagonist activity according to Arrang et al. [107]. It is possible that the improvement of mental functions of elderly patients is the result of this H_3-receptor blockage. Efforts were made by Stark et al. [114] to improve the H_3-receptor antagonist activity of betahistine by N^α-acylation, but unfortunately the affinity of this compound is strongly reduced compared with betahistine itself. The dimethylated derivative **8** is more lipophilic but accompanied by decreased H_1-receptor activity.

Table 2
H_1-, H_2- and H_3-receptor agonist activity of 2-(thiazol-2-yl)ethanamine and related thiazoles.

cpd.	Het–CH2–CH2–NR1R2 Het	R_1	R_2	H_1 (ileum) i.a.	rel.act.	H_2 (atrium) i.a.	rel.act.	H_3 (cortex) rel.act.	ref.
11	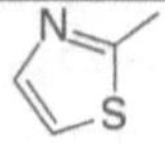 (thiazol-2-yl)	H	H	1.0	11.2[a]	0.6	2.2	<0.008	[6, 115]
12		CH3	H	0.8	10		n.d.	n.d.	[112]
13		CH3	CH3	0.7	8.2	0.2	1.6	n.d.	[112]
14	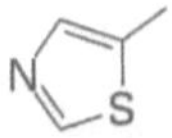 (thiazol structure)	H	H		0.01		0.1	n.d.	[104]
15	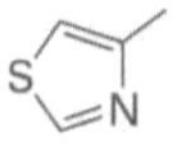 (isothiazol structure)	H	H		2		0.6[b] active[c]	n.d.	[116, 117]
16	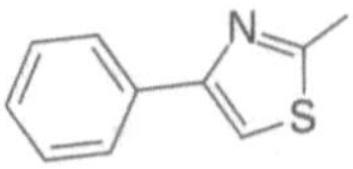 (phenyl-thiazole)	H	H	0.8	8.3		<0.13	n.d.	[112]
17	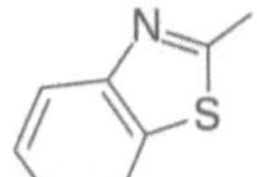 (benzothiazole)	H	H	0.5	48[d]		0[e]	n.d.	[112]
18		H	CH3	pA2 = 6.9			n.d.	n.d.	[112]

a) 20–33 [104].
b) cat blood pressure measured [117].
c) gastric acid secretion measured [118].
d) $pA_2 = 6.1$.
e) inactive, negative inotropic effect observed at high doses.

The most prominent compound in the class of thiazole analogues of histamine is 2-(thiazol-2-yl)ethanamine (**11**) which has been successfully used in pharmacological experiments [119–123]. However, the activity at H_1-receptors is controversial. Durant et al. [104] found a rel. act. of 26% (19.7–32.7%) in the presence of 1 µmol atropine, whereas according to

Steffens et al. [115] in the classical guinea-pig ileum assay only 11.2% (10.4–11.5%/40 determinations) could be determined. Interestingly mono- or dimethylation of the amine is not accompanied by a pronounced loss in activity. On the other hand the isomers of **11**, e.g. **14** and **15** are nearly inactive at H_1-receptors, which is supposed to be a consequence of the 2-aminoethane side-chain not being in "ortho position" to the nitrogen in the thiazole ring. Regarding lipophilic derivatives of **11**, **16** has reasonable H_1-receptor activity, whereas **17** is a partial agonist and **18** shows weak antagonist activity at H_1-receptors. From there it can be concluded that the replacement of the imidazole moiety by different five- or six-membered heterocycles, e.g. thiazole, pyridine or triazole, partly led to selective but only weak H_1-receptor agonists.

4.2   2-Alkylhistamines and analogues

For a long time now, interest has focused on structural modification of the histamine molecule itself. Shortening (**19**) or elongation (**29**) of the side-chain results in a complete or an extensive loss in activity. In contrast,

Table 3
H_1-, H_2- and H_3-receptor agonist activity of methyl congeners of histamine.

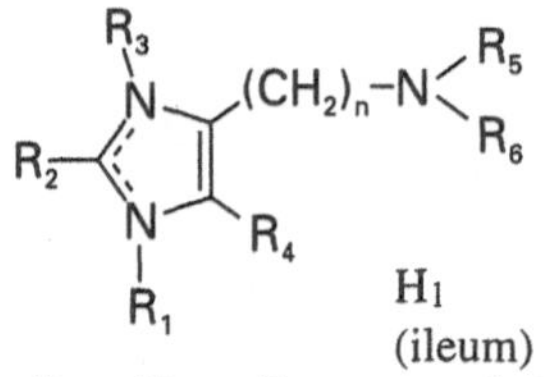

cpd.	n	R_1	R_2	R_3	R_4	R_5	R_6	H_1 (ileum)	H_2 (atrium)	H_3 (cortex)	ref.
								(relative activity)			
19	1	H	H	H	H	H	H	0	0.2	0	[78, 124, 125]
20	2	CH_3	H	H	H	H	H	0.4	<0.1[a]	<4	[6]
21	2	H	CH_3	H	H	H	H	14[b]	4	<0.08	[6, 127]
22	2	H	H	CH_3	H	H	H	<0.01	<0.1	<4	[6, 128]
23	2	H	H	H	CH_3	H	H	1	71	<0.008	[6, 96]
24	2	H	H	H	H	CH_3	H	72	74	270	[6]
25	2	H	H	H	H	CH_3	CH_3	44	51	170	[6]
26	2	H	CH_3	H	H	CH_3	H	35	3	n.d.	[129]
27	2	H	CH_3	H	H	CH_3	CH_3	18	1.9	n.d.	[129]
28	2	H	H	H	CH_3	CH_3	H	1.3	95	<0.06	[96, 106]
29	3	H	H	H	H	H	H	0.2[c]	0.4	<0.06[d]	[106, 125]

a) <0.01, determined by measuring gastric acid secretion in rat [128].
b) 16.5 [128].
c) unpublished.
d) $pA_2 = 6.0$ [78].

improvement of selectivity to one of the three receptor subtypes is possible by monomethylation, but often connected to a decrease of potency [105]. An overview is given in Table 3.

For the characterization of histamine receptors an important selective agonism could be demonstrated by methylation of the C-atoms of the imidazole nucleus. Methylation of C-2 (**21**) led to H$_1$-receptor selectivity, whereas by methylation of C-5 (**23**) a mainly H$_2$-receptor selective agonist could be obtained. These properties remain unchanged in the case of mono-(**26**) and dimethylation (**27**) of the N$^\alpha$-atom of **21** and in the case of monomethylation (**28**) of the N$^\alpha$-atom of **23**. Monosubstitution of the N$^\alpha$-atom with bulkier residues (*n*-propyl, *i*-propyl, *n*-butyl, *t*-butyl, hexyl, phenyl, benzyl, phenylethyl, phenyl-*n*-propyl or phenyl-*n*-butyl) resulted in very weak H$_1$-receptor agonists with different behaviour towards H$_2$-receptors [112]. Ringmethylation led to a complete loss of potency in the case of N$^\tau$-methylhistamine (**20**), the main metabolite of histamine, and also in the case of N$^\pi$-methylhistamine (**22**). Mono- (**24**) or dimethylation (**25**) of the N$^\alpha$-atom results in compounds with enhanced H$_3$-receptor activity (rank order: H$_3$ > H$_2$ > H$_1$) [6, 130].

After these important observations, efforts were made to synthesize compounds with higher H$_1$-receptor activity by introduction of longer alkyl

Table 4
H$_1$,-, H$_2$- and H$_3$-receptor agonist activity of some 2- or 5-substituted histamine derivatives.

cpd.	R$_1$	R$_2$	H$_1$ (ileum) i.a.	pD$_2$	rel.act.	H$_2$ (atrium) i.a.	pD$_2$	rel.act.	H$_3$ (cortex) rel.act.	ref.
30	C$_2$H$_5$	H	1.0	5.7	6.9	0.7	4.1	1.4	<0.06	[106, 127]
31	C$_3$H$_7$	H	0.8	4.3	0.3	0.3			<0.06	[106, 127]
32	C$_4$H$_9$	H	1.0	4.3$^{a)}$	0.5			n.d.	n.d.	[131]
33	CH(CH$_3$)$_2$	H	0.9	4.6	0.6	0.6			n.d.	[127]
34	CF$_3$	H	1.0	5.6$^{b)}$	7.4			n.d.	n.d.	[132]
35	NH$_2$	H	1.0	5.5$^{c)}$	1.4	1.0	5.2$^{d)}$	30	n.d.	[133]
36	NH$_2$	CH$_3$		0				<0.1$^{d)}$	n.d.	[133]
37	OH	H		0				0$^{d)}$	n.d.	[134]
38	SH	H		0				0$^{d)}$	n.d.	[134]

a) histamine standard (pD$_2$ = 6.6).
b) histamine standard (pD$_2$ = 6.7).
c) histamine standard (pD$_2$ = 7.3).
d) pD$_2$-determination on the isolated guinea-pig stomach, histamine standard (pD$_2$ = 5.7).

chains in position 2 of the imidazole ring. As a trend, it is obvious that **30–33** are less active compounds than 2-methylhistamine (**21**) but slightly more selective. Notable is also a slight improvement in activity in the case of 2-*i*-propylhistamine (**33**) compared with the isomer 2-*n*-propylhistamine (**31**). A compound with moderate H_1-receptor activity is the recently synthesized **34**. The introduction of strong polar groups in position 2 led to inactive compounds, e.g. 2-hydroxyhistamine (**37**), 2-mercaptohistamine (**38**), and 2-amino-5-methylhistamine (**36**) or to a compound with significant H_2-receptor agonist activity namely 2-aminohistamine (**35**). The complete loss of activity in **37** and **38** can be explained by the appearance of the tautomers 2-(2-oxo-4-imidazolin-4-yl)ethanamine or 2-(2-thio-4-imidazolin-4-yl)ethanamine. Compared with the imidazole system of histamine these tautomers show dramatic differences in ring geometry, which strictly inhibit interaction with H_1- or H_2-receptors.

4.3   2-Phenylhistamines

Initial studies by Dziuron et al. [131] proved that an aromatic moiety at C-2 of the imidazole ring lead to selective H_1-receptor agonists. Recently a great improvement in potency and clear structure-activity relationships could be realized by introduction of different residues into the phenyl ring.

The majority of the 2-phenylhistamine derivatives **39-72** possesses moderate to strong histamine H_1-receptor agonist activity. Substitution in ortho-position leads in the case of the halo derivatives **40** and **41** or the trifluoromethyl derivative **42** to a decrease in H_1-receptor agonist potency and to compounds which display lower activity than the unsubstituted parent molecule **39**. Substitution in ortho-position of the phenyl ring seems to be unsuitable for an improvement in H_1-receptor activity. Among the para-substituted derivatives only the fluoro (**56**) and the hydroxy derivative (**61**) possess more than 10% of the potency of histamine. Surprisingly the 4-chloro derivative (**57**) and its trifluoromethyl analogue (**58**) are only very weak H_1-receptor agonists. Therefore para-substituents which are bulkier than a hydroxy group lead to a drastic reduction of H_1-receptor activity. The same was observed in the case of a second substitution. Bulky residues bigger than two fluoro atoms are apparently not accepted by the receptor and lead like the 3,4-dichloro derivative (**67**) to weak H_1-receptor antagonists. However, the introduction of substituents in meta-position of the phenyl ring leads to a remarkable improvement of the histaminergic potency at H_1-receptors. With the exception of **50** and **51** all compounds of this type

Table 5

H$_1$-receptor agonist activity of different substituted 2-phenylhistamines.

cpd.	R$_1$	R$_2$	R$_3$	R$_4$	H$_1$ (guinea-pig ileum)			ref.
					i.a.	pD$_2$[a]	rel.act.	
39	H	H	H	H	1.0	5.7	12.6[b)c)d]	[131]
40	F	H	H	H	0.9	5.2	2.2	[135]
41	Cl	H	H	H	0.8	4.9	1.1	[135]
42	CF$_3$	H	H	H	0.3	4.5	0.6	[132]
43	H	F	H	H	1.0	6.79	87.1	[135]
44	H	Cl	H	H	1.0	6.76	81.3[e]	[135]
45	H	Br	H	H	1.0	6.90	112.2	[91]
46	H	I	H	H	1.0	6.68	96.0	[132]
47	H	CF$_3$	H	H	1.0	6.96	128.8	[91]
48	H	CH$_3$	H	H	1.0	6.3	29.5[f]	[135]
49	H	OCH$_3$	H	H	1.0	6.2	39.8	[136]
50	H	OC$_2$H$_5$	H	H	0.7	4.6	1.0	[136]
51	H	OC$_4$H$_9$	H	H	0.7	4.4	0.6	[136]
52	H	OCF$_3$	H	H	1.0	6.4	53.7	[132]
53	H	OH	H	H	1.0	5.4	6.3	[136]
54	H	NH$_2$	H	H	1.0	5.7	7.3[g]	[135]
55	H	NO$_2$	H	H	1.0	6.2	39.8	[136]
56	H	H	F	H	1.0	6.0	14.1	[135]
57	H	H	Cl	H	0.5	4.3	0.5	[136]
58	H	H	CF$_3$	H	0.2	4.6	0.7	[132]
59	H	H	CH$_3$	H	0.4[h]	4.2	0.4[i]	[136]
60	H	H	OCH$_3$	H		[j]		[136]
61	H	H	OH	H	1.0	5.8	15.9	[136]
62	H	H	NH$_2$	H	1.0[k]	5.2	2.6[l]	[135]
63	H	H	N(CH$_3$)$_2$	H	0			[135]
64	H	H	NO$_2$	H		[j]		[136]
65	H	H	NHCHO	H	0.7	4.5	0.6	[137]
66	F	F	H	H	0.7	5.4	3.6	[135]
67	H	Cl	Cl	H		pA$_2$ = 5.3[j]		[136]
68	H	O–CH$_2$–O		H		[j]		[136]
69	H	OCH$_3$	OCH$_3$	H		[j]		[136]
70	H	OH	OH	H	1.0	4.3	0.5	[136]
71	H	F	H	F	0.9	5.9	12.3	[135]
72	H	OCH$_3$	H	OCH$_3$		[j]		[136]

a) [131], [136]: histamine standard (pD$_2$ = 6.6); [132], [137]: histamine standard (pD$_2$ = 6.7).
b) 10.0 [136].   c) 19.1 [127].   d) 31.6 [91].   e) 15.9 [136].   f) 12.6 [136].   g) 2.5 [136].
h) 0.7 [136].   i) 0,3 [136].   j) inactive, (pD$_2$ < 4).   k) 0.7 [136].   l) 1.6 [136]

possess full intrinsic activity and the activities range from 0.6 up to 128% compared to histamine 100% but no consistent trends can be observed. A substitution in meta-position is well tolerated, independent of the electronical features of the residues (3-NO_2, 3-halo, but also 3-OCH_3, 3-CH_3). The compounds with the highest histamine H_1-receptor agonist potency are 2-[3-(trifluoromethyl)phenyl]histamine (**47**) and 2-(3-bromophenyl)histamine (**45**) and its halo analogues **43**, **44** and **46**. Among the halo series a maximum is reached when the phenyl nucleus is substituted with a bromo atom. There seems to be a limit with regard to the volume of the substituent, also observed in the phenolether series **49–52**. Outgoing from **43**, the introduction of an additional fluoro atom in 2- or 5-position (**66**, **71**) leads again to a marked decrease of potency. Thus it is obvious that the possibilities for further substitutions at the aromatic system are strongly limited.

Compounds **43–47** are the most potent H_1-receptor agonists known so far. For that reason it is interesting to look precisely at the pharmacological properties of these ligands. The concentration-response curves of **43–46** are not significantly different from the histamine standard, whereas **47** possesses significantly higher potency than histamine at H_1-receptors. The pA$_2$-values of the H_1-receptor antagonist diphenhydramine measured against **43** and **44** are nearly 8 (determined by Schild-plot analysis [138]). This is in good agreement with the value found by Marshall [139] with histamine. The same is valid for **45** to **47** with the exception that for mepyramine a depression of the maximum effect was observed with increasing concentrations. However, the pA$_2$-values are near by 9.1, which is in the same order of magnitude with the value determined in the same series of experiments for histamine. According to Schild-plot analysis, competitive behaviour was observed for diphenhydramine and mepyramine against **44–47** (slope nearly –1), whereas the slope of the *Schild-plot* regression of **43** is significantly different from unity (slope –0.71), thus indicating that the interaction diphenhydramine against **43** is non competitive. On the isolated guinea-pig right atrium for **43** and **44** slightly positive chronotropic and inotropic effects could be detected but these cannot be influenced by the H_2-receptor antagonist cimetidine nor by the β-adrenoceptor antagonist metoprolol. For the most potent H_1-receptor agonists **45** and **47** pD'$_2$-values [140] on the atrium of 3.4 and 3.8, respectively, were obtained [91]. In pithed and vagotomized rats **45** and **47** are devoid of an indirect sympathomimetic effect and at high doses they produce a vasodepressor response not mediated via histamine receptors [141]. Experiments concerning the interaction with H_3-receptors are available only for a few substances.

Lipp et al. [106] found a rel. act. < 0.06% (histamine 100%) for the unsubstituted 2-phenylhistamine (**39**). For **45** and **47**, the so far most potent H_1-receptor agonists, the -log K-values at the H_3-receptor guinea-pig ileum assay are smaller than 5.0 [132].

Recently for several 2-phenylhistamines direct interactions with pertussis-toxin-sensitive G-proteins in HL-60-leukemic cells were observed, which are interestingly not mediated by histamine H_1-receptors [142, 143]. The cationic amphiphilic 2-substituted histamine derivatives activate pertussis toxin sensitive the heterotrimeric regulatory guanine nucleotide-binding proteins (G-proteins) in HL-60 membranes (see tab. 6). The responses were determined by measurement of GTP hydrolysis. The activation of G-proteins was observed also in the presence of H_1-receptor antagonist indicating that the mechanism of these effects is H_1-receptor independent. The H_1-receptor activity of the 2-phenylhistamines does not correlate with GTP-hydrolysis. Compound **57**, a very weak H_1-receptor agonist, stimulates the GTP-hydrolysis with the same potency as the potent H_1-receptor agonists **44–46**.

Table 6
G-protein activation by 2-phenylhistamines.

cpd.	GTP-hydrolysis (HL-60 membranes)	
	rel.eff. [%]	pEC_{50}
39	36	3.5
40	31	3.7
41	36	–
43	38	–
44	75	3.5
45	80	3.7
46	80	3.8
56	35	–
57	80	3.4

Among the till now synthesized 2-phenylhistamines no simple correlation between lipophilicity (π), electronic influences (σ), or steric effects (E_s-constants [144]) on one hand and H_1-receptor agonist activity on the other hand could be observed. Therefore so far no quantitative structure-activity relationships are available. Semiquantitative methods according to Topliss [145, 146] are not applicable. In addition, the comparison of the results is strongly limited, because for the "same compounds" different pD_2-values are reported in literature, e.g. for the parent molecule 2-phenylhistamine

10–31.6%. Also problems with non-standardized procedures or with different animals breeds have to be taken into consideration.

4.4   Analogues of 2-phenylhistamine and related substances

Table 7 displays H_1- and H_2-receptor activity of some heterocyclic analogues of 2-phenylhistamine and related compounds.

Table 7
H_1- and H_2-receptor agonist activity of heterocyclic analogues of 2-phenylhistamine and related compounds.

cpd.	name	H_1 (ileum)			H_2 (atrium)	
		i.a.	pD2	rel. act.	i.a.	ref.
73	2-(2-thienyl)histamine	1.0	6.5	45.7	0[a)]	[91]
74	2-(3-thienyl)histamine	1.0	6.7	66.1	0[a)]	[91]
75	2-(5-bromo-3-thienyl)histamine	1.0	6.3	25.7	n.d.	[91]
76	2-(2-thienylmethyl)histamine	1.0	5.2	2.2	n.d.	[91]
77	2-(3-thienylmethyl)histamine	1.0	5.4	3.6	n.d.	[91]
78	2-(2-pyrrolyl)histamine	0.9	5.9[b)]	14.0	n.d.	[132]
79	2-(2-furanyl)histamine	1.0	6.4	34.7	0.4[c)]	[91]
80	2-(2-pyridyl)histamine	1.0	4.8	0.9	0.3	[127]
81	2-(3-pyridyl)histamine	1.0	5.9	11.0	0.3	[127]
82	2-(4-pyridyl)histamine	1.0	5.8	9.1	0.3	[127]
83	2-(5-bromo-3-pyridyl)histamine	1.0	6.5[b)]	69.2	n.d.	[132]
84	2-(2-piperidyl)histamine	0.6	4.7	0.7	0.2	[127]
85	2-(3-piperidyl)histamine	0.4	5.0	1.5	0.2	[127]
86	2-(4-piperidyl)histamine	0.5	4.9	1.2	0.2	[127]

a) 10^{-5} to 10^{-4} mol/l lead to transient positive chronotropic and inotropic effects, which are neither cimetidine nor metoprolol sensitive.
b) histamine standard (pD2 = 6.7).
c) transient positive chronotropic effects.

A marked increase in H_1-receptor activity of **39** was achieved by exchanging the phenyl ring for the bioisosteric thiophene moiety. The compound covering a 3-thienyl ring (**74**) is still more active than the compound with a 2-thienyl ring (**73**). 2-(2-Pyrrolyl)histamine **78** is significantly less active than 2-(2-furanyl)histamine **79** and 2-(2-thienyl)histamine **73**. Introduction of a methylene group between the thiophene heterocycle and histamine leads to the nearly equipotent compounds **76** and **77**. Both are much less active than **73** or **74**, compounds with a direct heterocyclic substitution of the histamine moiety. As can be seen for substance **75** (and also for **83**), it is not possible to improve H_1-receptor activity by bromo-substitution of the heterocyclic rings in meta position. Among the 2-pyridylhistamine derivatives **80–82** it is remarkable that the following rank order concerning the H$_1$-receptor activity was recognized: meta > para > ortho. This is in good agreement with the corresponding monofluorinated 2-phenylhistamine derivatives **40**, **43** and **56**. Conceivable for both series of compounds are H-bonds of the pyridine nitrogen or the fluorine atom with a proton donor group of the H$_1$-receptor. The hydrogenation of the pyridine moiety to the corresponding piperidine derivatives **84–86** leads to a strong decrease in potency, although the aforementioned rank order is valid again. On the isolated guinea-pig right atrium compounds **80–82** and **84–86** show intrinsic activities of 0.2–0.3, whereas **73** and **74** cause positive chronotropic and inotropic effects, which are as shown for **43** and **44** (see above) neither of histaminergic nor of adrenergic nature.

Some 2-phenylhistamines and their heterocyclic analogues were also screened on the isolated guinea-pig aorta. The H$_1$-receptor agonists and histamine itself contract the aorta rings with pEC$_{50}$-values generally smaller and intrinsic activities generally lower compared to the ileum values, but the results largely mirrored those seen previously and a linear relationship between pD$_2$-values on the ileum and pEC$_{50}$-values on the aorta was found [132]. For all agonists on the aorta a significant sensitiza-

Table 8
Histamine H$_1$-receptor agonist activity of some histamine derivatives on the guinea-pig aorta [132].

cpd.	2. curve i.a.	pEC$_{50}$	rel.act.	3. curve i.a.	ΔpEC$_{50}$	mepyramine pK$_B$ (pA$_2$),
1	1.1	5.9	105	1.1	0.1	(9.1)
11	1.0	5.2	18	1.1	0.1	(9.0)
39	0.9	5.2	19	0.9	0.3	9.1
43	0.8	5.4	30	0.9	0.3	(8.7)
44	0.7	5.7	59	0.8	0.4	9.0
45	0.7	5.6	49	0.8	0.5	(8.9)
46	0.5	5.6	47	0.7	0.6	9.1
47	0.8	5.9	94	0.9	0.2	9.0
73	0.5	5.0	12	0.8	0.5	8.8
74	0.4	5.2	19	0.6	0.5	9.0
75	0.6	4.9	11	0.8	0.4	8.6
76	0.5	3.8	0.8	0.7	0.4	a)
77	0.4	3.9	0.9	0.7	0.4	a)
78	0.5	5.3	23	0.6	0.4	9.3
79	0.7	5.0	12	0.8	0.4	9.3

a) blockable by 10^{-6} M mepyramine.

tion was observed for two successive curves. All contractile effects could be antagonized by mepyramine.

The H_1-receptor activity of different substituted 2-benzylhistamines is given in Table 9.

Table 9
H_1-receptor activity of different 2-benzylhistamines.

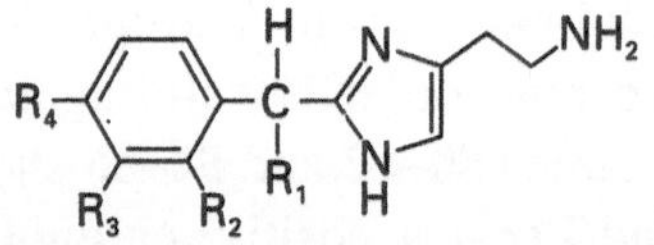

cpd.	R_1	R_2	R_3	R_4	i.a.	pD_2[a]	rel. act.	pA_2	ref.
87	H	H	H	H	0.9	5.0	2.5		[131]
88	CH_3	H	H	H	0.8	5.0	1.5		[147]
89	H	Cl	H	H	0.5	5.1	2.6		[132]
90	H	H	Cl	H	0.8	4.9	1.5		[132]
91	H	H	H	Cl	0.4	5.2	4.0		[131]
92	H	CF_3	H	H	0			3.6	[132]
93	H	H	CF_3	H	0.3	4.6	0.7		[132]
94	H	H	H	CF_3	0			4.5	[132]
95	H	H	H	OCH_3	0.4	4.2	0.4		[131]

The table above has the column "H_1 (guinea-pig ileum)" spanning i.a., pD_2, rel. act., pA_2.

a) [131]: histamine standard ($pD_2 = 6.6$), [132]: histamine standard ($pD_2 = 6.7$).

The introduction of a methylene (87) linkage between phenyl moiety and imidazole ring leads to a decrease of H_1-receptor activity. Compound 87 is comparable to 76 and 77 because of the bioisosteric aromatic ring systems. Indeed the compounds are nearly equipotent. Structural modification of 2-benzylhistamine (87) by introduction of a methyl group at the methylene bridge leads to the racemic compound 88, the activity of which is also in the same order of magnitude. Substitution of 87 with chloro (89–91), trifluoromethyl (92–94) or para-methoxy groups (95) leads to compounds showing lower activity than the parent 2-phenylhistamines, but the highest activity in each case was found in the meta series. The H_1-receptor activity of stronger modified 2-substituted histamines is given in Table 10.

As seen for 87, the introduction of a linkage between phenyl ring and imidazole moiety leads to a strong decrease of H_1-receptor activity (96). The alicyclic compounds 97 and 98 synthesized by hydrogenation of 87 and 96 are weak H_1-receptor antagonists, while 99 is nearly inactive at H_1-receptors. The combination of histamine with a diphenylmethyl moiety which is characteristic for H_1-receptor blockers leads to compound 100 showing

Table 10
H$_1$-receptor activity of 2-substituted histamine derivatives with aromatic or alicyclic structures.

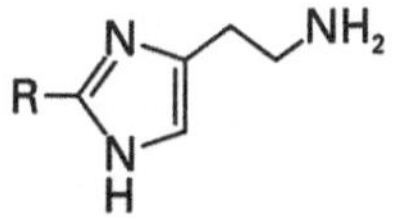

			H$_1$ (guinea-pig ileum)				
cpd.	R		i.a.	pD$_2$[a]	rel. act.	pA$_2$	ref.
96	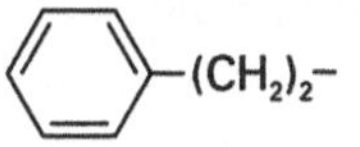 phenyl-(CH$_2$)$_2$-		0.9	5.1	3.2		[131]
97	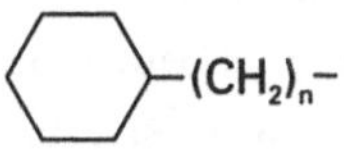 cyclohexyl-(CH$_2$)$_n$-	n = 1	0.1			5.7	[131]
98		n = 2	0			5.3	[131]
99	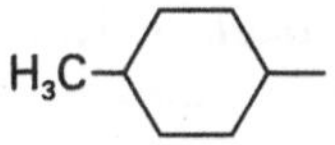 H$_3$C-cyclohexyl-		0.2				[131]
100	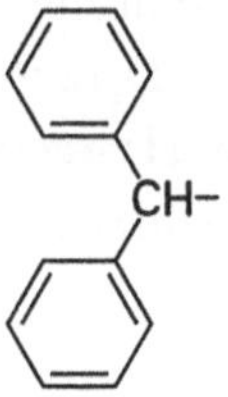 (diphenyl)CH-		0			6.5	[131]
101	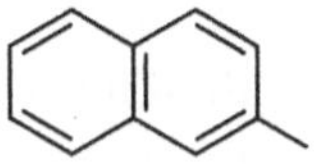 naphthyl		0.2	4.8	1.2		[132]
102	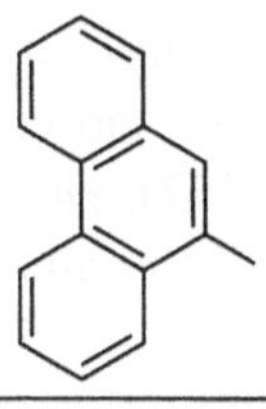 phenanthryl		0			4.7	[132]

a) [131]: histamine standard (pD$_2$ = 6.6), [132]: histamine standard (pD$_2$ = 6.7).

significant H$_1$-receptor antagonist activity. Introduction of more lipophilic residues (101: naphthyl or 102: phenanthryl) close to the imidazole nucleus also leads to a dramatic decrease in activity compared to 2-phenylhistamine (39). On the basis of these results it can be concluded that the structural modification of 39, realized by the introduction of different aromatic, heteroaromatic or alicyclic substituents in position 2 of the imidazole ring leads with a few exceptions to a more or less pronounced decrease in activity or alters the agonistic activity to H$_1$-receptor antagonism.

4.5   2-Substituted histamine derivatives with long, flexible
          side-chains

The introduction of aryloxyalkyl moieties with different chain lengths
(**103–105**) led to H_1-receptor antagonism. The same was observed for the
naphthoxy derivatives **106** and **107**. In analogy to the potent histamine
H_2-receptor agonist impromidine (a combination of a weak partial H_2-re-
ceptor agonist (SK&F 91486 [149]) with a cimetidine moiety (SK&F 92408
[150])), efforts were made to synthesize interesting compounds by combination of histamine with structural elements mediating H_2-receptor affinity,
e.g. a piperidinomethylphenoxyalkyl group. This moiety is the central
building block of highly potent H_2-receptor antagonists, e.g. lamtidine,
lavoltidine (formerly known as loxtidine) or *roxatidine acetate* (Roxit^R) and
interacts with a lipophilic areal of H_2-receptors [151].
Compounds **108–118** represent a new type of histamine H_1-receptor
agonists showing H_1-receptor agonist with combined H_2-receptor antagonist activity [148]. All substances of this type display H_1-receptor agonist
activity. Regarding the activity on the guinea-pig ileum, one should note'
that **109** is the most potent compound in this series and possesses 6.9% of
the activity of histamine. This lamtidine analogue differs from the known
H_2-receptor antagonist only in the replacement of the diaminotriazole
system by a histamine component. Variations in the length of the side-chain
of **109** are connected with a marked decrease in activity. Elongation to a
5-membered chain (**110**) between the imidazole and phenyl ring leads to a
full H_1-receptor agonist, whereas further lengthening or shortening of the
chain results in very weak partial agonists (**108, 111, 112**). Outgoing from
109, the variation of the basic function by exchange of the piperidine ring
with a dimethylamino substituent (**113**) is expressed by a drastic reduction
of H_1-receptor agonist activity, which is strengthened by the exchange of
the piperidine ring against a pyrrolidine ring (**114**). In this series the
piperidine ring seems to be the optimal substituent.
The conclusion might be drawn that a basically substituted side-chain of
H_2-receptor antagonists in position 2 of the imidazole ring is well tolerated.
In comparison to the 2-(aryloxyalkyl)histamines **103–105**, the lamtidine
analogues **109–111** are weak H_1-receptor agonists, whereas the appropriate
2-(aryloxyalkyl)histamines are H_1-receptor antagonists. The difference in
structure is only the additional piperidinomethyl residue in the meta-position of the phenyl ring. Therefore H_1-receptor agonist activity of lamtidine-
like compounds is the result of the basic piperidine ring.

Considering the pA2-values obtained on the guinea-pig right atrium for **108–118** and the relative activities compared with the known H2-receptor antagonist cimetidine, great differences compared with H1-receptor activity could be observed. All compounds except for the cimetidine analogues **115** and **116** possess histamine H2-receptor antagonist activity. In this series the lamtidine analogue **109** shows highest potency also on H2-receptors. The results given in Table 11 demonstrate that a piperidinomethylphenoxyalkyl

Table 11
H1-receptor activity of 2-substituted histamine derivatives with long, flexible side-chains and/or typical moieties of H2-receptor antagonists.

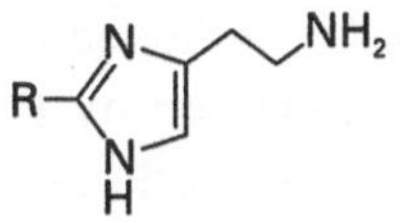

cpd.	R		H1 (ileum) i.a.	pD2	rel. act.	H2 (atrium) pA2	rel. act.[a]	ref.
103	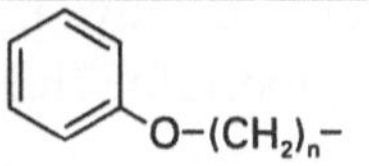	n = 3	0	pA2 = 4.7			n.d.	[147]
104		n = 4	0	pA2 = 5.9			n.d.	[147]
105	O–(CH2)n–	n = 5	0	pA2 = 5.5			n.d.	[147]
106	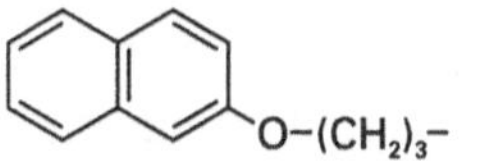 O–(CH2)3–		0	pA2 = 5.4			n.d.	[147]
107	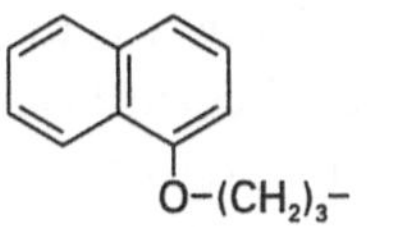		0	pA2 = 5.7			n.d.	[147]
108	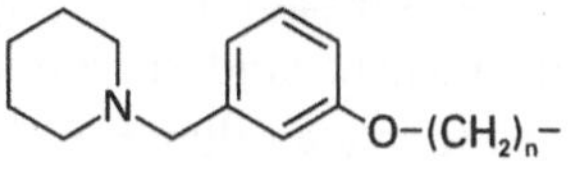	n = 1	0.1			4.8	2.5	[148]
109		n = 3	0.7	5.7	6.9	6.3	75.9	[148]
110	O–(CH2)n–	n = 4	1.0	4.2	0.2	5.9	34.7	[148]
111		n = 5	0.3			5.0	4.4	[148]
112		n = 6	0.3			5.9	31.6	[148]
113	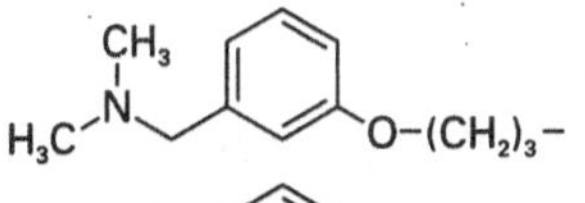 O–(CH2)3–		0.7	5.0	1.3	5.1	5.5	[148]
114	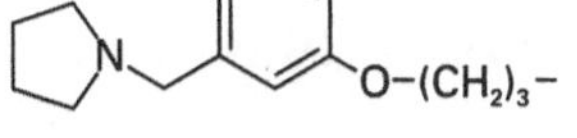 O–(CH2)3–		0.8	4.5	0.4	5.5	11.8	[148]
115 R1 = CH3	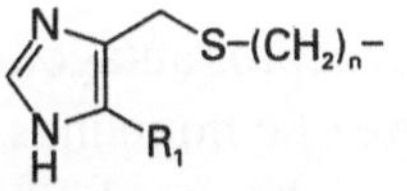 S–(CH2)n–	n = 3	0.5	4.3	0.3	b)		[148]
116 R1 = H		n = 4	0.6	4.2	0.2	b)		[148]
117	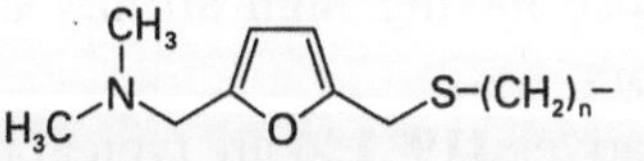	n = 3	0.7	4.8	0.8	4.8	2.4	[148]
118	S–(CH2)n–	n = 4	0.9	4.6	0.6	3.6	0.2	[148]

a) compared with cimetidine (pA2 = 6.4; rel. act. = 100 %).
b) inactive at H2-receptors up to $0.3 \cdot 10^{-3}$ mol/l.

residue can be combined with a [4-(2-aminoethyl)imidazol-2-yl] moiety, but that H_2-receptor antagonist activity decreases to the potency of cimetidine. Compared with lamtidine, compounds **109–112** also show a characteristic depression of the concentration-response curves, ranging from 5 to 15% [152]. The noncompetitive part increases simultaneously with H_2-receptor antagonist activity.

In this row an optimum of activity is reached with a four-membered chain between the phenyl and imidazole ring. This is in good agreement with [153], where elongation of the side-chain of lamtidine was accompanied by a decrease in H_2-receptor antagonist activity. Change of the basic function of **109** diminishes H_2-receptor antagonist activity in the case of the pyrrolidine derivative (**114**), which is strengthened for the dimethylamino derivative (**113**). Similar results were obtained by Bays et al. [154] with lamtidine analogues influencing the acid secretion of heidenhain pouched dogs (an in vivo model for the testing of H_2-receptor antagonists independent of vagal innervation [155]). The authors gave the following rank-order (the most active compound with the piperidine ring (lamtidine) is on the left, activity and duration of action decrease to the right): piperidine > pyrrolidine > ranitidine > dimethylamine. It has to be taken into account that ranitidine and lamtidine have different "polar groups", whereas the "H_2-receptor antagonists" **109**, **113**, **114**, **117** possess the same "polar group". This was unimportant in this comparison, because Bays et al. [154] could additionally demonstrate that the combination of a 3-[3-(piperidinomethyl)phenoxy]propyl residue with a nitroethenediamine (of ranitidine) resulted in a compound, which inhibits the gastric acid secretion of the anaesthetized rat [156] in a significantly stronger way than ranitidine. As mentioned above the cimetidine analogues **115** and **116** are devoid of H_2-receptor antagonist activity. Obviously the {[(5-methylimidazol-4-yl)methyl]thio}alkyl moiety acts very sensitively for variations considering the "polar group". This is in accordance with the observation that the replacement of the cyanoguanidine in this class is always accompanied by a significant decrease in activity.

The introduction of structural parts of H_2-receptor antagonists in H_1-receptor agonist moieties shows that the structure of compounds interacting with H_1-receptors are very different from those having high affinity but no intrinsic activity for histamine H_2-receptors.

The basically substituted histamine derivatives **119–126** are typical partial H_1-receptor agonists, except for **120** and **124–126**, which are weak H_1-receptor antagonists. Among the histamine derivatives with long-chained

Table 12

H$_1$-receptor activity of 2-substituted histamine derivatives with basic groups and typical moieties of H$_1$-receptor antagonists.

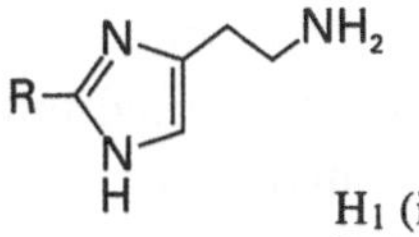

cpd.	R	n	H$_1$ (ileum)				H$_2$ (atrium)		ref.
			i.a.	pD$_2$	rel. act.	pA$_2$	pD$_2$	pA$_2$	
119	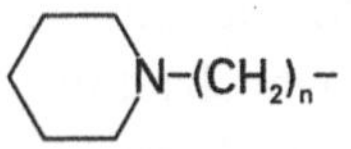 piperidino–(CH$_2$)$_n$–	n = 3	0.7	4.6	0.6		a)	n.d.	[157]
120		n = 4	0			3.4	n.d.	a)	[157]
121	morpholino–(CH$_2$)$_n$–	n = 5	0.1				3.3	a)	[157]
122		n = 6	0.5	4.6	0.5		n.d.	a)	[157]
123	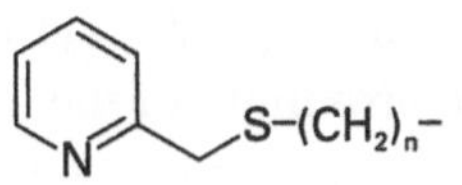 pyridyl–CH$_2$–S–(CH$_2$)$_n$–	n = 3	0.6	4.3	0.3		n.d.	a)	[157]
124		n = 4	0			5.1		3.1	[157]
125	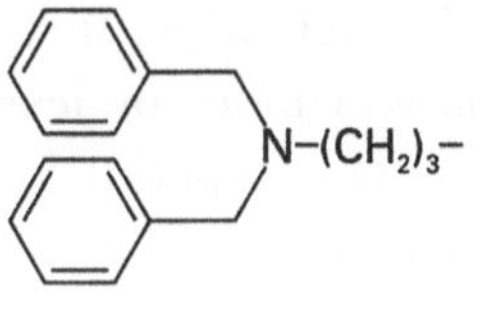 N–(CH$_2$)$_3$– (diphenylmethyl)		0			5.2		n.d.	[147]
126	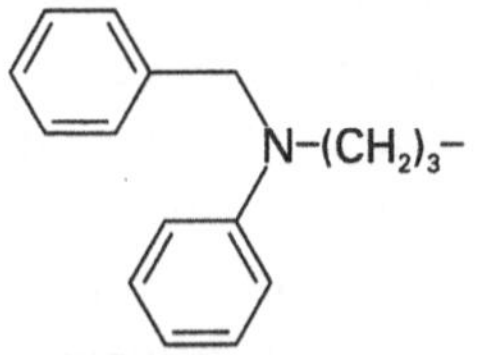 N–(CH$_2$)$_3$– (dibenzyl)		0			5.9		n.d.	[147]

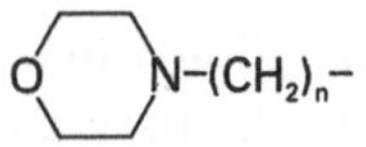

a) inactive up to 10^{-3} mol/l.

piperidino- or morpholinoalkyl residues, 119, a compound with a basic 3-piperidinopropyl moiety, showed a minor increase in activity compared to the above-mentioned 2-n-propylhistamine (31) (see Table 4). Elongation of the methylene chain of 119 leads to the H$_1$-receptor antagonist 120. Lengthening of the chain by an additional methylene group and exchange of the piperidine ring against a morpholine ring resulted in 121, a very weak H$_1$-receptor agonist. The same was noticed for 123, where the piperidine ring was exchanged against a pyridine ring and the side-chain elongation was performed by the introduction of a thioether linkage. In this context the cimetidine analogue 115 (see Table 11) is worth mentioning, because it is closely related to 123, where the (5-methylimidazol-4-yl) moiety is substituted by a pyridine ring. Both substances are nearly equipotent. Elongation of the side-chain between the basical function and the histamine moiety result in a strong increase of H_1-receptor agonist activity in case of the morpholine derivative **122**, whereas for the imidazole derivative **116** a slight decrease in activity was observed, which turned into H_1-receptor antagonism in the case of the pyridine derivative **124**.

One should note that regarding H_1-receptor agonist activity a long-chained substituent in position 2 of the imidazole ring is tolerated by H_1-receptors. That means that an amine function might be able to reach additional binding sites of the H_1-receptor. By comparing **119** with the basically substituted histamine analogues **125** and **126**, which carry additional lipophilic residues, a turnover to H_1-receptor antagonists is observed. This is strengthened when the basicity, as shown in the case of 2-[N-benzyl-(3-anilino)propyl]histamine **126**, is decreased due to the proximity of the nitrogen to the phenyl ring.

This effect is confirmed by the above mentioned observation, that all in position 2 basically substituted histamines possess a more or less pronounced H_1-receptor activity. In addition, this was also supported by the pharmacological behaviour of the 2-(aryloxyalkyl)histamines **103–105** (see Table 11) and the increase of H_1-receptor activity of the five-membered morpholine derivative (**121**) to the six-membered homologue (**122**). If the activity of the lamtidine-like compound **109** is caused by the piperidinomethyl substituent, a strong active H_1-receptor agonist of the 2-(piperidinoalkyl)histamine-type should contain a methylene chain of approx. 7–9 members. These considerations are speculative because the influence of the "chain fixing" aromatic system, which abolishes flexibility of the methylene chain in this position, is hard to estimate.

4.6   Miscellaneous H_1-receptor agonists

In the mid 80's, Steffens et al. [158] synthesized some bis(2,2'-histamines) carrying ethylene (**127**, see Table 13), tetramethylene (**128**), hexamethylene (**129**), or p-phenylene groups (**130**) between both histamine molecules. Unfortunately these compounds are devoid of H_1-and H_2-receptor activity except for **129**, which is a weak agonist on both H_1- and H_2-receptors.

Recently, Young et al. [112] introduced a second imidazolylethyl substituent at N^α. The resulting compound **131** is equivalently effective to histamine on both H_1- and H_2-receptors. In contrast, the dimer of **6** is a much weaker active compound (**136**) than the parent molecule. The same

Table 13
H₁- and H₂-receptor agonist activity of miscellaneous H₁-receptor agonists.

cpd.		H₁ (ileum) i.a.	rel. act.	H₂ (atrium) rel. act.	ref.
127	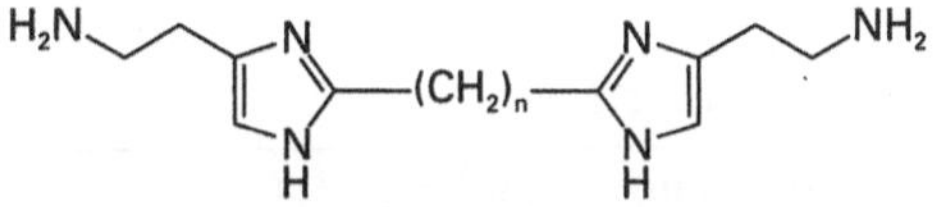 $n = 2$	0		0	[158]
128	$n = 4$	0		n.d.	[158]
129	$n = 6$	0.2		$0^{a)}$	[158]
130	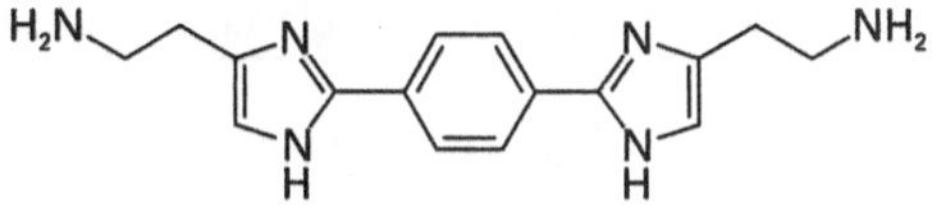	0		n.d.	[158]
131			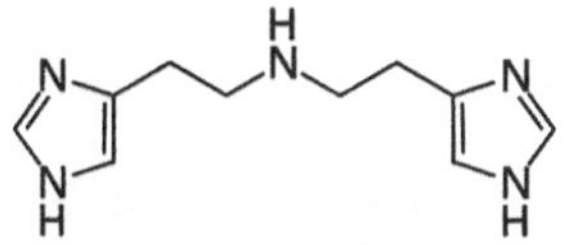 104	$94^{b)}$	[112]
132	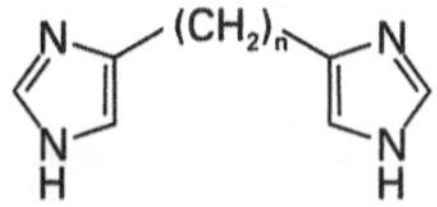 $n = 3$	$0^{c)}$		n.d.	[132]
133	$n = 4$	$0^{d)}$		n.d.	[132]
134	$n = 5$	$0^{e)}$		n.d.	[132]
135	$n = 6$	$0^{f)}$		n.d.	[132]
136	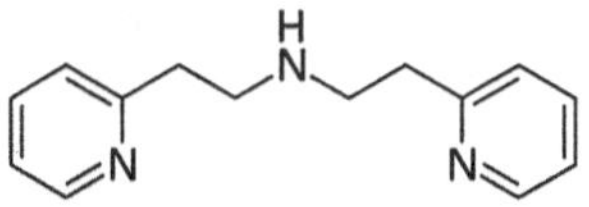	0.7	2.7	<0.13	[112]
137	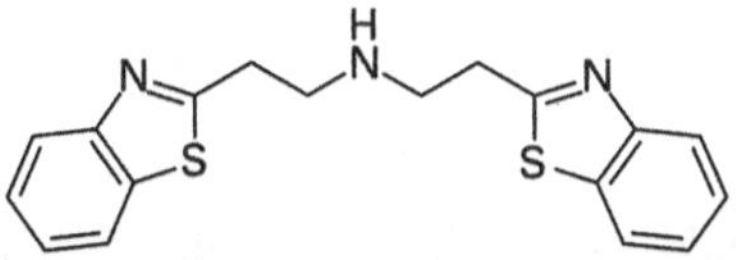	0.4	8.2	n.d.	[112]

a) i.a. = 0.2. b) i.a. = 0.9. c) pD′₂ = 4.56. d) pD′₂ = 4.46. e) pD′₂ = 4.72. f) pD′₂ = 4.98.

was observed for **137/17**. Two imidazole moieties each linked in postion 4 by a long, flexible methylene chain resulted in compounds showing very weak H₁-receptor activity (**132–135**).

4.7 Stereoselectivity of the H₁-receptor

Side-chain methylation of the histamine molecule in α- or β-position leads according to the stereochemical configuration predominantly to compounds with pronounced selectivity towards H₃-receptors in comparison to H₁-/H₂-receptors. Compound **138** is at present one of the most potent H₃-receptor agonists. It seems to be obvious that H₂- and H₃-receptors follow steric requirements even better than H_1-receptors, but one should note that the relative H_1-receptor agonist activity of **138–141** amounts to only 0.5–0.75% of the activity of histamine.

Table 14
Activity of chiral agonists on histamine receptor subtypes.

cpd.		H_1 (ileum)		H_2 (atrium)	H_3 (cortex)	
		conf.	rel. act.	rel. act.	rel. act.	ref.
138	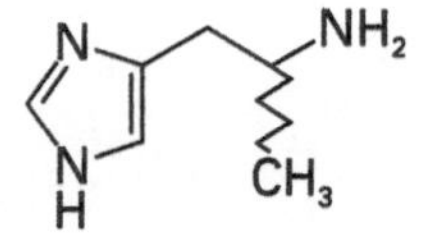	R	0.5	1.0	1550	[106]
139		S	0.5	1.7	13	[106]
140	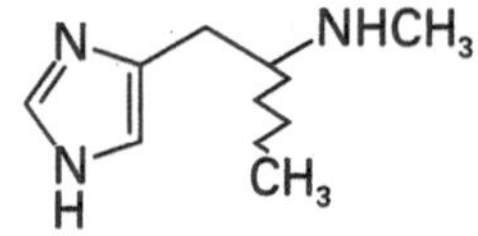	R	0.7	0.4	4.1	[159, 160]
141		S	0.7	1.0	0.1	[159, 160]
142	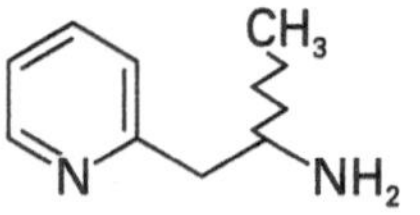	rac.	0.25	n.d.	n.d.	[161]
143		d	0.38	n.d.	n.d.	[161]
144		l	0.12	n.d.	n.d.	[161]
145	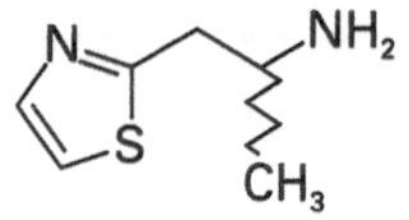	rac.	0.5	0[a]	n.d.	[115]
146	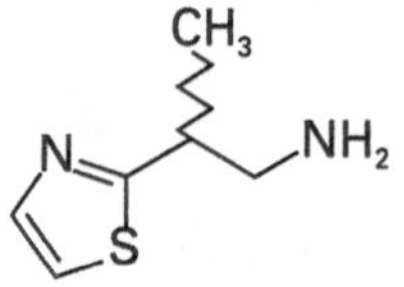	rac.	0.5	0[a]	n.d.	[115]
147	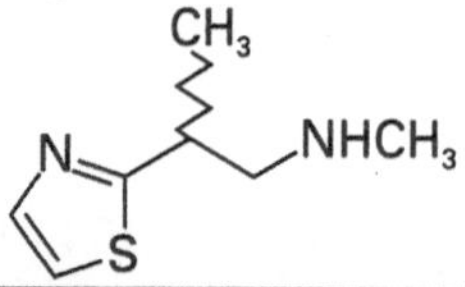	rac.	0.5	0[a]	n.d.	[115]

a) i.a. < 0.2.

Initial studies to evidence a possible stereoselectivity of histamine H_1-receptors were performed by Graham et al. [161]. Outgoing from the racemic **142** [162] both enantiomers were tested pharmacologically with the result that higher activity on the guinea-pig ileum was seen for the *d*-enantiomer **143** than for the *l*-enantiomer **144** and for the racemate. Nevertheless the H_1-receptor activity is substantially less pronounced compared with the non-methylated parent molecule 2-(pyridin-2-yl)ethanamine (**6**) (see

Table 1), and the pharmacological differences are negligible which makes a precise assessment doubtful.

Similar problems appeared with the side-chain methylation of 2-(thiazol-2-yl)ethanamine (11) (see Table 2) and N$^\alpha$-methyl-2-(thiazol-2-yl)ethanamine. Compounds 145–147 possess only 0.5% of the potency of histamine and therefore a separation of the racemates does not seem to be lucrative enough [115].

Thus, data concerning the stereospecificity of H$_1$-receptor agonists are at present very limited, whereas it could be demonstrated for certain H$_1$-receptor antagonists, e.g. dimethindene [163–165], chlorpheniramine [166], bromopheniramine, carbinoxamine, and mebrophenhydramine [167].

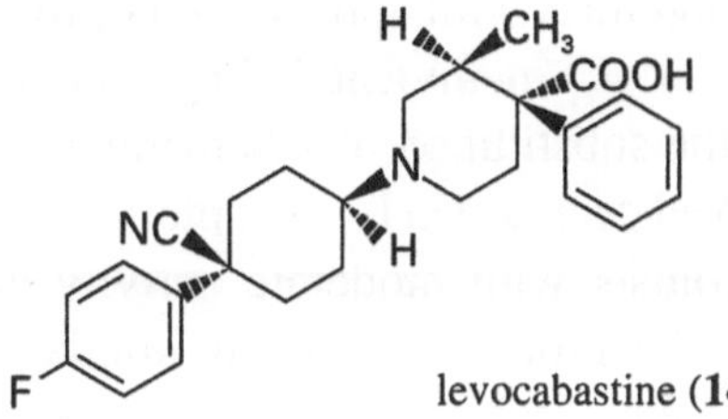

levocabastine (148)

Recently, levocabastine (Levocab^R) (148) [168], the first chiral H$_1$-receptor antagonist, was introduced as a pure enantiomer of 8 possible isomers for the local treatment of allergic conjunctivitis or rhinitis. Levocabastine was selected for clinical studies because of its low histamine-induced lethality compared to dextrocabastine and cabastine (an enantiomeric pair of levocabastine and dextrocabastine) [169]. In the case of the H$_1$-receptor antagonist triprolidine and analogues it was observed that E-isomers compared to Z-isomers always possess higher activity [170].

5   Conclusion

Summing up the results of structure-activity relationships obtained from different animal preparations, highest activity on the isolated guinea-pig ileum was found in the group of H$_1$-receptor agonists of the histamine-type substituted by a monocyclic aromatic ring at C-2 of the imidazole nucleus. Other residues in position 2 or heterocyclic analogues of histamine lead to compounds with weaker H$_1$-receptor activity.

The following conclusions might be drawn:

1. Lipophilic aromatic residues close to the imidazole ring represented by the class of 2-phenylhistamines lead to a strong increase in H_1-receptor activity which is influenced by the substitution pattern of the phenyl ring. Strongly active ligands were obtained in the meta substituted phenyl series, followed by para- and ortho-substituted analogues. A multiple substitution at the phenyl ring becomes apparent in a drastic decrease in activity. 2-[3-(Trifluormethyl)phenyl]histamine (47) and its halo analogues (43–46) are the most potent selective histamine H_1-receptor agonists so far known. Bulkier residues close to the imidazole moiety, e.g. naphthyl (101) or phenanthryl (102) lead to a dramatic decrease in activity compared to 2-phenylhistamines. Replacement of the phenyl ring e.g. by a bioisosteric thiophen moiety results in H_1-receptor agonists with approx. two thirds of the activity of histamine. The introduction of a methylene linkage between phenyl and imidazole moiety and also the substitution of 2-benzylhistamines with different residues lead to a marked decrease in H_1-receptor activity. 2-Alkylhistamines are H_1-receptor agonists with moderate activity and selectivity, whereas compounds with polar groups close to the imidazole ring, e.g. 2-hydroxyhistamine (37) or 2-mercaptohistamine (38) are devoid of H_1-receptor activity or possess H_2-receptor agonist activity as could be demonstrated for 2-aminohistamine (35).

2. Opposite effects were found in the group of the histamine derivatives carrying long flexible side-chains (minimum three methylene) at C-2. Lipophilic compounds like 2-(aryloxyalkyl)histamines (103–105) show H_1-receptor antagonist activity. This effect is intensified by stronger lipophilic compounds carrying two aromatic rings, e.g. 2-[N-benzyl-(3-anilino)propyl]histamine (126). In contrast, substances with strong basic substituents in the side-chain are generally weak H_1-receptor agonists. This could also be verified in the class of histamines carrying typical structural elements of H_2-receptor antagonists, which are in fact also long-chained basically substituted histamine derivatives. The observed H_1-receptor activity seems to be the result of weak, unspecific interactions of the basic function in the side-chain of the agonists with the receptor protein.

3. Among the heterocyclic analogues of histamine also the "classical H_1-receptor agonists" could be found, which have been used in numerous pharmacological experiments for a long time. The imidazole nucleus is not mandatory for selective H_1-receptor activity. The relative activity of these heterocyclic analogues is limited to a maximum of approx. 30% of histamine. Structural modifications, e.g. by methyl branching of the ethanamine

side-chain nearly lead to a complete loss of H_1-receptor activity. Heterocyclic analogues of histamine seem to possess no promising structures to enhance H_1-potency in the future.

Finally, it is to mention that among histamine H_1-receptor agonists an improvement of activity and selectivity could be reached first of all in the class of 2-phenylhistamines. The first successful synthesis of selective H_1-receptor agonists with a potency in the magnitude of histamine itself means a major step forward in histamine research, because strongly active agonists are at present only known in the field of H_2- [171, 172] and H_3-receptors [173–175]. Hitherto these highly potent and selective H_1-receptor agonists are not generally accepted as "pharmacological tools". Further studies are necessary to demonstrate the importance of these compounds.

References

1   H. H. Dale and P. P. Laidlaw: J. Physiol. (London) *41*, 318 (1910).
2   H. H. Dale and P. P. Laidlaw: J. Physiol. (London) *43*, 182 (1911).
3   H. H. Dale and P. P. Laidlaw: J. Physiol. (London) *52*, 355 (1919).
4   A. S. F. Ash and H. O. Schild: Br. J. Pharmacol. Chemother. *27*, 427 (1966).
5   J. W. Black, W. A. M. Duncan, G. J. Durant, C. R. Ganellin and M. E. Parsons: Nature (London) *236*, 385 (1972).
6   J. M. Arrang, M. Garbarg and J. C. Schwartz: Nature (London) *302*, 832 (1983).
7   H. Giertz and L. Flohé, in: W. Forth, D. Henschler and W. Rummel (Eds.): Allgemeine und spezielle Pharmakologie und Toxikologie, 5th edition, p. 176, Bibliographisches Institut Wissenschaftsverlag, Mannheim (1987).
8   J. C. Garrison, in: A. Goodman Gilman, T. W. Rall, A. S. Nies and P. Taylor (Eds.): Goodman and Gilman's The Pharmacological Basis of Therapeutics, 8th edition, p. 575, Pergamon Press, New York (1990).
9   D. Bovet and A. M. Staub: C. R. Soc. Biol. *124*, 547 (1937).
10   B. N. Halpern: Arch. Int. Pharmacodyn. Ther. *68*, 339 (1942).
11   R. Scherkl, A. Hashem and H. H. Frey, in: H. Timmerman and H. van der Goot (Eds.): New Perspectives in Histamine Research, Agents Actions Suppl. Vol. 33, p. 85, Birkhäuser Verlag, Basel (1991).
12   L. Tuomisto and U. Tacke: Neuropharmacology *25*, 955 (1986).
13   H. Yokoyama, K. Onodera, K. Maeyama, K. Yanai, K. Iinuma, L. Tuomisto and T. Watanabe: Naunyn-Schmiedeberg's Arch. Pharmacol. *346*, 40 (1992).
14   J. F. Schwartz and J. H. Patterson: Am. J. Dis. Child. *132*, 37 (1978).
15   K. Iinuma, H. Yokoyama, T. Otsuki, K. Yanai, T. Watanabe, T. Ido and M. Itoh: Lancet *341*, 238 (1993).
16   H. Yokoyama, K. Onodera, K. Iinuma and T. Watanabe: Pharmacol. Biochem. Behav. *47*, 503 (1994).
17   R. Leurs, M. J. Smit, A. Bast and H. Timmerman: Eur. J. Pharmacol. *196*, 319 (1991).

18   R. Leurs, M. J. Smit, M. M. Brozius, W. Jansen, A. Bast and H. Timmerman, in: H. Timmerman and H. van der Goot (Eds): New Perspectives in Histamine Research, Agents Actions Suppl. Vol. 33, p. 393, Birkhäuser Verlag, Basel (1991).
19   D. R. Bristow, P. C. Banford, I. Bajusz, A. Vedat and J. M. Young: Br. J. Pharmacol. *110*, 269 (1993).
20   N. Toda: Circ. Res. *61*, 280 (1987).
21   K. Matsuyama, H. Yasue, K. Okumura, K. Matsuyama, H. Ogawa, Y. Morikami, N. Inotsume and M. Nakano: Circulation *81*, 65 (1990).
22   T. Ishikawa, J. R. Hume and K. D. Keef: J. Physiol. (London) *468*, 379 (1993).
23   R. Oishi, N. Adachi and K. Saeki: Eur. J. Pharmacol. *237*, 155 (1993).
24   W. Schunack: Z. Klin. Med. *46*, 1603 (1991).
25   R. W. Brimblecombe, W. A. M. Duncan, G. J. Durant, J. C. Emmett, C. R. Ganellin and M. E. Parsons: J. Int. Med. Res. *3*, 86 (1975).
26   M. Deakin and J. G. Williams: Drugs *44*, 709 (1992).
27   G. J. Durant, W. A. M. Duncan, C. R. Ganellin, M. E. Parsons, R. C. Blakemore and A. C. Rasmussen: Nature (London) *276*, 403 (1978).
28   G. Baumann, B. Permanetter and A. Wirtzfeld: Pharmacol. Ther. *24*, 165 (1984).
29   S. B. Felix, A. Buschauer and G. Baumann, in: H. Timmerman and H. van der Goot (Eds.): New Perspectives in Histamine Research, Agents Actions Suppl. Vol. 33, p. 257, Birkhäuser Verlag, Basel (1991).
30   A. Buschauer: J. Med. Chem. *32*, 1963 (1989).
31   J. C. Schwartz: ISI Atlas of Science 2, 185 (1988).
32   A. Philippu and H. Prast: Agents Actions *33*, 124 (1991).
33   J. C. Schwartz, J. M. Arrang, M. Garbarg, H. Pollard and M. Ruat: Phys. Rev. *71*, 1 (1991).
34   J. C. Schwartz, J. M. Arrang, M. Garbarg and M. Korner: J. Exp. Biol. *124*, 203 (1986).
35   H. Wada, N. Inagaki, N. Itowi and A. Yamatodani, in: H. Timmerman and H. van der Goot (Eds.): New Perspectives in Histamine Research, Agents Actions Suppl. Vol. 33, p. 11, Birkhäuser Verlag, Basel (1991).
36   T. Watanabe, A. Yamatodani, K. Maeyama and H. Wada: Trends Pharmacol. Sci. *11*, 363 (1990).
37   P. J. Barnes and M. Ichinose: Trends Pharmacol. Sci. *10*, 264 (1989).
38   B. J. O'Connor and P. J. Barnes: Am. Rev. Resp. Dis. *141*, A361 (1990).
39   I. M. Mazurkiewicz-Kwilecki and S. Nsonwah: Can. J. Physiol. Pharmacol. *67*, 75 (1989).
40   K. Yanai, T. Watanabe, K. Meguro, H. Yokoyama, I. Sarto, H. Sasano, M. Itoh, R. Iwata, T. Takahashi and T. Ido: NeuroReport *3*, 433 (1992).
41   K. Yanai, T. Watanabe, H. Yokoyama, J. Hatazawa, R. Iwata, K. Ishiwata, K. Meguro, M. Itoh, T. Takahashi, T. Ido and T. Matsuzawa: J. Neurochem. *59*, 128 (1992).
42   M. Yamashita, H. Fukui, K. Sugama, Y. Horio, S. Ito, H. Mizuguchi and H. Wada: Proc. Natl. Acad. Sci. USA *88*, 11515 (1991)
43   K. Fujimoto, Y. Horio, K. Sugama, S. Ito, Y. Q. Liu and H. Fukui: Biochem. Biophys. Res. Commun. *190*, 294 (1993).
44   Y. Horio, Y. Mori, I. Higuchi, K. Fujimoto, S. Ito and H. Fukui: J. Biochem. *114*, 408 (1993).
45   E. Traiffort, R. Leurs, J. M. Arrang, J. Tardivel-Lacombe, J. Diaz, J. C. Schwartz and M. Ruat: J. Neurochem. *62*, 507 (1994).

46   M. D. De Backer, W. Gommeren, H. Moereels, G. Nobels, P. Van Gompel, J. E. Leysen and W. H. M. L. Luyten: Biochem. Biophys. Res. Commun. *197*, 1601 (1993).

47   I. Gantz, M. Schäffer, J. DelValle, C. Logsdon, V. Campbell, M. Uhler and T. Yamada: Proc. Natl. Acad. Sci. USA *88*, 429 (1991).

48   R. A. Shapiro, N. M. Scherer, B. A. Habecker, E. M. Subers and N. M. Nathanson: J. Biol. Chem. *263*, 18397 (1988).

49   S. J. Hill and J. Donaldson, in: J. C. Schwartz and H. L. Haas (Eds.): The histamine receptor, p. 109, Wiley-Liss, Inc., New York (1992).

50   M. J. Berridge and R. F. Irvine: Nature (London) *312*, 315 (1984).

51   M. J. Berridge and R. F. Irvine: Nature (London) *341*, 197 (1989).

52   Y. Yuan, H. J. Granger, D. C. Zawieja, D. V. DeFily and W. M. Chilian: Am. J. Physiol. *264*, H1734 (1993).

53   R. Leurs, M. M. Brozius, W. Jansen, A. Bast and H. Timmerman: Biochem. Pharmacol. *42*, 271 (1991).

54   E. Richelson: Science *201*, 69 (1978).

55   T. T. Quach, A. M. Duchemin, C. Rose and J. C. Schwartz: Mol. Pharmacol. *17*, 301 (1980).

56   Y. Nishizuka: Nature (London) *334*, 661 (1988).

57   Y. Nishizuka: Nature (London) *308*, 693 (1984).

58   M. I. Kotlikoff, R. K. Murray and E. E. Reynolds: Am. J. Physiol. *253*, C561 (1987).

59   R. K. Murray, C. F. Bennett, S. J. Fluharty and M. I. Kotlikoff: Am. J. Physiol. *257*, L209 (1989).

60   S. P. H. Alexander, S. J. Hill and D. A. Kendall: Br. J. Pharmacol. *98*, 832P (1989).

61   D. Rotrosen and J. I. Gallin: J. Cell. Biol. *103*, 2379 (1986).

62   M. Kuno and P. Gardner: Nature (London) *326*, 301 (1987).

63   R. Penner, G. Matthews and E. Neher: Nature (London) *334*, 499 (1988).

64   A. P. Morris, D. V. Gallacher, R. F. Irvine and O. H. Peterson: Nature (London) *330*, 653 (1987).

65   R. F. Irvine and R. M. Moor: Biochem. Biophys. Res. Commun. *146*, 284 (1987).

66   C. W. Taylor: Trends. Pharmacol. Sci. *11*, 269 (1990).

67   J. M. Berridge: Nature (London) *361*, 315 (1993).

68   R. Leurs, E. Traiffort, J. M. Arrang, J. Tardivel-Lacombe, M. Ruat and J. C. Schwartz: J. Neurochem. *62*, 519 (1994).

69   L. R. Hegstrand, P. D. Kanof and P. Greengard: Nature (London) *260*, 163 (1976).

70   J. C. Schwartz, G. Barbin, A. M. Duchemin, M. Garbarg, J. M. Palacios, T. T. Quach and C. Rose, in: G. Pepeu, M. J. Kuhar and S. J. Enna (Eds.): Receptors for Neuro-transmitters and Peptide Hormons, p. 169, Raven Press, New York (1980).

71   J. Donaldson, S. J. Hill and A. M. Brown: Mol. Pharmacol. *33*, 626 (1988).

72   C. Gulat-Marnay, A. Lafitte, J. M. Arrang and J. C. Schwartz: J. Neurochem. *52*, 248 (1989).

73   C. Gulat-Marnay, A. Lafitte, J. M. Arrang and J. C. Schwartz: J. Neurochem. *53*, 519 (1989).

74   S. J. Hill and R. M. Straw: Br. J. Pharmacol. *95*, 1213 (1988).

75   S. J. Hill and C. S. Young: Br. J. Pharmacol. *93*, 90P (1988).

76   C. Gulat-Marnay, A. Lafitte, J. M. Arrang and J. C. Schwartz: J. Neurochem. *55*, 47 (1990).

77   J. M. Arrang, M. Garbarg and J. C. Schwartz: Neuroscience *15*, 553 (1985).

78   R. Leurs and H. Timmerman, in: E. Jucker (Ed.): Progress in Drug Research, vol. 39, p. 127, Birkhäuser Verlag, Basel (1992).

79   J. M. Arrang, J. Roy, J. L. Morgat, W. Schunack and J. C. Schwartz: Eur. J. Pharmacol. *188*, 219 (1990).

80   P. Cumming, C. Shaw and S. R. Vincent: Synapse *8*, 144 (1991).

81   E. Schlicker, K. Fink, G. Molderings and M. Göthert: J. Neurochem. *57*, S37 (1991).

82   J. P. Trzeciakowski: J. Pharmacol. Exp. Ther. *243*, 874 (1987).

83   K. Tamura, J. M. Palmer and J. D. Wood: Neuroscience *25*, 171 (1988).

84   M. Ichinose and P. J. Barnes: Eur. J. Pharmacol. *163*, 383 (1989).

85   M. Ichinose, C. D. Stretton, J. C. Schwartz and P. J. Barnes: Br. J. Pharmacol. *97*, 13 (1989).

86   W. Schunack: Arch. Pharm. (Weinheim) *306*, 934 (1973).

87   J. C. Castillo and E. J. de Beer: J. Pharmacol. Exp. Ther. *90*, 104 (1947).

88   D. F. Hawkins: Br. J. Pharmacol. *10*, 230 (1955).

89   D. Bovet and F. Walthert: Ann. Pharm. Franc. (Suppl. *2*), 1 (1944).

90   M. Rocha e Silva, A. Antonio, in: M. Rocha e Silva (Ed.): Histamine II and Anti-His-taminics, Handbuch der experimentellen Pharmakologie, Vol. XVIII/2, p. 381, Springer-Verlag, Berlin (1978).

91   C. Leschke, S. Elz and W. Schunack: XIIth International Symposium on Medicinal Chemistry, Poster P-126.A, Basel (1992).

92   G. J. Menkveld and H. Timmerman: Eur. J. Pharmacol. *186*, 343 (1990).

93   G. Morini, J. F. Kuemmerle, M. Impicciatore, J. R. Grider and G. M. Makhlouf: J. Pharmacol. Exp. Ther. *264*, 598 (1993).

94   E. J. Ariens: Arzneim.-Forsch./Drug Res. *16*, 1376 (1966).

95   J. M. van Rossum: Arch. Int. Pharmacodyn. Ther. *143*, 299 (1963).

96   H. G. Lennartz, M. Hepp and W. Schunack: Eur. J. Med. Chem. Chim. Ther. *13*, 229 (1978).

97   H. J. Roth, K. Eger and R. Troschütz: Pharmazeutische Chemie II Arzneistoffanalyse, 2nd edition, p. 408, Georg Thieme Verlag, Stuttgart (1985).

98   J. W. Black and C. R. Ganellin: Experientia *30*, 111 (1974).

99   C. R. Ganellin, in: C. R. Ganellin and M. E. Parsons (Eds.): Pharmacology of histamine receptors, p. 10, Wright PSG, London (1982).

100   A. Windaus and W. Vogt: Ber. Dtsch. Chem. Ges. *40*, 3691 (1907).

101   L. A. Walter, W. H. Hunt and R. J. Fosbinder: J. Am. Chem. Soc. *63*, 2771 (1941).

102   D. G. Cooper, R. C. Young, G. J. Durant and C. R. Ganellin, in: C. Hansch (Ed.): Histamine receptors in Comprehensive Medicinal Chemistry, Vol. 3, Membranes & receptors, p. 324, Pergamon Press, Oxford (1990).

103   C. R. Ganellin: J. Med. Chem. *16*, 620 (1973).

104   G. J. Durant, C. R. Ganellin and M. E. Parsons: J. Med. Chem. *18*, 905 (1975).

105   C. R. Ganellin, in: J. C. Schwartz and H.L. Haas (Eds.): The histamine receptor, p. 1, Wiley-Liss, Inc., New York (1992).

106   R. Lipp, H. Stark and W. Schunack, in: J. C. Schwartz and H. L. Haas (Eds.): The histamine receptor, p. 57, Wiley-Liss, Inc., New York (1992).

107   J. M. Arrang, M. Garbarg, T. T. Quach, M. D. Trung Tuong, E. Yeramian and J. C. Schwartz: Eur. J. Pharmacol. *111*, 73 (1985).

108   P. R. Gater, S. E. Webber, G. P. H. Gui, C. C. Jordan, N. A. Hayes, J. J. Ashford and J. C. Foreman: Agents Actions 18, 342 (1986).

109 D. Ackermann and W. Wasmuth: Hoppe Seylers Z. Physiol. Chem. *259*, 28 (1939).

110 A. Buschauer, K. Wegner and W. Schunack: Arch. Pharm. (Weinheim) *317*, 9 (1984).

111 E. C. Kornfeld, L. Wolf, T. M. Lin and I. H. Slater: J. Med. Chem. *11*, 1028 (1968).

112 R. C. Young, C. R. Ganellin, R. Griffiths, R. C. Mitchell, M. E. Parsons, D. Saunders and N. E. Sore: Eur. J. Med. Chem. *28*, 201 (1993).

113 C. Niemann and J. T. Hays: J. Am. Chem. Soc. *64*, 2288 (1942).

114 H. Stark, R. Lipp, W. Schunack, J. M. Arrang, N. Defontaine and J. C. Schwartz: Arch. Pharm. (Weinheim) *323*, 729 (1990).

115 R. Steffens and W. Schunack: Arch. Pharm. (Weinheim) *317*, 771 (1984).

116 H. Erlenmeyer and M. Müller: Helv. Chim. Acta. *28*, 922 (1945).

117 H. M. Lee and R. G. Jones: J. Pharmacol. Exp. Ther. *95*, 71 (1949).

118 M. I. Grossman, C. Robertson and C. E. Rosiere: J. Pharmacol. Exp. Ther. *104*, 277 (1952).

119 T. A. Bökesoy and H. O. Onaran: Eur. J. Pharmacol. 197, *49* (1991).

120 N. Inagaki, H. Fukui, S. Ito, A. Yamatodani and H. Wada: Proc. Natl. Acad. Sci. USA *88*, 4215 (1991).

121 L. Jennings, N. Malek, A. Gimeno, M. J. Pozo, J. Singh, G. M. Salido and J. S. Davison: J. Physiol. *446*, 195P (1992).

122 H. A. Bull, P. F. Courtney, M. H. A. Rustin and P. M. Dowd: Br. J. Pharmacol. *107*, 276 (1992).

123 B. Malinowska and E. Schlicker: Naunyn-Schmiedeberg's Arch. Pharmacol. *347*, 55 (1993).

124 B. N. Craver, W. Barrett, A. Cameron and E. Herrold: Arch. Int. Pharmacodyn. Ther. *87*, 33 (1951).

125 G. J. Sterk, H. van der Goot and H. Timmerman: Arch. Pharm. (Weinheim) *319*, 624 (1986).

126 C. R. Ganellin, G. N. J. Port and W. G. Richards: J. Med. Chem. *16*, 616 (1973).

127 M. Hepp, P. Dziuron and W. Schunack: Arch. Pharm. (Weinheim) *312*, 637 (1979).

128 G. J. Durant, J. C. Emmett, C. R. Ganellin, A. M. Roe and R. A. Slater: J. Med. Chem. *19*, 923 (1976).

129 M. Hepp: PhD thesis, Mainz 1981.

130 A. Buschauer, W. Schunack, J. M. Arrang, M. Garbarg, J. C. Schwartz and J. M. Young, in: M. Williams, R. A. Glennon and P. B. M. W. M. Timmermans (Eds.): Receptor Pharmacology and Function, p. 293, Marcel Dekker, Inc., New York (1989).

131 P. Dziuron and W. Schunack: Eur. J. Med. Chem. Chim. Ther. *10*, 129 (1975).

132 C. Leschke: PhD thesis, Freie Universität Berlin 1994.

133 M. Impicciatore, G. Morini, M. Chiavarini, P. V. Plazzi, F. Bordi and F. Vitali: Agents Actions *18*, 134 (1986).

134 P. V. Plazzi, F. Bordi and M. Impicciatore: Farmaco Sci. Ed. *40*, 218 (1985).

135 V. Zingel, S. Elz and W. Schunack: Eur. J. Med. Chem. *25*, 673 (1990).

136 J. G. Koper, A. van der Vliet, H. van der Goot and H. Timmerman: Pharm. Weekbl. Sci. Ed. *12*, 236 (1990).

137 J. G. Koper, H. van der Goot and H. Timmerman: 18th Meeting of the European Histamine Research Society, Abstract p. 54, Breda (1989).

138 O. Arunlakshana and H. O. Schild: Br. J. Pharmacol. *14*, 48 (1959).

139 P. B. Marshall: Br. J. Pharmacol. Chemother. *10*, 270 (1955).

140 E. J. Ariens and J. M. van Rossum: Arch. Int. Pharmacodyn. Ther. *110*, 275 (1957).

141   B. Malinowska, C. Leschke, S. Elz, W. Schunack and E. Schlicker: Agents Actions (Special Conference Issue) *38*, C257 (1993).

142   R. Seifert: Naunyn-Schmiedeberg's Arch. Pharmacol. *345*, R49 (1992).

143   R. Seifert, A. Hagelüken, A. Höer, D. Höer, L. Grünbaum, S. Offermans, I. Schwaner, V. Zingel, W. Schunack and G. Schultz: Mol. Pharmacol. *45*, 578 (1994).

144   E. Kutter and C. Hansch: J. Med. Chem. *12*, 647 (1969).

145   J. G. Topliss: J. Med. Chem. *15*, 1006 (1972).

146   J. G. Topliss: J. Med. Chem. *20*, 463 (1977).

147   R. Steffens and W. Schunack: Arch. Pharm. (Weinheim) *320*, 135 (1987).

148   V. Zingel, S. Elz and W. Schunack: Arch. Pharm. (Weinheim) *326*, 143 (1993).

149   M. E. Parsons, R. C. Blakemore, G. J. Durant, C. R. Ganellin and A. C. Rasmussen: Agents Actions *5*, 464 (1975).

150   G. J. Durant, J. C. Emmett, C. R. Ganellin, P. D. Miles, M. E. Parsons, H. D. Prain and G. R. White: J. Med. Chem. *20*, 901 (1977).

151   C. R. Ganellin, in: C. R. Ganellin and J. C. Schwartz (Eds.): Frontiers in Histamine Research, p. 47, Pergamon Press, Oxford (1985).

152   V. Zingel: PhD thesis, Freie Universität Berlin 1990.

153   Glaxo Group Ltd. (J. Bradshaw, J. W. Clitherow, M. J. W. MacFarlane, R. Hayes and L. Carey, inv.), EP 29306 (27.5.81); CA *95*, 132900q (1981).

154   D. E. Bays and B. J. Price, in: R. Dahlbom and J. L. G. Nilsson (Eds.): VIIIth International Symposium on Medicinal Chemistry, Proceedings Vol. 2, p. 183, Swedish Pharmaceutical Press, Stockholm (1985).

155   H. Troidl, W. Lorenz, H. Barth, H. Rohde, G. Feifel, A. Schmal, K. Goecke, A. Reimann-Huhnd and W. Seidel: Agents Actions *3*, 157 (1973).

156   M. N. Ghosh and H. O. Schild: Br. J. Pharmacol. Chemother. *13*, 54 (1958).

157   V. Zingel, S. Elz and W. Schunack: Pharmazie *47*, 746 (1992).

158   R. Steffens and W. Schunack: Arch. Pharm. (Weinheim) *318*, 582 (1985).

159   W. Schunack, A. Buschauer, S. Büyüktimkin, P. Dziuron, S. Elz, G. Gerhard, E. Lebenstedt, H. G. Lennartz, S. Schwarz, M. Spitzhoff and R. Steffens, in: R. Dahlbom and J. L. G. Nilsson (Eds.): VIIIth International Symposium on Medicinal Chemistry, Proceedings Vol. 2, p. 169, Swedish Pharmaceutical Press, Stockholm (1985).

160   J. M. Arrang, J. C. Schwartz and W. Schunack: Eur. J. Pharmacol. *117*, 109 (1985).

161   J. D. P. Graham and R. S. Tonks: Arch. Int. Pharmacodyn. Ther. *106*, 457 (1956).

162   N. B. Chapman and J. F. A. Williams: J. Chem. Soc. (London) *1953*, 2797.

163   U. Borchard, D. Hafner and R. Heise: Naunyn-Schmiedeberg's Arch. Pharmacol. *330*, Suppl. R9 (1985).

164   R. Towart, M. Sautel, E. Moret, E. Costa, M. Theralauz and A. F. Weitsch, in: H. Timmerman and H. van der Goot (Eds.): New Perspectives in Histamine Research, Agents Actions Suppl. Vol. 33, p. 403, Birkhäuser Verlag, Basel (1991).

165   J. Leuschner, B. W. Neumann, H. Brunnauer and D. Rehn: Agents Actions, Special Conference Issue, C431 (1992).

166   A. N. Nicholson, P. A. Pascoe, C. Turner, C. R. Ganellin, P. M. Greengrass, A. F. Casy and A. D. Mercer: Br. J. Pharmacol. *104*, 270 (1991).

167   A. F. Casy, A. F. Drake, C. R. Ganellin, A. D. Mercer and C. Upton: Chirality *4*, 356 (1992).

168   F. Awouters, C. J. E. Niemegeers, T. Jansen, A. A. H. P. Megens and P. A. J. Janssen: Agents Actions *35*, 12 (1992).

169   G. Vanden Bussche: Drugs Future *11*, 841 (1986).

170   A. F. Casy, C. R. Ganellin, A. D. Mercer and C. Upton: J. Pharm. Pharmacol. *44*, 791 (1992).

171   H. van der Goot, A. Bast and H. Timmerman, in: B. Uvnäs (Ed.): Histamine and histamine antagonists, Handbook of Experimental Pharmacology, Vol. 97, p. 573, Springer-Verlag, Berlin (1991).

172   A. Buschauer and G. Baumann, in: H. Timmerman and H. van der Goot (Eds.): New Perspectives in Histamine Research, Agents Actions Suppl. Vol. 33, p. 231, Birkhäuser Verlag, Basel (1991).

173   J. M. Arrang, M. Garbarg, J. C. Schwartz, R. Lipp, H. Stark, W. Schunack and J. M. Lecomte, in: H. Timmerman and H. van der Goot (Eds.): New Perspectives in Histamine Research, Agents Actions Suppl. Vol. 33, p. 55, Birkhäuser Verlag, Basel (1991).

174   R. Lipp, J. M. Arrang, M. Garbarg, P. Luger, J. C. Schwartz and W. Schunack: J. Med. Chem. *35*, 4434 (1992).

175   R. C. Vollinga, J. P. de Koning, F. P. Jansen, R. Leurs, W. M. P. B. Menge and H. Timmerman: J. Med. Chem. *37*, 332 (1994).

Progress in Drug Research, Vol. 44 (E. Jucker, Ed.)
© 1995 Birkhäuser Verlag, Basel (Switzerland)

Antifungal chemotherapy

By Paul D. Hoeprich

1007 Colby Drive, Davis, CA 95616-1757, USA

1   Introduction

Mycoses are almost always conditioned in occurrence by some pre-existing, nonfungal ailment – a predisposing condition that in some way disables one or more host defense mechanisms. Thus, mycoses are facilitated by abrogation of mechanical barriers (maceration of the skin, burns, major surgical operations), immunodeficiencies (malignancies and their treatments; transplantation of organs and antirejection therapies; the acquired immunodeficiency syndrome [AIDS]), metabolic derangements (diabetes mellitus; hypercorticism), and suppression of competitor microorganisms (application of multiagent antibacterial therapy). Possibly because they are often not amenable to correction, immunodeficiencies appear to be the most important contributors to the current burgeoning of the deep mycoses. Indeed, immunodeficient patients with deep mycoses highlight the need for agents that are perorally and parenterally administrable, systemically active, nontoxic, and fungicidal. Currently available drugs fall short of these ideal characteristics. However, it is useful to consult recent reviews of antifungal chemotherapy [1–3] and assess the current situation in this chapter as we work toward optimal antifungal chemotherapy.

2   Topical agents

A host of topical therapies is applied in the treatment of superficial mycoses (fungal infections of the skin, mucous membranes, and dermal appendages, without penetration into the subcutaneous or submucosal tissues). As these therapies are quite often effective, and the infections are not usually life-threatening [4], it is sufficient to note that: 1) some agents unsafe or inappropriate for systemic therapy have congeners that are useful and safe for topical application, e.g., topical nystatin *cf.* intravenously injected amphotericin B, topical clotrimazole *cf.* perorally administered ketoconazole; and 2) the newer topical agents, amorolfine and two allylamines, naftifine and terbinafine, have special characteristics that merit consideration.

2.1   Amorolfine

The development of derivatives of the cyclic amine, 2,6-dimethylmorpholine, as agrifungicides in the 1960s [5] and 1970s [6] led to the synthesis

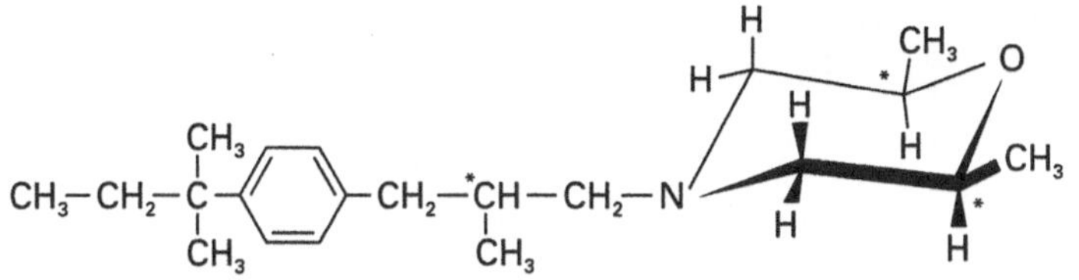

Fig. 1
Amorolfine is a synthetic, morpholone derivative that is antifungal as a result of coupling the (+)S-enantiomorph of the phenylpropyl function to the *cis*-form of the 2,6-dimethylmorpholine nucleus (* identifies the site of optical activity).

of amorolfine (AMF), a phenylpiperidine compound (Fig. 1) that was shown in the early 1980s to be active against fungi pathogenic for humans [7]. For antifungal activity, the *cis*-form of the 2,6-dimethylmorpholine nucleus must be coupled with the (+)-S-enantiomeric phenylpropyl side chain characteristic of AMF [8].

The antifungal morpholines interfere with the biosynthesis of ergosterol by inhibiting Δ^{14}-reductase and Δ^{8}——Δ^{7}-sterol isomerase ([9]; Fig 2). As a result, ergosterol is depleted, unnatural demethylsterols (especially, ignosterol) and lanosterol accumulate, the synthesis and deposition of chitin becomes abnormal, and there is hyperfluidity of destabilized cell membranes with changes in permeability [9,10]. Fungistasis is the usual effect, but some pathogenic fungi are killed by high concentrations of AMF. Development of resistance has not been observed in susceptible fungi exposed to AMF, possibly because it acts at two sites in an essential synthetic pathway.

AMF is active against the dermatophytes, *Candida* spp., *Cryptococcus neoformans*, dematiaceous fungi, *Histoplasma capsulatum, Coccidoides immitis, Blastomyces dermatitidis, Sporothrix schenckii*, and *Pseudallescheria boydii* with minimal inhibitory concentrations (MICs) of 0.01–0.55 µg/ml [7, 10, 11]. The *Aspergillus* spp., *Fusarium* spp., and the Zygomycetes are resistant.

AMF-hydrochloride is a colorless solid that is soluble in water. Peroral administration is of no benefit. Topical application is effective, as concentrations in skin and nails peak 2–5 hours after application, declining slowly to suboptimal concentrations over 48–50 hours [12]. A concentration of 0.25% amorolfine in a cream vehicle, applied once daily for 3–4 weeks, is as effective as azole preparations (cure rates ≥80%) in the treatment of dermatophytoses [13]. For treating onychomycoses, lacquer (5%, applied once or twice weekly for 6–12 months – longer for toenails) is curative in

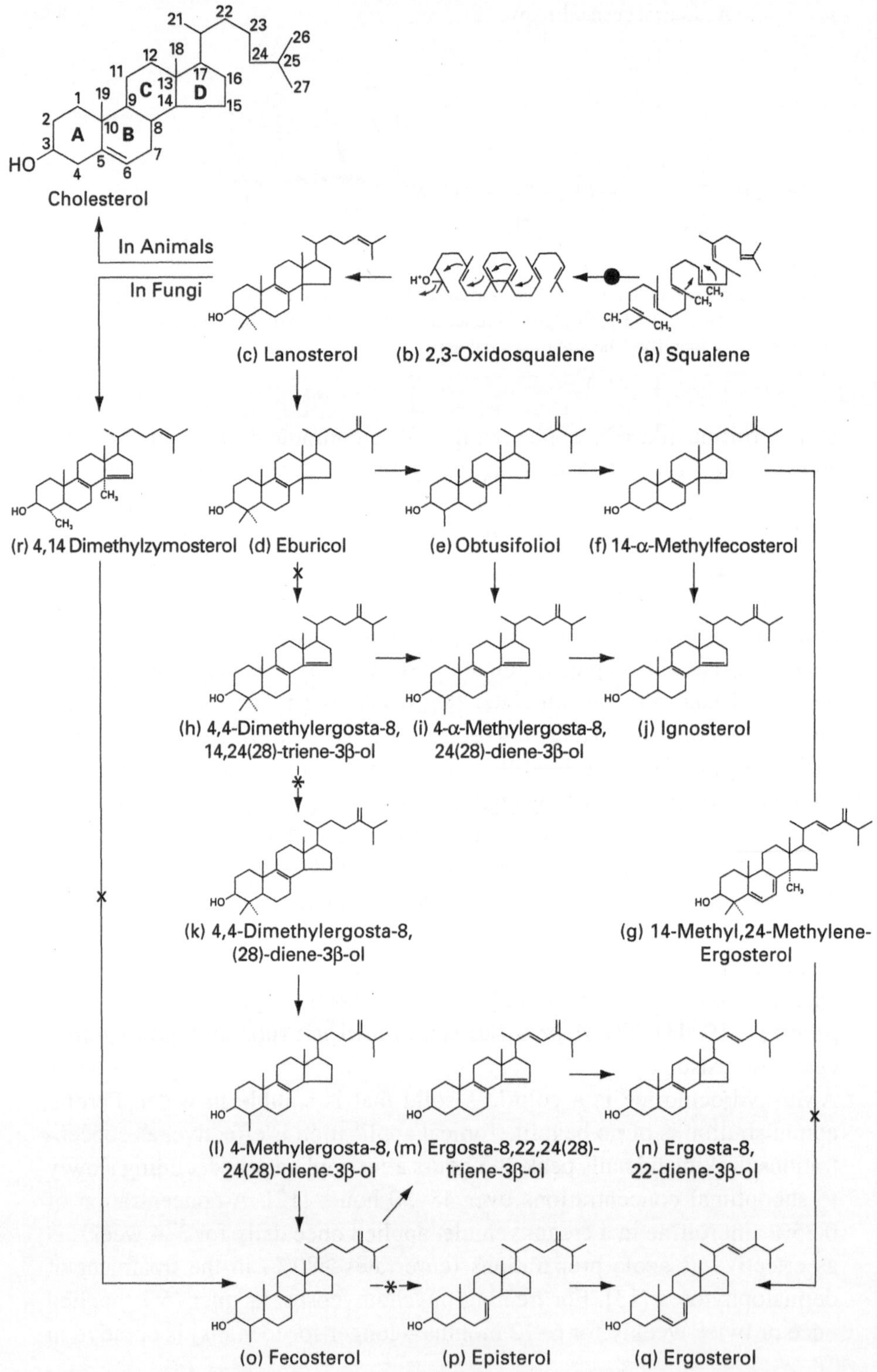

Cholesterol

In Animals

In Fungi

(c) Lanosterol   (b) 2,3-Oxidosqualene   (a) Squalene

(r) 4,14 Dimethylzymosterol   (d) Eburicol   (e) Obtusifoliol   (f) 14-α-Methylfecosterol

(h) 4,4-Dimethylergosta-8,   (i) 4-α-Methylergosta-8,   (j) Ignosterol
14,24(28)-triene-3β-ol   24(28)-diene-3β-ol

(k) 4,4-Dimethylergosta-8,   (g) 14-Methyl,24-Methylene-
(28)-diene-3β-ol   Ergosterol

(l) 4-Methylergosta-8,   (m) Ergosta-8,22,24(28)-   (n) Ergosta-8,
24(28)-diene-3β-ol   triene-3β-ol   22-diene-3β-ol

(o) Fecosterol   (p) Episterol   (q) Ergosterol

≥ 50% of patients [13]. Tablets for single-dose treatment of candidal vulvovaginitis (50 mg and 100 mg) are as effective as clotrimazole tablets (500 mg) yielding a cure in ≥90% of patients [14]. The amorolfine preparations are well tolerated.

2.2 Allylamines

The antifungal allylamines are a group of highly lipo- and keratinophilic compounds that were derived from heterocyclic spironaphthalenones in a program for developing drugs active in the central nervous system (CNS). Antifungal activity was found in 1981 [15], as a result of general screening of novel compounds for bioactivity. The allylamines are antifungal only if the double bond of the side chain has the *trans* orientation ([16]; Fig 3). Inhibition of squalene 2,3-epoxidase (Fig 2) is the primary mechanism of the antifungal activity of the allylamines [17]. Susceptible fungi become depleted of ergosterol and accumulate squalene [18]; the result is failure growth, and cell death with some fungi [15]. The hepatic squalene epoxidases of rats and guinea pigs are 2–3 orders of magnitude less sensitive to inhibition than the epoxidases of *Candida* spp. [18]. The cytochrome P450 enzymes are unaffected by the allylamines [19].

2.2.1 Naftifine
The dermatophytes are susceptible to naftifine (NAF) with MICs of 0.05–0.50 μg/ml [15, 20]. Other pathogenic fungi are relatively resistant, e.g., 50.0–≥100.0 μg/ml for *Candida albicans* [21].
Absorption from the gut is inadequate for systemic therapy. However, on topical application, NAF penetrates and accumulates in the outer layers of the skin and mucous membranes [22].
Once daily application of 1% cream or gel for 3–5 weeks yields mycologic cure of dermatophytoses in 50–90% of patients [23]. Candidal dermatitis responds in ≥70% of patients. Local adverse reactions of irritation are uncommon, and systemic reactions have not been reported.

<

Figure 2. Correlation of the pathways for synthesis of ergosterol in fungi with the sites of inhibition by antifungal antimicrobics: allylamines, ●; amorolfine, ✳; azoles, ✕ and ✳. (From Hoeprich, P.D.: Antifungal Chemotherapy, Chapter 23, in P.D. Hoeprich, M.C. Jordan and A.R. Ronald (Eds.), *Infectious Diseases*. J.B. Lippincott Company; Philadelphia (1994). p. 59).

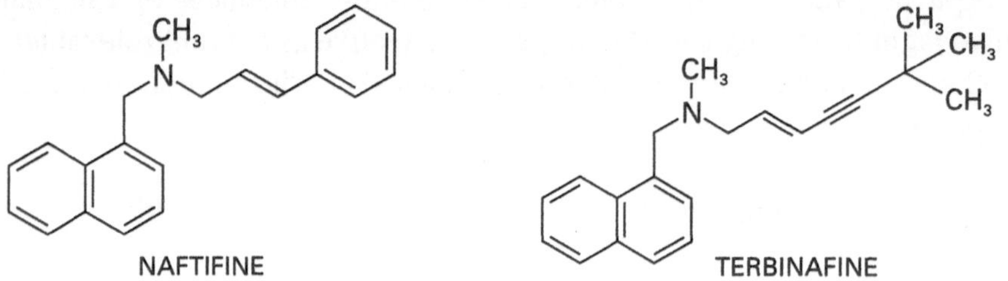

NAFTIFINE
M.W. 287.4

TERBINAFINE
M.W. 291.4

Fig. 3
Naftifine and terbinafine are synthetic allylamine derivatives that have come to clinical use.

2.2.2   *Terbinafine*

The presence of an acetylene function in the side chain of terbinafine (TER) is unique among biologically active compounds ([24]; Fig. 3). By testing in vitro, the dermatophytes are much more susceptible to TER than to NAF with MICs of 0.003–0.01 µg/ml [16, 20, 21, 24]. Moreover, some isolates of *Aspergillus* spp., S. *schenckii, Candida* spp., and *Malassezia furfur* are inhibited by concentrations low enough to pique clinical interest.

As with NAF, the topical application of TER results in excellent penetration and retention in the skin and mucous membranes, with local or systemic adverse reactions comparably uncommon [25]. When applied once daily as a 1% cream or gel, TER achieves overall mycologic cure rates of 85–93% in dermatomycoses, candidosis, and in tinea versicolor [25, 26]. In comparative clinical trials, TER was more rapidly effective and yielded marginally better cure rates than clotrimazole or bifonazole [25, 26]. There are no reports of comparative clinical evaluations of topically applied TER and NAF.

Unlike NAF, however, peroral administration of TER is therapeutically useful [25, 26]. Bioavailability is not influenced by eating, and 70–80% of a dose is absorbed from the gut [25]. Two hours after the usual dose of 250 mg, the concentration of TER in the plasma peaks at 0.9 µg/ml with an elimination halflife of about 11 hours [25]. However, the drug accumulates in the skin and nails, achieving as much as 3 mg/kg in the stratum corneum [27], and 0.25–0.55 µg/gm of nails [28].

Using 250 mg once daily for periods of 2–12 weeks brought about mycologic cure of dermatophyte infections of the skin in 80–90% of patients [26, 29]. With onychomycoses, treatment periods of 12 weeks to as long as 6 months may be necessary for mycologic cure [26, 30].

Cutaneous candidosis and sporotrichosis may respond to treatment with TER [26], but rigorous evaluation is yet to be reported.
Peroral administration of TER is only occasionally associated with gastro-intestinal disturbances [26, 29]. No adverse effect was detected on steroidal or peptide hormones [25].

3 Systemic agents

3.1 Amphotericin B

Although hundreds of macrolide polyenic compounds are elaborated by actinomycetes, only amphotericin B (AmB) is used in the systemic therapy of mycoses. It was discovered in 1953 [31], and is produced by certain strains of *Streptomyces nodosus*. The structure of AmB (Fig. 4) was deduced

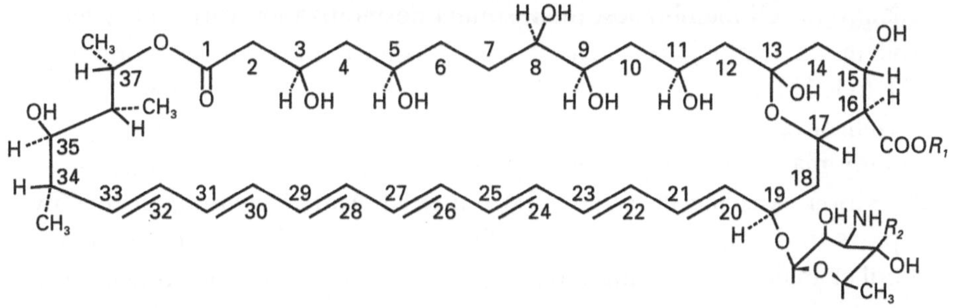

AMPHOTERICIN B: R_1–H; R_2–H
M.W. 924.10

N-ACETYL AMPHOTERICIN B: R_1–H; R_2–C(=O)–CH_3
M.W. 966.14

DAPEG-AMPHOTERICIN B: R_1–H; R_2–C(=N–CH_2–CH_2–CH_2–N(CH_3)$_2$)–NH–CH_2–CH_3
M.W. 1078.33

AMPHOTERICIN B METHYL ESTER: R_1–CH_3; R_2–H
M.W. 938.13

D-ORNITHYL AMPHOTERICIN B METHYL ESTER: R_1–CH_3; R_2–C(=O)–CH(NH_2)–CH_2–CH_2–CH_2–NH_2
M.W. 1052.28

Fig. 4
Amphotericin B is a naturally occurring antifungal, heptaenic polyene; several semisynthetic derivatives have been prepared.

in 1970 [32]. It is a heptaene because of seven conjugated double bonds in that portion of the rod-like molecule called the chromophore. The chromophore endows AmB with a deep yellow color, planar rigidity, lipophilicity, and susceptibility to degradation by extremes of pH, light, heat, and oxygen. An oxygen bridge links the chromophore to a flexible, polyhydroxylated, lipophobic region that is fused with a microlactone ring subtending the one carboxyl of the compound at C-16. The aminosugar mycosamine (also present in other antifungal polyenes, e.g., nystatin) is glycosidically linked to the hydroxyl at C-19 on the macrolactone ring. Amphotericity results from the carboxyl at C-16 and the primary amine of mycosamine. While the carboxyl is not essential to antifungal activity, a primary amine function must be present (the water-soluble N-acetyl derivative was markedly diminished in antifungal activity [33]).

Amphotericin B, and presumably other polyenes, is bioactive through combination with sterols in the cell membranes of eukaryotic cells and certain prokaryotic organisms, e.g., *Acholeplasma* spp. [34, 35]. With eukaryotic cell membranes, the resultant destabilization varies in severity from minimal injury, causing reversible leakage of intracellular cations [36, 37], to lethal injury from the loss of large molecules, such as nucleic acids. Certain enveloped viruses are susceptible to AmB [38]; the sites of antiviral activity may be envelope sterols derived from the host cell membrane as the virion exits the host cell. The utility of AmB to antifungal therapy appears to depend on stronger binding by ergosterol, the cell membrane sterol characteristic of fungi, than by cholesterol, the cell membrane sterol characteristic of human cells.

3.1.1   Deoxycholate formulation

Amphotericin B is insoluble in water at physiologic pH, and a formulation that enables absorption from the gut of humans has yet to be devised. Indeed, therapeutic trials were delayed until 1955 when an AmB-deoxycholate suspension was developed that could be injected intravenously [31]. The commercial preparation now in use consists of 50 mg of AmB, 11 mg of sodium deoxycholate, and 25.2 mg of sodium phosphates in glass, rubber-stoppered vials sealed under nitrogen. The addition of 10 ml of sterile water for injection yields, with shaking, a clear yellow, stably dispersed, colloidal suspension of amphotericin B-deoxycholate complex (AmB-DC). In some countries, 2-aminoglucose is used instead of deoxycholate.

By testing in vitro [39–50], the usual MICs of AmBDC are ≤1.5 µg/ml for

B. dermatitidis, Candida spp., *C. immitis, C. neoformans, Histoplasma* spp., *S. schenckii*, the Zygomycetes, and some *Aspergillus* spp. However, many strains of *Aspergillus* spp. are not susceptible; *Candida lusitaniae* are generally resistant, whereas the other pathogenic *Candida* spp. are usually susceptible; and *Fusarium* spp., *Geotrichum* spp., *P. boydii* and many of the dematiaceous fungi are often resistant. Typically, the minimal lethal concentrations (MLCs) of AmB-DC are only modestly higher than the MICs. However, lethal concentrations are not generally attained in patients. Susceptible fungi rarely develop resistance during therapy [51]. In one carefully studied case [52], acquisition of resistance was associated with the disappearance of ergosterol from the fungal cell membrane, a reduction in the binding of AmB by the fungal cell membrane, and a decrease in pathogenicity (as tested in hypercorticoid mice).

AmB-DC is usually administered by intravenous (IV) injection; the drug is too irritating to be given by subcutaneous (SC), intramuscular (IM), or intraperitoneal (IP) injection, and is poorly absorbed from the gut. As penetration from the blood into the cerebrospinal fluid (CSF), the central nervous system (CNS), and the eye is inadequate for therapy [53], itrathecal (IT), subconjunctival, and intravitreal injections are necessary for treatment. Direct injection into serous cavities, joint spaces, and the urinary bladder may provide fungicidal concentrations.

Using doubly-labelled AmB-DC (^{3}H-AmB complexed with ^{14}C-DC), distribution was studied in rhesus monkeys 24 hours after IV injection of 1 mg/kg [54]. The complex dissociated with the DC collecting in the liver and bile. The AmB went to kidneys, liver, spleen, adrenals, lungs, thyroid, heart, somatic muscle, pancreas, brain, and bone (in descending order of concentrations). The concentration of AmB in the urine was very low, and the drug was barely detectable in the CSF, CNS, and aqueous and vitreous humors.

In normal sheep, passage from the blood (after IV injection of 1 mg/kg) into the interstitium of the lungs, and thence into the pulmonary lymph, was not hampered by either the colloidal state of AmB-DC or binding by plasma proteins [55]. AmB appeared promptly in pulmonary lymph, and disappeared at an approximately exponential rate from both pulmonary lymph and venous blood.

In humans, about 5% of AmB-DC appears in the urine as antifungally active drug during the 24 hours postdose [53], as was found in rhesus monkeys [56]. The major route of excretion appears to be the bile [54]. After IV administration of AmB-DC to the adult human, the halflife in the blood is about 24 hours [57]), an observation that provides pharmacokinetic support for alternate day (inpatients) or thrice weekly (outpatients) administration. It is presumed that the toxicity of AmB-DC results mainly from perturbations of the regulatory functions of cell membranes damaged by cholesterol-AmB [58]. However, deoxycholate is a detergent capable of deranging cell membranes [59, 60], an effect that may be of importance following IT injection into CSF, a relatively static, fixed and confined volume of liquid. Adverse reactions are virtually always caused by the administration of AmB-DC. IV injection causes:

1) *Reversible reactions*, most commonly as chills, fever, headache, nausea, and vomiting. Hypotension is uncommon, usually asymptomatic, and usually does not occur after the first or second dose. With prolonged therapy, anorexia and malaise may accompany the other adverse reactions; loss of body weight may become prominent. With alternate day or thrice weekly administration, surcease from these reactions enables PO replenishment of electrolytes, water, and calories [61].

2) *Anemia*, develops in about 75% of patients, sometimes with thrombocytopenia. Renal failure may be contributory, but direct suppression of erythropoiesis (and platlet formation) is the usual cause. Hemolysis from AmB-DC is unlikely to be important because much higher concentrations than are attained in therapy are required by testing in vitro [58]. The potential value of giving erythropoietin has not been carefully evaluated. Repair of anemia follows cessation of treatment with AmB-DC.

3) *Nephropathy* virtually always results from treatment with AmB-DC, varies in severity from patient to patient [58, 62, 63], but is also dose-dependent [63]. Hypokalemia, hyposthenuria, and diminished capacity to excrete acid result from tubular injury; decreased creatinine clearance, with or without azotemia, reflects a fall in glomerular filtration and decreased renal blood flow [64]. The major histopathology in kidneys rendered afunctional from AmB-DC is necrosis and calcification of the renal tubules [65–67]. Renal blood flow is reduced within minutes after beginning IV injection of AmB-DC, an effect that occurs with every dose [64, 68], and is not correlated with the blood pressure. Renal hypoperfusion has particular impact in the relatively poorly vascularized medulla, the very region of the kidney where oxygen-requiring transport enzymes are pushed to maximal activity to conserve cations, especially Na^+. Anoxic necrosis of renal tubular epithelium may result from the combination of decreased renal blood flow, increased demand on O_2-requiring functions, and AmB-damaged cell membranes [69]. Alternate day or thrice weekly treatment, in

providing periodic relief of anoxia, may enable repair of injury [61]. Making certain that the patient is eunatremic appears to mitigate nephrotoxicity [70]. Possibly, the co-administration of a calcium-channel blocker will prevent injury [71].

4. *Neurotoxicity* from the IV injection of AmB-DC may take the form of hyperthermia, hypotension, confusion, incoherence, delerium, depression, obtundation, psychotic behavior, tremors, convulsions, blurring of vision, loss of hearing, flaccid quadriparesis with degeneration of the myelin in the brachial plexus, akinetic mutism, and diffuse cerebral leukoencephalopathy [58, 72, 73]. With intrathecal injection, radiculitis, arachnoiditis, pareses (mono- or para-), hypesthesias, paresthesias, urinary retention, fever, impairment of vision, loss of hearing, and delerium have been reported [58, 72]. No preventive measures have been suggested.

5) *Other* applications, such as injection into serous cavities, joint spaces, or the urinary bladder, or topical application to skin or mucous membranes, do not usually cause adverse reactions.

Adverse effects are virtually obligatory consequences of parenteral therapy with AmB-DC. Over the years, a lore has accumulated regarding the treatment and prevention of such reactions that is not always based on rigorous evaluations. However, there is support for maintaining eunatremia [70], alternate day administration (thrice weekly to outpatients), and injection of each dose over a period of 30–45 minutes [61, 74]. A protocol for the administration of AmB-DC that incorporates these measures has been published [2].

3.1.2   Lipoidal formulations

The chemical structure of AmB is not altered in any of the many lipoidal formulations that have been investigated as carriers for the delivery of AmB. The AmB is complexed to various lipids; thus, the kinds of lipids and their physicochemical arrangement determine both the content of AmB and the size of the particles characteristic of particular preparations (Table 1). Lipoidal formulations are generally administered IV as suspensions of particles.

The particles are adsorbed to phagocytic cells and internalized by endocytosis primarily in the mononuclearphagocyte system (MPS – formerly called the reticuloendothelial system) and by circulating macrophages [82, 83]. The MPS is targeted because the particles are too large to pass through either continuous or fenestrated capillary endothelium but pass freely through the discontinuous endothelium of the liver, spleen, bone marrow,

Table 1. Some properties of five lipoidal formulations of amphotericin B [75-81]

Formulation	mol% AmB	Particle Shape and Size
Multilamellar vesicles (MLV) of dimyristoylphosphatidylcholine: dimyristoylphostidylglycerol, 7:3 molar ratio	5	Spherical, 0.25–6.0 μm in diameter
Small unilamellar vesicles (SW) of hydrogenated soy phosphatidylcholine: cholesterol: distearoylphosphatidylglycerol, 10:5:4 ratio	10	Spherical, ≤0.2 μm in diameter
Lipid complex (ABLC) with dimyristolyphosphatidylcholine: dimyristoylphosphatidylglycerol, 7:3 ratio	33	Rod-like
Cholesterol-3-sulfate complex (ABCD), equi-molar with AmB	32–38	Disc-like, 4 nm thick by 122 nm in diameter
Fat emulsion, 20% (Intralipid® 20%, consisting of 20% soybean oil, 50% linoleic acid, 26% oleic acid, 10% palmitic acid, 9% linolenic acid, 3.5% stearic acid, 1.2% egg phospho-lipids and 2.25% glycerol), plus AmB-DC to yield a final concentration of 2 mg of AmB per ml	0.7	Spherical, 0.4–0.5 μm in diameter

and, to some extent, lungs and lymph nodes [82–84]. In the MPS, particles are taken up by the resident phagocytes (there may be some congregation of particles in the extracellular spaces of the MPS, especially if the phago-cytes are sated). Indeed, the phagocytic capacity of the MPS is finite and large doses of particulates, especially if repeated, will saturate, in sequence, the liver, the spleen, and then the bone marrow – i.e., impaired function of the MPS by blockade is a potential hazard of zealous therapy [85]. Distri-bution to non-MPS organs/tissues is minor. Circulating macrophages that have engulfed particles may migrate to extravascular sites, e.g., in response to inflammation [84, 85].

Since lipoidal preparations of AmB are taken up primarily by the MPS, their therapeutic utility may be limited to the treatment of infectious diseases caused by organisms that are: 1) susceptible to AmB; and 2) localized either facultatively or obligatorily inside the cells of the MPS [85]. Examples include visceral leishmaniasis and the hepatosplenic candidosis that may complicate general candidosis. Preparations that target non-MPS sites of mycoses are not available.

Abating the toxicity of AmB is the primary goal of lipoidal formulations, and, indeed, cloaking AmB in lipids reduces (but does not eliminate) acute toxicity and avoids nephrotoxicity. Apparently, the release of AmB from lipoidal particulates into the non-MPS extracellular space is so slow that the classic toxicity of AmB is avoided. Comparative evaluations of the many lipoidal formulations with each other have not been carried out in regard to either toxicity or efficacy in the treatment of mycoses. Moreover, evaluations of clinical efficacy controlled by comparing lipoidal formulations with AmB-DC, and assessments of toxicity from long-term treatment with lipoidal formulations have yet to be reported.

3.1.2.1   Liposomal amphotericin B

Liposomes are microscopic, spherical vesicles that enclose an aqueous core. They were originally used as models of biological membranes [86]. The lipid bilayer structure of liposomal walls resembles that of cell membranes and is also permeable to water but relatively impermeable to solutes [86, 87]. Liposomes have many characteristics [82–85, 87] that vary from preparation to preparation: 1) size – 20 to ≥5000 nm in diameter, effecting both toxicity (larger usually more toxic than smaller), and pharmacokinetics (larger are more rapidly eliminated); 2) number of concentric walls (lamellae) per vesicle – multilamellar vesicles (MLVs) are generally used for delivery of antimicrobial agents as they release drugs more slowly than unilamellar vesicles; 3) constituents – either natural lipids, i.e., compounds normally present in the cell membranes of eukaryotes, or synthetic lipids; 4) charge; 5) stability – both in storage (change in size and lamellation; leakage of constituents) and in the body (rates of degradation and release of drugs); 6) efficiency of incorporation of drugs; and 7) methods of manufacture – batch to batch variation.

Liposomal formulations of amphotericin B (L-AmB) depend on the incorporation of AmB into the walls of liposomes. Natural constituents used to prepare L-AmB commonly include phosphatidylethanolamine (no charge), phosphatidylserine (negative charge), phosphatidylcholine (no charge), and sphingomyelin (no charge); synthetic phospholipid constituents include dipalmitoylphosphatidylcholine, stearylamine, and dicetylphosphate derivatives [82, 83, 87]. Other compounds that may be added to the mix include sterols (cholesterol or ergosterol – both reduce permeability, increase stability and lamellarity, but may inhibit the release of AmB [82]), fatty acids, glycolipids, and proteins [83, 84, 87]. As amphotericin B (without DC) is amphoteric, it intercalates into the walls of liposomes during their preparation. Theoretically, adsorption of L-AmB on fungi could permit transfer of the AmB from the wall of the liposome to the fungal cell membrane to interact with fungal ergosterol [82].

The MLV preparation described in Table 1 was administered IV to patients in doses as high as 5 mg/kg/day, but did not come to commercial production because of difficulties with batch to batch variation in content of AmB, stability, and homogeneity [75, 81].

The SUV (small unilamellar vesicle) preparation (Table 1) has been licensed for use in some countries as it is a replicable formulation. Doses as high as 5 mg/kg/day may yield peak concentrations of AmB in the blood of 25–29 µg/ml. The second phase halflife in the blood is about 32 hours, possibly as a consequence of inclusion of distearoylphosphatidylglycerol as a component [78].

After IV injection, liposomes made with natural lipids are immediately coated with plasma proteins. These are either opsonins that facilitate removal from the blood by phagocytosis, or are high density lipoproteins that mediate destabilization of liposomal bilayers [84].

Liposomes prepared with certain gangliosides have surfaces that mimic the' composition of the outer leaflet of erythrocyte membranes [88]. Such preparations yielded much longer halflives in the blood of mice with increased distribution into non-MPS tissues. Specific targeting by attaching the antigen-specific Fab portion of antibodies, or glycoprotein or glycolipid ligands, appears to be promising [84, 88].

L-AmB preparations are not nephrotoxic and cause less severe immediate and short-term adverse reactions than AmB-DC. However, long-term evaluation of toxicity, especially neurotoxicity, using well-characterized, replicable preparations of L-AmB, has yet to be carried out.

3.1.2.2   Non-liposomal amphotericin B
The non-liposomal formulations of AmB that have come to evaluation in humans are also suspensions of particles (Table 1), that distribute primarily to the MPS [75–81]. Clinical experience is inadequate for informed judgement as to the efficacy and safety of these preparations in the treatment of mycoses.

3.1.3   *Chemical derivatives*
Actual modification of the chemical structure of AmB by the semisynthesis of derivatives was undertaken to provide solubility in water and decreased toxicity, with preservation of antifungal activity. Of the derivatives depicted

in Fig. 4, only amphotericin B methyl ester (AME) came to clinical trial [72]. Experience in treating experimental animals and 53 patients with a variety of mycoses revealed that AME caused less severe immediate adverse reactions, was virtually non-nephrotoxic, and was equal to AmB-DC in clinical efficacy [72].

However, it was suggested that AME was more neurotoxic for patients than AmB-DC [89], a view not supported when the neurohistopathology of specimens from recipients and non-recipients of AME was evaluated by observers who were blind as to the origin of the specimens [90]. The matter was confused further by the fact that none of the 53 patients was treated with pure AME. All of the preparations used in therapy were mixtures containing 35–67% AME, with 2–8% AmB, and various amounts of six to seven multimethylated derivatives [72].

The importance of contamination of AME with AmB was demonstrated in subsequent work employing rat glial cells in culture [91], direct injection into rat peripheral nerves [92], and both IV and intraventricular injections into intact rats [93]. It was shown that: 1) AmB-DC is at least 10 times more neurotoxic than pure AME; and 2) contamination of pure AME with 10% AmB (w/w, using the commercial deoxycholate formulation employed in treating humans) resulted in neurotoxicity equal to that of AmB-DC. Confirmation and extension of these results may lead to clinical evaluation of pure AME.

3.2   Azole compounds

The antifungal azole derivatives are less toxic than AmB, and are active against several genera of fungi [94, 95]. Susceptible fungi are blocked from replication through azole-mediated inhibition of the microsomal cytochrome P450-dependent lanosterol 14-alpha-demethylase system ([96–98]; see Fig. 2). The cytochrome P450 enzymes are a superfamily of hemoproteins [99] that catalyze oxidative reactions [100, 101]. Membrane-bound and often substrate-inducible, they are present in prokaryotes as well as eukaryotes (plant and animal). Regardless of source, all P450 enzymes share a highly conserved heme-cysteine region and hydrophobicity. Except for erythrocytes and skeletal muscles, all cells of humans contain P450 enzymes with highest concentrations in the liver. P450s are vital to eliminating or disabling virtually any undesirable molecule that gains entry into the cell. It is truly an adventure in comparative biochemistry to design, discover and develop azole compounds that are orders of magnitude less avid for the 25–30 different P450s of humans than for the fungal P450 enzymes, while steering clear of subtle and/or long-term adverse effects. The carcinogenicity of genaconazole (derivative from fluconazole) and the tumorogenicity of saperconazole (derivative from itraconazole) are testimony to the keen sensitivity of the problem.

Inhibition of fungal P450 enzymes decreases the biosynthesis of ergosterol and causes accumulation of 14-methylated intermediary sterols (Fig 2). As a result, the liquidity and the permeability of the fungal cell wall/membrane complex is decreased, the activity of surface enzymes (chitin synthetase, lipid metabolism, oxidative enzymes) is disturbed, and metabolites (e.g., glucose) are retained [96–98]. Growth at sites of abcission of buds in yeast fungi, and hyphal tips and septa in mycelial fungi, is dramatically reduced as chitin synthetase activity is shut down. The fungi are not killed, but are morphologically abnormal [102] and may be more susceptible to destruction by phagocytes. Depletion of ergosterol reduces cell membrane sites for the interaction of polyenic antifungal agents; i.e., the azoles may antagonize AmB (see discussion in 3.6, below).

At concentrations relevant to therapy, the antifungal azoles are fungistatic' [2], a distinct therapeutic limitation. Fungicidal therapy is often critical to successful treatment since most systemic fungal infections are facilitated by defective host defenses.

When susceptible fungi are exposed to an azole drug, fungistasis is not immediately expressed but is delayed until cellular reserves of ergosterol are exhausted. One result is lack of clarity of endpoints in tests of susceptibility in vitro with the azole compounds. Moreover, unidentified constituents of conventional undefined culture media block the antifungal activity of azoles, an effect that can be avoided by using defined, synthetic culture media for testing [103]. Lack of correlation between results of conventional testing in vitro with activity in vivo and with clinical effectiveness may be related phenomena; the problem is particularly severe with fluconazole. Overall, when appropriate methods of testing in vitro are applied, the antifungal azoles are active against *C. neoformans, C. albicans* (but less active against non-*albicans Candida* spp. and *Torulopsis glabrata), C. immitis, B. dermatitidis* (not miconazole) *H. capsulatum, Paracoccidioides brasiliensis, P. boydii, S. schenckii,* and the dermatophytes. Up to one-third of *Aspergillus* spp. are susceptible, with itraconazole more active than the other azoles [94, 104–106].

Since introduction into clinical use in 1960, the antifungal azole drugs have been improved remarkably in potency, ease of administration, and adverse

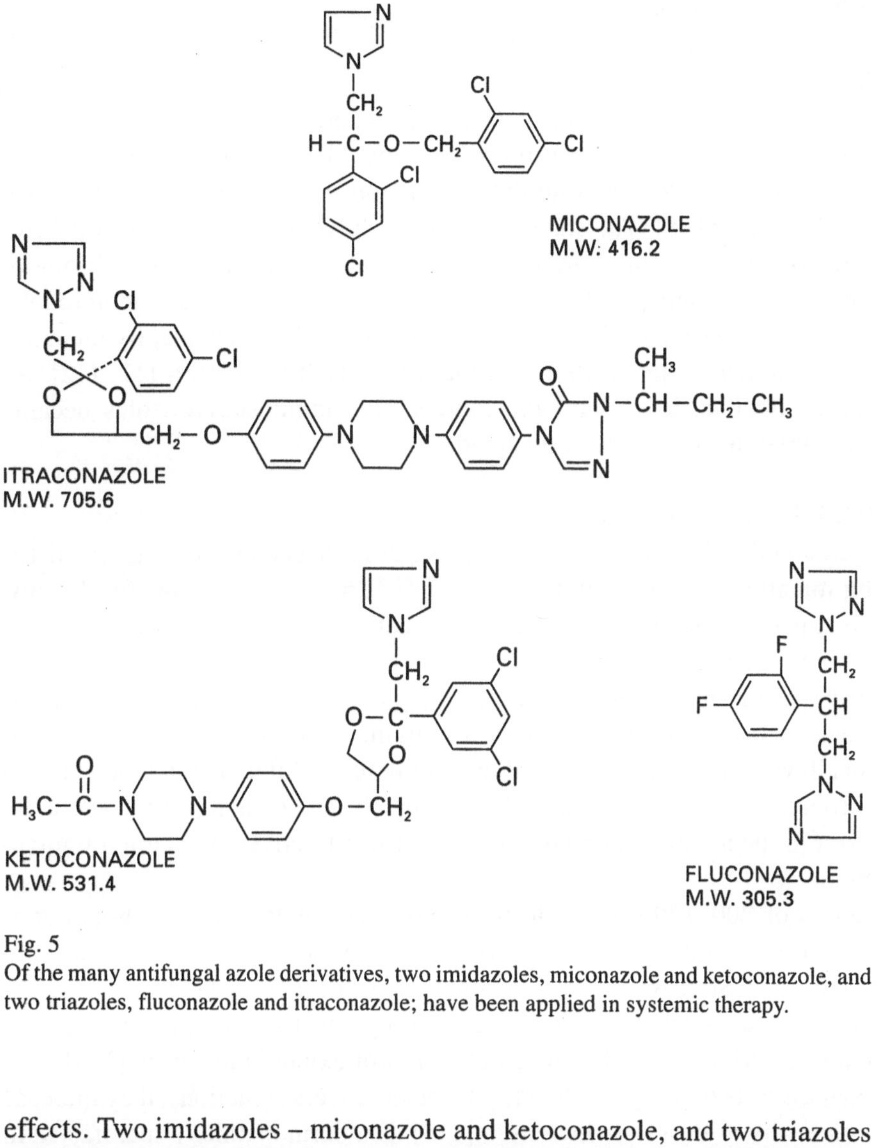

Fig. 5
Of the many antifungal azole derivatives, two imidazoles, miconazole and ketoconazole, and two triazoles, fluconazole and itraconazole; have been applied in systemic therapy.

effects. Two imidazoles – miconazole and ketoconazole, and two triazoles – fluconazole and itraconazole (Fig. 5) have been applied widely in the systemic treatment of mycoses. Miconazole is now obsolete and ketoconazole is obsolescent, leaving the less toxic and pharmacologically advantageous fluconazole and itraconazole as the dominant azole drugs.

104   Paul D. Hoeprich

3.2.1   *Imidazoles*

3.2.1.1   Miconazole

Synthesized in the late 1960s [107], miconazole (MON) was the first azole drug applied in systemic antifungal therapy. MON is formulated solely for IV administration as a colloidal suspension in water that is stable ≥ one week at 37C [108]. The stabilizing agent, polyethoxylated castor oil (Cremophor EL^R), is a mixture of substances that frequently cause thrombophlebitis, rouleauxing of erythrocytes, hyperlipidemia, and, uncommonly, anaphylaxis [109, 110]. Pruritus, anemia, thrombocytopenia, hyponeutremia, and nausea are attributed to the MON itself [104, 109, 111, 112]. As more effective, less toxic, and more easily administered azoles became available, the use of MON declined.

3.2.1.2   Ketoconazole

Ketoconazole (KET) was the first azole drug that achieved systemic distribution after PO administration – the only form made available for therapy. As it is insoluble in water at physiological pH, but dissolves in 0.1 N HCl, patients with achlorhydria, and those rendered functionally hypochlorhydric or achlorhydric by medications, may not respond to therapy with KET. Such patients may be treated by dissolving each dose in 0.1 N HCl, and swallowing it quickly (to avoid damaging teeth) after sucking the solution through a glass or plastic straw. Foregoing all antacid therapy for 8–12 hours prior to the administration of a dose may be effective, but is often impractical.

Doses of 200–1200 mg yield peak blood concentrations 2–4 hours after ingestion of 2–20 µg/ml; the halflife in the blood is 6–10 hours. Entry into the urine, CSF, CNS, and eye is too meager for therapy [113].

KET is catabolized in the liver, yielding inactive compounds that are excreted primarily in the bile and to a minor extent in the urine [113].

Nausea and vomiting are the most frequent adverse reactions; they increase in severity as doses are increased [113]. Endocrinopathies – manifested in males as gynecomastia, loss of libido, and oligospermia, and in females as irregular menses and amenorrhea – are also dose-related in severity [114]. Hepatitis is rare, usually reversible, but may be lethal [115]. KET also affects other drugs on coadministration, increasing the concentrations in the blood of cyclosporine, phenytoin, terfenidine, and astemizole, while the concentration of KET in the plasma is decreased by isoniazid and rifampin [95].

KET was particularly useful in the treatment of chronic mucocutaneous candidosis, an application that required indefinitely continued therapy for maintenance of remission [116]. Primary histoplasmosis responded quite satisfactorily [117]. However, use of KET in other systemic mycoses was not uniformly endorsed. Accordingly, the advent of the more effective and less toxic triazoles will eclipse KET.

3.2.2   Triazoles

3.2.2.1   Fluconazole

Fluconazole (FLU) entered clinical trials in 1986 shortly after therapeutic efficacy was demonstrated in experimental fungal infections [118–125]. Excellent reviews provide summaries of work carried out with FLU by several investigators in many countries [106, 126–128].

Properties of FLU that are unique among the azole antifungal agents [129–137] include: 1) solubility in water and 0.9% NaCl solution to the extent of 6 and 4 g/l, respectively; 2) relative resistance to catabolism with ≤4% of a dose detectable as metabolites; 3) virtually quantitative absorption from the gut (PO = IV dosage) without regard to gastric acidity or intake of food; 4) distribution in all body water as antifungally active drug, *n.b.*, there is no CNS, CSF or ocular barrier, and there is accumulation in the skin and nails; 5) excretion primarily in the urine, with ≤80% of the dose unchanged drug and ≤11% as metabolites (about 10% is passed in the feces as active drug); 6) only about 11% binding to plasma proteins; and 6) a halflife of 30–36 hours, permitting one dose/day therapy.

Tablets containing 50, 100, or 200 mg of FLU are available for PO administration, and an isosmotic solution containing 2 mg/ml is available for IV administration. Maximal concentration in the blood are attained 2–4 hours after ingestion of a dose [129, 135, 136] and are roughly proportional to the size of the dose. With daily administration, a steady state is reached after 6--10 days [129, 136, 137], a delay that may be avoided by doubling the initial dose. At steady state, 400 mg/day yields 1830 µg/ml in the blood of adults [106]. If renal function is reduced, the manufacturer suggests reducing the dose according to the creatinine clearance (C_{cr}): C_{cr} ≥50 ml/min, normal dose; C_{cr} 21–50 ml/min, 50% of normal dose; C_{cr} 11–20 ml/min, 25% of normal dose [138]. As FLU is dialyzable, a normal dose should be given after each dialysis.

FLU does not undergo hepatic catabolism [129]. While asymptomatic elevations of hepatocellular enzymes occur in ≤1% of patients [139], severe hepatotoxicity is rare [140]. Interference with steroidogenesis has not been detected [141]. Other adverse reactions are infrequent (nausea in 3.7%, vomiting in 1.7%, abdominal pain in 1.7%, diarrhea in 1.5%, headache in 1.9%, and skin rash in 1.8%) and trivial e.g., lead to discontinuing therapy in 1.5% of patients [138]. FLU influences the pharmacokinetics of several drugs on co-administration [142–144]: with coumadin, increase in the prothrombin time; with phenytoin, increased concentrations of phenytoin, with cyclosporine, increased concentrations of cyclosporine; with sulfony-lurea agents, hypoglycemia; and with rifampin, increased concentrations of FLU.

By conventional susceptibility testing in vitro, FLU usually appears to have little therapeutic potential. However, if a totally defined, synthetic, liquid culture medium is used [103], and testing is carried out by experienced personnel, the MIC values are generally consistent with the efficacy of FLU as demonstrated in experimental mycoses and clinical experience [145].

Evaluations of the efficacy of FLU based on controlled clinical trials comparing FLU with non-azole or other azole antifungal agents are gener-ally lacking. Indeed, only two studies have been reported that compared FLU with AmB (regimens with or without concomitant flucytosine). In the first controlled trial [146], 194 previously untreated patients with crypto-coccal meningitis complicating AIDS received either FLU (200 or 400 mg/day, usually PO, but IV in some patients) or AmB [(median dose of 0.4–0.5 mg/kg/day, IV), plus flucytosine in some patients (150 mg/kg/day, PO)] for 10 weeks. The regimens appeared to be equally effective with regard to mortality. However, both left a residuum of about one-quarter of the patients who were improved but continued to yield C. neoformans in cultures of their CSF. The authors concluded that single drug therapy with FLU was most effective in patients at low risk for failure of treatment.

In the second controlled trial [147], 236 non-neutropenic, clinically ill patients with candidemia, usually associated with an intravascular device, were treated for 14 days with either FLU (400 mg/day, PO) or AmB (0.5 mg/kg/day, IV). Intravascular access devices were changed before, or at the start of, therapy. The regimens appeared to be equally effective.

Many reports of open trials offer testimony to the effectiveness of treatment of a variety of mycoses with FLU. A sampling includes: 1) cryptococcosis (meningeal (FLU alone [148, 150]; FLU plus flucytosine [151]); nonmen-ingeal [139, 150, 152]); 2) candidosis (oropharyngeal [139, 153–161]; vulvovaginal [162, 163]; skin and nails [139, 164, 165]); candidemia [166–168]; deep (hepatosplenic [169, 170]; post-transplantation [139,

171]); 3) blastomycosis [172]; 4) histoplasmosis [173]; 5) coccidioidomycosis (meningeal [174–178], non-meningeal [173, 178]); 6) paracoccidioidomycosis [173]; sporotrichosis [173]; dermatomycoses [164]; aspergillosis [152, 178)] and miscellaneous mycoses [152–173]. While these reports are generally favorable, they do not provide data that enable selection
among available drugs, judgement as to regimens, or definition of the place
of FLU in antifungal therapy.

The use of FLU to prevent recurrences of cryptococcal meningitis complicating AIDS was evaluated in patients who had negative cultures of their
CSF following primary therapy [179]. Daily administration of FLU (200
mg, PO) was more effective and better tolerated than weekly AmB (1 mg/kg,
IV). Life-long application of FLU in a dose of 200–400 mg/day is recommended in such patients [180, 181].

Prevention of mycoses complicating acute leukemia, either newly diagnosed or in first relapse, was attempted in 54 patients who had severe
granulocytopenia [182]. Either FLU (50 mg, PO, once/day) or AmB (200
mg in suspension plus 200 mg in tablets, PO, 4 times/day) was given until
granulocyte counts exceed 500/µl. While the regimens were equally effective in preventing severe local or deep mycoses, the study has little value
because of the dose of FLU (too low) and the peroral (non-systemic)
administration of AmB.

Non-comparative prophylactic use of FLU has been reported in patients
without fungal infections who are infected with the human immunodeficiency virus (HIV) [183], and in recipients of bone marrow transplants
[184]. It is not possible to assess the preventive value of FLU from these
reports alone.

3.2.2.2   Itraconazole

The itraconazole (ITR) in clinical use is a 1:1:1:1 racemic mixture of two
enantionmeric pairs, each with three chiral centers (Fig. 5). All components
are strongly lipophilic and virtually insoluble in water [105]. The pharma-
cotherapeutic properties of ITR have been extensively investigated since
the early 1980s; several reviews provide summaries of this work [94, 95,
105, 185, 186].

Nominally the successor of ketoconazole, ITR partakes of several of the
undesirable features of KET, namely: requirement for an acid pH in the
stomach for absorption (see discussion under 3.2.1.2, Ketoconazole,
above), although ingestion with food aids absorption [187, 188]; and
meager, therapeutically insignificant penetration into the eye, CSF, CNS,

tracheobronchial secretions, sputum and urine [187, 189]. However, ITR has significant offsetting advantages over KET: greater activity against *Aspergillus* spp. and dematiaceous fungi by testing in vitro [190, 191]; a longer halflife (in volunteers [192] 16–26 hours after a single dose of 200 mg; 32–96 hours after 200 mg 12-hourly, for 15 days) enabling once or twice a day dosage; no effect on the endogenous synthesis of steroidal hormones after one or more months of treatment with doses ≤400 mg/day [193, 194], but suppression at doses ≥600 mg/day [195]; and accumulation in pus, fat, and keratin – ITR is excreted in sebum and sweat [187, 196].

ITR is formulated only for PO administration in capsules containing 50 and 100 mg. In normal volunteers, peak concentrations in the blood after ingestion of a single dose of 200 mg with food were 0.15–0.32 µg/ml [192]. Daily doses of 200 mg led to a steady state in 10–14 days with peak concentrations of 0.16–0.42 µg/ml [187]. Increasing the dose to 200 mg 12-hourly yielded peak concentrations of 1.8–2.8 µg/ml [192]. Thus, catabolism appears to be a saturable process, and initiation of therapy by giving 200 mg, 8-hourly, for 3 days, then dropping to 200 mg 12-hourly, will speed attainment of steady state therapy in patients with severe mycoses [95].

ITR binds to plasma proteins and erythrocytes so extensively that only about 0.2% of the drug in the blood is free [187]. ITR is not dialyzable, the dose need not be reduced because of either renal or hepatic failure [187].

ITR is eliminated primarily in the bile and urine as metabolites that result from non-inducible hepatic catabolism [187]. Hydroxyitraconazole is a major metabolite and is antifungally active; although it is eliminated more rapidly than ITR, at steady state the concentration of hydroxyitraconazole is almost twice that of ITR in the blood [188].

Asymptomatic abnormalities of hepatic function occur in 0.3–2.7% of patients treated with ITR [192]. Reversible, apparently idiosyncratic, hepatitis is very rare. Other adverse effects are usually trivial, leading to cessation of therapy in 3–10% of patients [192]. Nausea is most common at 2.4–10.6% of patients; less common are vomiting (0.8–5.1%); abdominal pain (1.4–1.5%), diarrhea (0.6–3.3%), headache (1.5–3.8%), and skin rashes (1.1–8.6%). The administration of ITR with certain other drugs has pharmacokinetic consequences: decrease in the concentration of ITR in the blood when co-administered with rifampin [187, 197], or phenytoin and phenobarbitone [197, 198]; increase in the concentration of cyclosporine [199–201], and digoxin [202] when co-administered with ITR.

Susceptibility testing in vitro with ITR suffers not only from the limitations common to all antifungal azole derivatives (see earlier discussion), but also from its virtual insolubility in water. Reliability of testing is favored when experienced personnel follow a set protocol and use a totally defined, synthetic culture medium. Given these demurrers, ITR appears to be more active than either KET or FLU; moreover, ITR is inhibitory to some *Aspergillus* spp. and many of the dematiaceous fungi [190, 191, 203].

Because of the vagaries of testing in vitro, assessment of activity in experimental mycoses may be of greater value. ITR was effective in experimental dermatophytoses, candidosis, cryptococcosis, coccidioidomycosis, histoplasmosis, blastomycosis, paracoccidioidomycosis, sporotrichosis, chromoblastomycosis, and aspergillosis (summarized in [94, 95, 105, 186, 187, 190]).

Most of the clinical trials of ITR have been uncontrolled and non-comparative; they testify to the effectiveness of ITR in various forms of: superficial fungal infections [161, 194, 198, 204], candidosis [171, 204, 205], cryptococcosis [194, 196, 204, 206–210], coccidioidomycosis [194, 195, 204, 211–214], histoplasmosis [204, 215–222], blastomycosis [204, 219], aspergillosis [194, 204, 206, 209, 223–231], paracoccidioidomycosis [204, 217, 237], sporotrichosis [194, 204, 232, 233], chromoblastomycosis [204, 234], and mycoses caused by dematiaceous fungi [195, 208, 235]. Indeed, ITR may be the agent of choice for the primary therapy of histoplasmosis, blastomycosis, and mycoses caused by dematiaceous fungi. However, these studies are not based on head-to-head comparative trials and do not permit conclusions as to the efficacy and toxicity of ITR relative to other antifungal agents. Moreover, the optimal regimens of therapy with ITR for particular mycoses have yet to be established.

ITR was compared with AmB in two trials. In the first [236], neutropenic (<500 neutrophils/μl) patients with proved or suspected mycoses were treated either with ITR [16 patients; 200 mg, 12-hourly for 20 days (mean period of therapy)] or AmB [0.6 mg/kg/day alone in 11 patients, or 0.3 mg/kg/day plus flucytosine (150 mg/kg/day in 5 patients) for 13 days (mean period of therapy)]. The regimens were equally effective in securing a good response, usually in association with restoration of neutrophils (13 of 15 patients). Of the 17 patients with persistent neutropenia, six had a favorable clinical response (equally divided as to regimen). The number of patients in this interesting study was too small to support preference for one regimen over the other.

The second comparative evaluation [237] was carried out in patients with cryptococcal meningitis complicating AIDS. Treatment was continued for

6 weeks either with ITR (200 mg, 12-hourly; 12 evaluable patients), or AmB (0.3 mg/kg/day) plus flucytosine (150 mg/kg/day) – 10 evaluable patients. Five patients treated with ITR had a complete response whereas all 10 patients who received AmB-flucytosine responded. All patients were given ITR (200 mg/day) as post-therapy maintenance treatment; 7 initially treated with ITR and 2 initially treated with AmB-flucytosine suffered relapse or recrudescence. The numbers of patients were small, but ITR was inferior to AmB-flucytosine in the acute disease, and was not effective in preventing reactivation. Other trials of ITR in chemoprophylaxis have yet to be reported.

3.3   Flucytosine

Flucytosine (5-fluorocytosine, 5FC) is a mock pyrimidine that is soluble in water to the extent of 15 g/l [238]. In aqueous systems at physiologic pH, 5FC is tautomeric (Fig. 6). Among pathogenic fungi, only yeast form genera are usefully susceptible to 5FC.

Susceptibility testing in vitro requires use of a defined culture medium that does not contain either cytosine or uridine as both will nullify the activity of 5FC [239, 240]. Overall, about 10–15% of clinical isolates of *C. albicans* [48, 241–247] and about 3–5% of isolates of *C. neoformans* [239, 241, 245, 247–249] are relatively resistant to 5FC, i.e., they will grow in the presence of ≥25 µg/ml. However, with both genera, native resistance varies from one geographic region to another. With *C. albicans,* there is also serogroup relationship, with about 15% of Group A and about 95% of Group B strains natively resistant [250]; with *C. neoformans*, no serogroup relationship to resistance has been found [251]. Susceptibility/resistance among non-*albicans Candida* spp. is unpredictably variable [247, 252]. 5FC is usually fungistatic in action against susceptible fungi. However, most isolates of *T. glabrata* are killed at clinically relevant concentrations, excepting about 5% of isolates that are natively resistant [243, 247]. Other pathogenic fungi are generally resistant to 5FC.

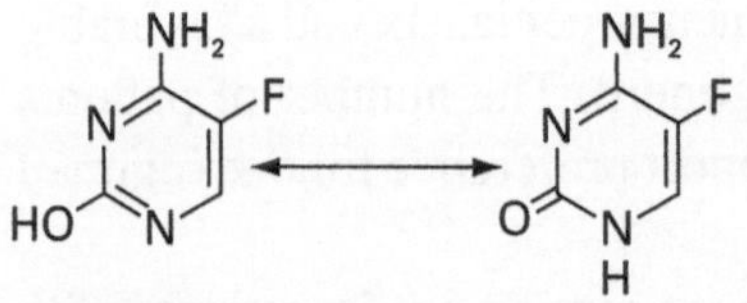

5-FLUOROCYTOSINE
M.W. 129.1

Fig. 6
Flucytosine (5FC; 5-fluorocytosine) is a synthetic pyrimidine derivative that is tautomeric under physiologic conditions.

Flucytosine itself has no cytotoxicity. Intracellular conversion to 5-fluorouracil through the action of cytosine deaminase is essential to antibiotic effect as was shown with *Salmonella typhimurium* [253], *Saccharomyces cerevisiae* [254, 255], and *C. albicans* [256]. The phosphorylated forms of 5-fluorouracil are cytotoxic through: 1) inhibition of thymidylate synthase thus inhibiting DNA synthesis by 5-fluorodeoxyuridine formed through the action of uridine monophosphate pyrophosphorylase on 5-fluorouracil [257]; and 2) the synthesis of abnormal proteins or the blockage of protein synthesis as a result of faulty instruction by RNA altered by containing either fluorouridine diphosphate or fluorocytidine triphosphate [254, 258]. As humans lack cytosine permease [259] and cytosine deaminase [260, 261], 5FC is non-toxic. However, the normal enteric bacterial flora (the Enterobacteriaceae, and perhaps other bacteria) are capable of deaminating 5FC [262]; the resultant 5-fluorouracil is poorly absorbed from the normal colon.

Native and acquired resistance to 5FC may result from absence, dysfunction, or deletion of one or more of three enzymes not essential to fungal survival: most often, uridine monophosphate pyrophosphorylase [256, 263, 264], cytosine permease [255, 263], and cytosine deaminase [264, 265]. Endogenous overproduction of pyrimidines may also lead to resistance to 5FC [255, 256]. Given this background, the development of resistance when 5FC is used alone in therapy is not surprising. The phenomenon was illustrated in a patient treated only with 5FC for infective endocarditis caused by *Candida parapsilosis;* mutational deletion of cytosine deaminase resulted in massive, one-step resistance [265].

5FC for PO administration is available in tablets containing either 0.25 or 0.50 g. For IV administration, 1.0% 5FC in 0.9% NaCl solution may be used. In patients with normal renal function, the usual dose is 150–200 mg/kg/day given in four equal portions, 6-hourly, as the halflife in the blood is about 3 hours [266, 267]. The PO and IV doses are the same since 5FC is quantitatively absorbed from the small bowel. Dosage should be individualized by measurement of concentrations in the serum. The desired predose concentration is 25–35 µg/ml; lower concentrations favor the development of resistance [268–270]. Peak concentrations should be 85–100 µg/ml; at concentrations $\geq$125 µg/ml, the frequency of adverse reactions increases [270, 271].

While the distribution of 5FC is general, i.e., into all body water, the concentrations measured in various liquids may be lower than in serum because of the temporal lag of equilibration. Typical values, expressed as percent of concentrations in contemporaneous serum, are: peritoneal fluid, 100% [273]; CSF, 75% [274]; synovial fluid 60% [275]; aqueous humor, 20% [276]; and bronchial secretions 76% [277].

About 90% of a PO dose of 5FC is excreted as unchanged drug [96, 266, 278] by glomerular filtration without tubular secretion or resorption [279]. Accordingly, the dose must be reduced when there is decreased renal function [266, 273, 279, 280]. Trimming the dose in direct proportion to the creatinine clearance is generally appropriate, but the reduced dose must be validated by measurement of concentrations in the blood. As 5FC is removed by dialysis, replenishment, e.g., administration of a single dose of 20 mg/kg, PO, after each treatment [281], is necessary.

Metabolites of 5FC also appear in the urine. About 1% of a PO dose of ^{14}C-labelled 5FC given to volunteers was detected in the urine in the form of alpha-fluorobeta-ureido-propionic acid [267]. This metabolite most likely resulted from catabolism of 5-fluorouracil absorbed from the gut after deamination of 5FC by enteric microorganisms.

Anorexia, nausea, vomiting, diarrhea, and/or abdominal pain occur in about 6% of patients given 5FC.

Hepatic disturbances such as elevations of transaminases, alkaline phosphatase, and, quite rarely, hyperbilirubinemia, may occur with or without hepatomegaly in about 5% of patients. The bone marrow suppression reported in about 5% of patients [270] occurred when dosage was not monitored by serial measurements of 5FC in the blood, or when concentrations exceeded 100 µg/ml for long periods [282]. Moreover, patients who require 5FC often have compromised function of the gut, liver, and bone marrow, or have been treated with drugs that injure these organs. Also, concomitant treatment with nephrotoxic drugs, e.g., AmB, impairs the excretion of 5FC and its metabolites. As slowed enteric motility causes shift of the colonic microflora mouthward [283], microbial intraenteric deamination of 5FC to yield 5-fluorouracil is favored. Injury to the enteric mucosa will facilitate absorption of 5-fluorouracil, increasing the probability of toxicity. However, even in such patients 5FC may be used safely and effectively [259]. Neither bone marrow aplasia, enterocolitis, hepatitis, nor death from 5FC occurred in 17 myelosuppressed patients when dosage was controlled by use of serial measurements of concentrations in the serum [259].

Flucytosine remains a useful agent for the treatment of certain systemic mycoses. However, the application of 5FC is constrained to coadministration with another drug, also proved active against the infecting fungus by testing in vitro. Laboratory support is also necessary for surveillance of dosage by serial measurements of concentrations in the blood.

3.4   Griseofulvin

Griseofulvin (GRI) is a water-insoluble, phenol-ether compound (Fig. 7) elaborated by at least six species of *Penicillium* [284]. First isolated in 1939 [285], GRI was used against fungal infections of plants and cattle prior to clinical trial in humans in 1958 [286]. GRI was the first perorally administrable, systemically distributed antifungal agent. However, griseofulvin is now obsolescent. It was of value only to treat the dermatophytoses, an application for which more effective drugs are now available [4].

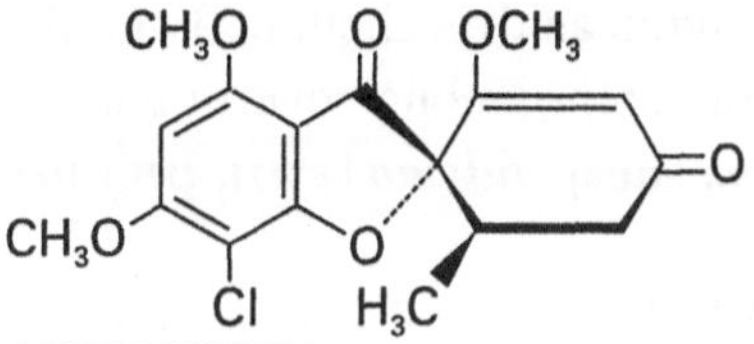

GRISEOFULVIN
M.W. 352.5

Fig. 7
Griseofulvin is a naturally occurring, antifungal phenol-ether compound that is active only against the dermatophytes.

Through unknown mechanisms, GRI is antimitotic to actively growing dermatophytes, producing multinucleate giant cells [287]. After PO administration, GRI is delivered to the stratum corneum in eccrine sweat, whence it is taken up by keratin-producing cells, and deposited in the forming keratin [288]. Since eccrine sweat functions as a vehicle for delivery of GRI, various formulations have been tested for topical therapy, with some success [289].

Griseofulvin is available only for PO administration. Absorption from the gut is inefficient but is favored by using tablets prepared from ultramicrosized crystals (mean diameter, about 2 μm [290] and partially dissólved in polyethylene glycol) and administration with a fatty meal [291].

Adverse reactions are uncommon, not life-threatening, and usually disappear as treatment is continued [292].

3.5   Other antifungal agents

3.5.1   Cilofungin

Cilofungin (CIL), a semisynthetic, amphiphilic lipopeptide derived from echinocandin B [293], came to clinical trial, but was abandoned because of lack of a safe vehicle for delivery. CIL is insoluble in water; formulation with polyethylene glycol for IV administration was associated with severe metabolic acidosis [294].

CIL was of great interest because its fungicidal activity was uniquely selective for *C. albicans* and *Candida tropicalis* [293, 295]. The synthesis of the beta 1,3 glucan component of the cell wall was inhibited, causing cell death through lysis [293].

3.5.2   Ambruticin

Ambruticin (BRT), a cyclopropyl-polyene-pyran acid, is chemically unlike other antifungal agents [296]. A major component among several antimicrobics produced by *Polyangium cellulosum,* subsp. *fulvum* [296], BRT has yet to be administered to humans.

By susceptibility testing in vitro [297, 298], the MICs of BRT against *C. immitis, B. dermatitidis, S. schenckii,* dematiaceous fungi, the dermatophytes, and zygomycetes were lower than, or the same as, those of AmB. With *H. capsulatum, Aspergillus* spp., and *P. boydii* the MICs were higher than those of AmB. The yeast-like fungi were generally resistant to BRT. Experimental murine coccidioidomycosis [299] and histoplasmosis [300] were cured by treatment with BR given PO.

BRT did not appear to affect fungal cell walls or membranes, although it was fungicidal. Suggested mechanisms include interference with the synthesis of RNA, inhibition of the uptake of amino acids, and blockage carbohydrate metabolism.

Peroral administration of BRT to mice was followed by rapid absorption and general distribution, except for lack of entry into either the CSF or CNS. BRT was eliminated principally in the bile. In mice the acute LD_{50} was >1000 mg/kg, and doses of 150 mg/kg/day, PO, were tolerated [297]. Further development of BRT·was halted as BRT was not active against *C. albicans* [301].

3.5.3   Saramycetin

Saramycetin (SAR) is an unstable, cyclic thiazolyl peptide product of *Streptomyces saramyceticus* with a molecular weight of 1,452 [302]. Despite lack of activity by conventional testing of susceptibility in vitro, and the absence of basic pharmacologic data, SAR was injected SC in doses of 3–17 mg/kg/day (given in four equal portions, 6-hourly, for 6–8 weeks) in the treatment of 57 patients [303]. Blastomycosis, histoplasmosis, sporotrichosis, aspergillosis, paracoccidioidomycosis (but not coccidioidomycosis) and zygomycosis were reported to have improved. Inflammation at the sites of SC injection, eosinophilia, and fever were noted, but the primary adverse reaction was hepatic dysfunction that was not associated with distinct hepatic histopathology [304].

Work with SAR ceased in 1963 as the commercial potential was considered dour [303].

3.5.4 Hamycin

Hamycin (HAM) is a water-insoluble (physiologic pH), heptaenic polyene that was discovered in 1961 [305]; it is elaborated by a strain of *Streptomyces pimprina*. HAM mimics AmB in antifungal spectrum and in action on susceptible fungi.

In limited studies, various preparations of HAM have been applied topically, given perorally, and injected.

Meager and variable absorption may have been a factor in the limited effectiveness of HAM in the treatment of 10 patients [306]. Nausea, vomiting, diarrhea and abdominal pain were the major adverse effects. The most recent formulation, JAI-hamycin, may prove to be advantageous [307].

3.6   Combinations

Combinations of antifungal drugs may be useful if the components of a combination: are active against the fungus; have different mechanisms of action; and have good access to the site(s) of the mycosis. Relatively few combinations have been studied thoroughly.

3.6.1   Amphotericin B plus flucytosine

Using AmB in combination with flucytosine (5FC) was undertaken to reduce toxicity from AmB and avoid the development of resistance to 5FC. When patients with cryptococcal meningitis were treated either with AmB alone (at a lower dose than is ordinarily used in monotherapy) or with AmB plus 5FC [308], there was no statistically significant difference in outcome. However, there was no pre-therapy susceptibility testing to detect infecting strains of *C. neoformans* that were natively resistant to 5FC – important as infection with 5FC-resistant strains might lead to failure of treatment with the combination. In one report of the treatment of cryptococcal meningitis complicating the acquired immunodeficiency syndrome (AIDS), a high frequency of occurrence of toxicity attributed to 5FC led to abandoning the combination in favor of monotherapy with AmB [180].

Extra-CNS systemic candidosis might benefit by treatment with AmB in combination with 5FC. While the combination is often applied (e.g., reference [259]), reports of such use are anecdotal and have not been verified by prospective, controlled evaluations.

3.6.2   Amphotericin B

As the activity of AmB depends on interaction with ergosterol in the fungal cell membrane, concomitant application of another antifungal agent that depletes the fungal cell of ergosterol will diminish the target for AmB. Assessments in vitro have yielded conflicting results, probably reflecting variables such as the culture media, the inocula, the order of addition of the drugs, and the length of incubation.

Evaluations in experimental murine mycoses have provided evidence of antagonism in candidosis (AmB plus either KET [309, 310] or ITR [310]), in cryptococcosis (AmB plus KET [311]), and in aspergillosis (AmB plus KET [309, 312]).

Both amorolfine and terbinafine should also antagonize AmB as they effect depletion of ergosterol. However, no reports of trials with such combinations are available.

3.6.3   Flucytosine

The antifungal activity of 5FC plus an azole was beneficial in murine candidosis [310]. In experimental murine cryptococcal meningitis, 5FC plus FLU was synergistic [313].

3.6.4   Others

Combinations of amorolfine with griseofulvin, terbinafine, fluconazole, or itraconazole were synergistic in experimental murine dermatophytosis [314].

Other combinations that merit examination include: antifungal azoles plus an allylamine – synergism should result in lethality as these drugs act at different sites in the biosynthetic sequence leading to the elaboration of ergosterol (Fig. 2).

References

1   A. Polak and P.G. Hartman: Progress in Drug Research *37*,181 (1991).
2   P.D. Hoeprich: Infectious Diseases, 5th edition, Chapter 23 "Antifungal Chemother-
     apy". J.B. Lippincott, Philadelphia (1994), p. 59.
3   W.E. Dismukes: Trans. Am. Clin. Climatol. Assoc. *104*, 1661 (1992).
4   B.E. Elewski and L. Nagashima-Whalen: Infectious Diseases, 5th edition, Chapter 121
     "Superficial Fungal Infections". Lippincott, Philadelphia (1994), p. 1029.
5   E.-H. Pommer and J. Kradel: Meded Rijksfac. Landbouwwetensch Gent. *32*, 735
     (1967).
6   K. Bohnen and A. Pfinner: Meded Rijksfac. Landbourwwetensch Gent. *44*, 487 (1979).
7   A. Polak: Sabouraudia. *21*, 205 (1983).
8   H.P. Isenring: Recent Trends in the Discovery, Development and Evaluation of Anti-
     fungal Agents. R.A. Fromtling (ed.), J.R. Prous Science Publishers, S.A., Barcelona
     (1987) p. 543.
9   A. Kerkenaar: Recent Trends in the Discovery, Development and Evaluation of
     Antifungal Agents. R.A. Fromtling (ed.), J.R. Prous Science Publishers, S.A., Bar-
     celona (1987) p. 523.
10   A. Polak: Dermatol. *184* (Suppl. 1), 3 (1992).
11   A. Polak and D.M. Dixon: Recent Trends in the Discovery and Development and
     Evaluation of Antifungal Agents. R.A. Fromtling (ed.), J.R. Prous Science Publishers,
     S.A., Barcelona (1987) p. 555.
12   T.J. Franz: Dermatol. *184* (Suppl. 1), 18 (1992).
13   M. Zaug and M. Bergstraesser: Clin. Exp. Dermatol. *17* (Suppl 1), 61 (1992).
14   A. del Palacio, F. Sanz, M. Garcia-Bravo, C. Gimeno, S. Cuetara, P. Miranda and A.R.
     Noriega: Mycoses *34*, 85 (1991).
15   A. Georgopoulos, G. Petranyi, H. Mieth and J. Drews: Antimicrob. Agents Chemother.
     19, 386 (1981).
16   A. Stutz and G. Petranyi: J. Med. Chem. *27*, 1543 (1984).
17   G. Paltauf, G. Daum, G. Zuder, G. Hogenauer, G. Schulz and G. Seidl: Biochim.
     Biophys. Acta *712*, 268 (1982).
18   N.S. Ryder: Ann. N.Y. Acad. Sci. *544*, 208 (1988).
19   I. Schuster: Xenobiotica *15*, 529 (1985).
20   S. Shadomy, A. Espinel-Ingroff and R.J. Gebhart: J. Med. Vet. Mycol. *32*, 125 (1985).
21   G. Petranyi, A. Stutz, N.S. Ryder, J.G. Meingassner and H. Meith: Recent Trends in
     the Discovery and Development and Evaluation of Antifungal Agents. R.A. Fromtling
     (ed.), J.R. Prous Science Publishers S.A., Barcelona. (1987) p. 441.
22   R.B. Stoughton, J. Sefton and L. Zeleznick: Cutis *44*, 333 (1989).
23   J. Monk and N. Brogden: Drugs *42*, 659 (1991).
24   G. Petranyi, N.S. Ryder and A. Stutz. Science *224*, 1239 (1984).
25   A. Stephen, R. Czok and O. Male: Recent Trends in the Discovery and Development
     and Evaluation of Antifungal Agents. R.A. Fromtling (ed.), J.R. Prous Publishers, S.A.,
     Barcelona. (1987) p. 511.
26   R.A. Fromtling: Drugs of Today. *28*, 501 (1992).
27   J. Faergemann, H. Zehender and T. Jones: Acta Dermatol. Venerol. *71*, 322 (1991).
28   A.Y. Finlay, L. Lever, R. Thomas and P.J. Dykes: J. Dermatol. Treat. *1* (Suppl. 2), 51
     (1990).

29   J.E. White, P.J. Perkins and E.G.V. Evans: Brit J. Dermatol. 125, *260* (1991).

30   M.J.D. Goodfield, N.R. Rowell, R.A. Forster, E.G.V. Evans and A. Raven: Brit. J. Dermatol. *121*, 753 (1989).

31   J.D. Dutcher: Dis. Chest *54* (Suppl.), 296 (1968).

32   W.Mechlinski, C.P. Schaffner, P. Ganis and G. Avitabile: Tetrahedron Lett. *44*, 3873 (1970).

33   H. Lechevalier, E. Borowski, J.O. Lampen and C.P. Schaffner: Antibiot. Chemother. *11*, 640 (1961).

34   S.C. Kinsky: Antibiotics I, Mechanisms of Action. Springer Verlag, New York (1967) p. 122.

35   A.W. Norman, A.M. Spielvogel and R.G. Wong: Adv. Lipid Res. *14,* 127 (1976).

36   W.A. Zygmunt: Appl. Microbiol. *14*, 953 (1966).

37   E.R. Block, J.E. Bennett, L.G. Livoti, W.J. Klein, R.R. MacGregor and L. Henderson: Ann. Intern. Med. *80*, 613 (1974).

38   C.P. Schaffner, O.J. Plescia, D. Potani, D. Sun, A. Thornton, R.C. Pandey and P.S. Sarin: Biochem. Pharmacol. *35*, 4110 (1986).

39   W. Gold, H.A. Stout, J.F. Pagano and R. Donovick: Antibiot. Ann. (1956), p. 579.

40   C. Halde, V.D. Newcomer, E.T. Wright and T.H. Sternberg: J. Invest. Dermatol. *28*, 217 (1957).

41   M.L. Littman, P.L. Horowitz and J.G. Swadeyo: Am. J. Med. *24*, 568 (1958).

42   H. Lechevalier: Antibiot. Ann. (1956), p. 614.

43   H. Seabury and H.E. Dascomb: Ann. N.Y. Acad. Sci. *89*, 202 (1960).

44   D. Artis and G.L. Baum: Antibiot. Chemother. *11*, 373 (1961).

45   G. Hildick-Smith, G.H. Blank and I. Sarkany: Little Brown & Co., Boston (1964).

46   E. Drouhet: Systemic Mycoses, G.E.W. Wolstenholm and R. Porter (eds.), Little Brown & Co., Boston (1967), p. 206.

47   S. Shadomy, H.J. Shadomy, J.A. McCay and J.P. Utz: Antimicrob. Agents Chemother. (1969), p. 452.

48   J.M.T. Hamilton-Miller: Sabouraudia. *10*, 276 (1972).

49   P.D. Hoeprich and A.C. Huston: J. Infect. Dis. *132,* 133 (1975).

50   A.C. Huston and P.D. Hoeprich: Antimicrob. Agents Chemother. *13*, 905 (1978).

51   J.M.T. Hamilton-Miller: Microbios. *10A*, 91 (1974).

52   R.A. Woods, M. Bard, I.E. Jackson and D.J. Drutz: J. Infect. Dis. *129*, 530 (1974).

53   D.B. Louria: Antibiot. Med. Clin. Ther. *5*, 295 (1958).

54   F.A. Jagdis, P.D. Hoeprich, R.M. Lawrence and C.P. Schaffner: Antimicrob. Agents Chemother. *12*, 582 (1977).

55   P.D. Hoeprich, J.M. Merry, R.A. Gunther and C.E. Franti: Antimicrob. Agents Chemother. *31*, 1234 (1987).

56   P.D. Hoeprich: Ann. Rev. Toxicol. *18*, 205 (1978).

57   P.D. Hoeprich: J. Infect. *20*, 173 (1990).

58   C.P. Schaffner: Macrolide Antibiotics. Chemistry, Biology and Practice. Academic Press, New York (1984).

59   R.C Beesley and R.G. Faust: Biochem. J. *190*, 731 (1980).

60   F. Bode, K. Baumann and R. Kinne: Biochem. Biophys. Acta. *433*, 294 (1976).

61   P.D. Hoeprich: Clin. Infect. Dis. *14* (Suppl. 1), S114 (1992).

62   W.T. Butler, J.E. Bennett and D.W. Aling: Ann. Intern. Med. *61*, 175 (1964).

63   W.A. Winn: Med. Clin. N. Am. *47*, 1144 (1963).

64   J.L. Burgess and R. Birchall: Am. J. Med. *53*, 77 (1972).
65   D.B. Bhathena, W.E. Bullock, C.E. Nuttall and R.G. Luje: Clin. Nephrol *9*, 10-3 (1978).
66   P.T. Westlake, W.T. Butler, G.J. Hill, II and J.P. Utz: Am. J. Path. *43*, 449 (1963).
67   E.S. Reynolds, Z.M. Tomkiewicz and G.J. Dammin: Med. Clin. N. Am. *47*, 1149 (1963).
68   W.T. Butler, G.J. Hill, II, C.F. Szwed and V. Knight: Jn Pharmacol. Exp. Ther. *143*, 47 (1964).
69   M. Brezis, S. Rosen, P. Silva, K. Spokes and F.H. Epstein: Science. *224*, 66 (1984).
70   H. Heidemann, J.F. Gerkins, W.A. Spickard, E.K. Jackson and R. Branch: Am. J. Med. *75*, 476 (1983).
71   B.H. Brouhard and B. Baetz-Greenwalt: Cleve. Clin. J. Med. *59*, 263 (1992).
72   P.D. Hoeprich, N.M. Flynn, M.M. Kawachi, K.K. Lee, R.M. Lawrence, L.K. Heath and C.P. Schaffner: Ann. N. Y. Acad. Sci (1988).
73   O. Devinsky, W. Lemann, A.C. Evans, J.R. Moeller and D.A. Rottenberg: Arch. Neurol. *44*, 414 (1987).
74   G.A. Sarosi: Postgrad Med. *88*, 151 (1990).
75   C. Gates and R.J. Pinney: J. Clin. Pharm. Ther. *18*, 147 (1993).
76   R. Jangknegt, S. de Marie, I.A.J.M. Bakker-Woudenberg and D.J.A. Crommehn: Clin. Pharmacokinet. *23*, 279 (1992).
77   G. Lopez-Berenstein, R. Mehta, R.L. Hopfer, K. Mills, L. Kasi, K. Mehta, V. Fainstein, M. Luna, E.M. Hersh and R. Juliano: J. Infect. Dis. *147*, 939 (1983).
78   J.A. Gondal, R.P. Swartz and A. Rahman: Antimicrob. Agents Chemother. *33*, 1544 (1989).
79   A.S. Janoff, L.T. Boni, M.C. Popescu, S.R. Minchey, P.R. Cullis, T.D. Madden, T. Taraschi, S.M. Gruner, E. Shyamsunder, M.W. Tate, R. Mendelsohn and D. Bonner: Proc. Natl. Acadn Sci. USA. *85*, 6122 (1988).
80   T.F. Patterson, P. Miniter, J. Dijkstra, F.C. Szoka Jr., J.L. Ryan and V.T. Andriole: J. Infect. Dis. *159*, 717 (1989).
81   R. Kirsh, R. Goldstein, J. Tarloff, D. Parris, J. Hook, N. Hanna, P. Bugelski and G. Poste: J. Infect. Dis. *158*, 1065 (1988).
82   M.J. Ostro: Sci. Am. *256*, 102 (1987).
83   J.A. Karlowsky and G.G. Zhanel: Clin. Infect. Dis. *15*, 654 (1992).
84   G. Gregoriadis: J. Antimicrob. Ther. *28* (Suppl. B), 39 (1991).
85   G. Poste: Biol. Cell. *47*, 19 (1983).
86   A.D. Bangham, M.M. Standish and J.C. Watkins: J. Mol. Biol. *13*, 238 (1965).
87   J. De Gier, J.G. Mandersloot and L.L.M. Van Deenen: Biochim. Biophys. Acta *150*, 666 (1968).
88   T.M. Allen, C. Hansen and J. Rutledge: Biochim. Biophys. Acta *981*, 27 (1989).
89   W.G. Ellis, R.A. Sobel and S.L. Nielsen: J. Infect. Dis. *146*, 125 (1982).
90   P.D. Hoeprich: J. Infect. Dis. *146*, 173 (1982).
91   S.P. Racis, O.J. Plescia, H.M. Geller and C.P. Schaffner: Antimicrob. Agents Chemother. *34*, 1360 (1990).
92   B.G. Gold, M.T. Ryzlak and C.P. Schaffner: J. Neuropath. Exptl. Neurol. *49*, 292 (1990).
93   K.R. Reuhl, M. Vapiwala, M.T. Tuzlak and C.P. Schaffner: Antimicrob. Agents Chemother. *37*, 419 (1993).
94   M.S. Saag and W.E. Dismukes: Antimicrob. Agents Chemother. *32*, 1 (1988).

95   J.A. Como and W.E. Dismukes: New Eng. J. Med. *330*, 263 (1994).
96   H. Vanden Bossche, G. Willemsens, P. Marichal, W. Cools and W. Lauwers: Mode of Action of Antifungal Agents. Cambridge University Press, Cambridge, 1984.
97   H. Vanden Bossche: Curr. Top. Med. Mycol. *1*, 313 (1985).
98   H.O. Sisler and N.N. Ragsdale: Mode of Action of Antifungal Agents. Cambridge University Press, Cambridge, 1984.
99   F.J. Gonzalez: Pharmac. Ther. *45*, 1 (1990).
100   J. George and G.C Farrell: Aust. N. Z. J. Med. *21*, 356 (1991).
101   F.P. Guengerich: Toxicol. Lett. *70*, 133 (1994).
102   R.D. Cannon and D. Kerridge: J. Med. Vet. Mycol. *26*, 57 (1988).
103   P.D. Hoeprich and A.C. Huston: J. Infect. Dis. *134*, 336 (1976).
104   P.D. Hoeprich and E. Goldstein: J. Am. Med. Assoc. *230*, 1153 (1974).
105   S.M. Grant and S.P. Clissold: Drugs *37*, 310 (1989).
106   S.M. Grant and S.P. Clissold: Drugs *391*, 877 (1990).
107   E.F. Godefroi, J. Heeres, J.M. Van Cutsem and P.A.J. Janssen: J. Med. Chem. *12*, 784 (1964).
108   P.D. Hoeprich and A.C. Huston: J. Infect. Dis *137*, 87 (1978).
109   P.D. Hoeprich and E. Goldstein: Clin. Res. *23*, 133A (1975).
110   H.B. Neld: New Eng. J. Med. *296*, 1479 (1977).
111   J.P. Sung, J.G. Grendahl and H.B. Levine: West. J. Med. *126*, 5 (1977).
112   D.A. Stevens, H.B. Levine and S.C. Deresinski: Am. J. Med. *60*, 191 (1976).
113   First International Symposium on Ketoconazole: Rev. Infect. Dis. *2*, 250 (1980).
114   J.R. Graybill: Sem. Resp. Dis. *1*, 53 (1986).
115   J.H. Lewis, H.J. Zimmerman, G.D. Benson and K.G. Ishak: Gastroenterol. *86*, 503 (1984).
116   E.A. Peterson, D.W. Alling and C.H. Kirkpatrick: Ann. Intern. Med. *93*, 791 (1980).
117   National Institute of Allergy and Infectious Diseases Mycoses Study Group (1985). Ann. Intern. Med. *103*, 861 (1985).
118   K. Richardson, K.W. Brammer, M.S. Marriott, and P.F. Troke: Antimicrob. Agents Chemother. *27*, 832 (1985).
119   P.F. Troke, R.J. Andrews, K.W. Brammer, M.S. Marriott and K. Richardson: Antimicrob. Agents Chemother. *28*, 815 (1985).
120   C.A. Lyman, A.M. Sugar and R.D. Diamond: Antimicrob. Agents Chemother. *29*, 161 (1986).
121   J.R. Perfect, D.V. Savani and D.T. Durack: Antimicrob. Agents Chemother. *29*, 579 (1986).
122   T.E. Roger and J.N. Galgiani: Antimicrob. Agents Chemother. *30*, 418 (1986).
123   J.R. Graybill, S.H. Sun and J. Ahrens: J. Med. Vet. Mycol. *24*, 113 (1986).
124   J.R. Graybill, E. Palou and J. Ahrens: Am. Rev. Resp. Dis. *134*, 768 (1986).
125   E.P. de Fernandez, M.M. Patino, J.R. Graybill and M.H. Tarbit: J. Antimicrob. Chemother. *18*, 261 (1986).
126   S.F. Kowalsky and D.M. Dixon: Clin. Pharm. *10*, 179 (1991).
127   A.M. Sugar, E.J. Anaissie, J.R. Graybill and T.F. Patterson: J. Med. Vet. Mycol. *30* (Suppl. 1), 201 (1992).
128   D. Debruyne and J.-P. Ryckelynck: Clin. Pharmacokinet. *24*, 10 (1993).
129   M.J. Humphrey, S. Jevons and M.H. Tarbit: Antimicrob. Agents Chemother. *28*, 648 (1985).

130 K.W. Brammer and M.H. Tarbit: Recent Trends in the Discovery, Development and Evaluation of Antifungal Agents, R.A. Fromtling (Ed.). J.R. Prous Science Publishers, S.A., Barcelona. 1987, p. 141.

131 D.V. Savani, J.R. Perfect, L.M. Cobo and D.T. Durack: Antimicrob. Agents Chemother. *31*, 6 (1987).

132 R.M. Tucker, P.L. Williams, E.G. Arathoon and B.E. Levine: Antimicrob. Agents Chemother. *32*, 369 (1988).

133 R.J. Hay: Ann. N. Y. Acad. Sci. *544*, 580 (1988).

134 K. Shiba, A. Saito and T. Miyahara: Jap. J. Antibiot. *42*, 1-7 (1989).

135 S. Milliken, R. Powles, A. Jones and G. Helenglass: Transplant. Proceed. *21*, 306 (1989).

136 E.T. Huang, O. Chappatte, O. Bryne, P.V. Macrae and J.E. Thorpe: Antimicrob. Agents Chemother. *34*, 909 (1990).

137 G. Foulds, C. Wajszczuk, D. Weidler, D.C. Garg and P. Gibson: Ann. N. Y. Acad. Sci. *544*, 427 (1988).

138 Roerig Division, Pfizer Incorporated: Physicians' Desk Reference, 48th edition. Medical Economics, Montvale, NJ (1994), p. 1978.

139 J.W. Van't Wout, H. Mattie and R. van Furth: J. Antimicrob. Chemother. *21*, 665 (1988).

140 C. Wells and A.M.L. Lever: J. Infect. *24*, 111 (1992).

141 D.P. Hanger, S. Jevons and J.T.B. Shaw: Antimicrob. Agents Chemother. *32*, 646 (1988).

142 J.D Lazar and K.D. Wilner: Rev. Infect. Dis. *12* (Suppl. 3), S327 (1990).

143 G. Apseloff, D.M. Hillgoss, M.J. Gardner, E.B. Henry, P.B. Inskeep, N. Gerber and J.D. Lazar: J. Clin. Pharmacol. *31*, 358 (1991).

144 J.A. Lopez-Gil: Ann. Pharmacother. *27*, 427 (1993).

145 H. Yamaguchi, K. Uchida, K. Kawasaki and T. Matsunaga: Jap. J. Antibiot. *42*, 1 (1989).

146 M.S. Saag, W.G. Powderly, G.A. Cloud, P. Robinson, M.H. Grieco, P.K. Sharkey, S.E. Thompson, A.M. Sugar, C.U. Tuazon, J.F. Fisher, N. Hyslop, J.M. Jacobson, R. Hafner, W.E. Dismukes and the NIAID Mycoses Study Group and the AIDS Clinical Trials Group: New Engl. J. Med. *326*, 83 (1992).

147 J.H. Rex, J.E. Bennett, A.M. Sugar, P.G. Pappas, C.M. Van der Horst, J.E. Edwards, R.G. Washburn, W.M. Scheld, A.W. Karchmer, J.C. Neu, J.J. Stern, C.U. Tuazon, A.P. Dine, M.J. Levenstein, C.D. Webb, the NIAID MSG and the Candidemia Study Group: Program and Abstracts of the 33rd Interscience Conference on Antimicrobial Agents and Chemotherapy, New Orleans, October 17–20, 1993. Washington, DC: American Society for Microbiology, 1993. p. 267 (abstract 805).

148 P.D. Jones, D. Marriott and B.R. Speed: Diagn. Microbiol. Infect. Dis. *12*, 235S (1989).

149 A.J. Berry, M.G. Rinaldi and J.R. Graybill: Antimicrob. Agents Chemother. *36*, 690 (1992).

150 H. Ikemoto: Diagn. Microbiol. Infect. Dis. *12*, 239S (1989).

151 E. Milefchik, M. Leal, R. Haubrich, D. See, S. Bozzette and R. Larsen: Abstracts of the IXth International Conference on AIDS, IVth STD World Congress, Berlin, June 6–11, 1993. Abstract WS-B12-5, p. 55.

152 S. Yagi, M. Watanabe, M. Nakajima, K. Tsukiyama, O. Moriya, J. Hino, Y. Niki and R. Soejima: Jap. J. Antibiot. *42*, 144 (1989).

153 B. Dupont and E. Drouhet: J. Med. Veterin. Mycol. *26*, 67 (1988).

154   J.P. Chave, A. Cajot, J. Bille and M.P. Glauser: J. Infect. Dis. *159*, 806 (1989).

155   A. Cirelli, F. Rossi and M. Ciardi: Curr. Ther. Res. *47*, 81 (1990).

156   J.P. Chave, R. Francioli, B. Hirschel and M.P. Glauser: AIDS *4*, 1034 (1990).

157   R. Esposito, A. Castagua and C.U. Foppa: AIDS *4*, 1033 (1990).

158   S.L. Koletar, J.A. Russell, F.J. Fass and J.F. Plouffe: Antimicrob. Agents Chemother. *34*, 2267 (1990).

159   A.M. Ansari, I.M. Gould and J.G. Douglas: J. Antimicrob. Chemother. *25*, 720 (1990).

160   V. Kremery Jr., I. Koza, M. Hormikova, P. Fuchsberger, S. Spanik, J. Mardiak, J. Sufliarsky. M. Blajova, Y. Savko and Ch. Mignon: Chemother. *37*, 343 (1991).

161   P. van der Bijl and T.M. Arendorf: Ann. Dent. *52*, 12 (1993).

162   G.M. Andersen, J. Varrat, T. Bergan, K.W. Brammer, J. Cohen and P. Dellenbach: Brit. J. Obstet. Gynecol. *96*, 226 (1989).

163   O.O. Adetoro: Curr. Ther. Res. *48*, 275 (1990). S.L.

164   J.M. Naeyert, J. de Bersaques, C. de Cuyper, Ph. Hindryckx, H. van Landuyt and B. Gordts: Recent Trends in the Discovery, Development and Evaluation of Antifungal Agents. R.A. Fromtling (Ed.). J.R. Prous Science Publishers, Barcelona. 1987, p. 157.

165   B. Coldiron: Arch. Dermatol. *128*, 909 (1992).

166   C. Viscoli, E. Castagnola, F. Fioredda, B. Ciravegna, G. Barigione and A. Terragna: Antimicrob. Agents Chemother. *35*, 365 (1991).

167   J.E. Edwards Jr. and S.G. Filler: Clin. Infect. Dis. *14* (Suppl. 1), S106 (1992).

168   J. Nolla-Salas, C. Leon, J.M. Torres-Rodriguez, E. Martin and A. Sitges-Serra: Clin. Infect. Dis. *14*, 952 (1992).

169   C.A. Kauffman, S.F. Bradley, S.C. Ross and D.R. Weber: Am. J. Med. *91*, 137 (1991).

170   E. Anaissie, G.P. Bodey, H. Kantarjian, C. David, K. Barnett, E. Bow, R. Defelice, M. Dowms, T. File, G. Karam, D. Potts, M. Shelton and A. Sugar: Am. J. Med. *91*, 142 (1991).

171   C.V. Paya: Clin. Infect. Dis. *16*, 677 (1993).

172   P.G. Pappas, R.W. Bradsher, S.W. Chapman, C. Kauffman, A. Feldman, G.A. Cloud, W.E. Dismukes and the NIAID Mycoses Study Group: Program and Abstracts 31st Interscience Conference on Antimicrobial Agents and Chemotherapy, Chicago, September 29–October 2, 1991. American Society for Microbiology, Washington, DC, 1991, p. 292, abstract 1159.

173   M. Diaz, R. Negroni, F. Montero-Gei, L.G.M. Castro, S.A.P. Sampaio, D. Borelli, A. Restrepo, L. Franco, J.L. Gran, E.G. Arathoon, D.A. Stevens and other investigators of the Fluconazole Pan-American Study Group: Clin. Infect. Dis. *14* (Suppl. 1), S68 (1992).

174   D.C. Classen, J.P. Burke and C.B. Smith: J. Infect. Dis. *158*, 903 (1988).

175   R.M. Tucker, D.W. Denning, B. Dupont and D.A. Stevens: Ann. Intern. Med. *112*, 108 (1990).

176   J.N. Galgiani, A. Catanzaro, G.A. Cloud, J. Higgs, B.A. Friedman, R.A. Larsen, J.R. Graybill and the NIAID Mycoses Study Group: Ann. Intern. Med. *119*, 28 (1993).

177   A. Catanzaro, J. Fierer and P.J. Friedman: Chest *97*, 666 (1990).

178   J.R. Graybill: Europ. J. Clin. Microbiol. Infect. Dis. *8*, 402 (1989).

179   W.G. Powderly, M.S. Saag, G.A. Cloud, P. Robinson, R.D. Meyer, J.M. Jacobson, J.R. Graybill, A.M. Sugar, V.J. McAuliffe, S.E. Follansbee, C.U. Tuazon, J.J. Stern, J. Feinberg, R. Hafner, W.E. Dismukes and the NIAID AIDS Clinical Trials Group, and the NIAID Mycoses Study Group: New Engl. J. Med. *326*, 793 (1992).

180   S.L. Chuck and M.A. Sande: New Engl. J. Med. *321*, 794 (1989).
181   S.A. Bozzette, R.A. Larsen, J. Chiu, M.A.E. Leal, J. Jacobsen, R. Rothman, P. Robinson, G. Gilbert, J.A. McCutchan, J. Tilles, J.M. Leedom, D.D. Richman and the California Collaborative Treatment Group: New Engl. J. Med. *324*, 580 (1991).
182   M. Rozenberg-Arska, A.W. Dekker, J. Branger and J. Verhoef: J. Antimicrob. Chemother. *27*, 369 (1991).
183   S.D. Nightingale, S.X. Cal, D.M. Peterson, S.D. Loss, B.A. Gamble, D.A. Watson, C.M. Manzone, J.E. Baker and J.D. Jockusch: AIDS 6, 191 (1992).
184   J.L. Goodman, D.J. Winston, R.A. Greenfield, P.H. Chandrasekar, B. Fox, H. Kaizer, R.K. Shadduck, T.C. Shea, P. Stiff, D.J. Friedman, W.G. Powderly, J.L. Silber, H. Horowitz, A. Lichtin, S.N. Worff, K.F. Mangan, S.M. Silver, D. Weisdorf, W.G. Ho, G. Gilbert and D. Buell: New Engl. J. Med. *326*, 845 (1992).
185   E.M. Bailey, D.J. Krakovsky and M.J. Rybak: Pharmacother. *10*, 146 (1990).
186   A.M. Sugar: Curr. Clin. Topics Infect. Dis. *13*, 74 (1993).
187   J. Heykants, M. Michiels, W. Meuldermans, J. Monbaliu, K. Lavrijsen, A. Van Peer, J.C. Levron, R. Woestenborghs and G. Cauwenbergh: Recent Trends in the Discovery, Development and Evaluation of Antifungal Agents, R.A. Fromtling (Ed.). J.R. Prous Science Publishers, Barcelona. 1987, p. 223.
188   J.A. Barone, J.G. Koh, R.H. Bierman, J.L. Colazzi, K.A. Swenson, M.C. Gaffer, B.L. Moskowitz, W. Mechlinski and V. Van De Velde: Antimicrob. Agents Chemother. *37*, 778 (1993).
189   M.A. Viviani, A.M. Tortorano, R. Woenstenborghs and G. Cauwenbergh: Mykosen *30*, 233 (1987).
190   J. Van Cutsem, F. Van Gerven and P.A.J. Janssen: Recent Trends in the Discovery, Development and Evaluation of Antifungal Agents, R.A. Fromtling (Ed.). J.R. Prous Science Publishers, Barcelona 1987, p. 177.
191   F.C Odds, A. Cockayne, J. Hayward and A.B. Abbott: J. Gen. Microbiol. *131*, 2581 (1985).
192   Jannsen Pharmaceutica Incorporated: Physicians' Desk Reference, 48th edition. Medical Economics, Montvale, NJ (1994), p. 1097.
193   H. Van Couteren, J. Heykants, R. De Coster and G. Cauwenbergh: Rev. Infect. Dis. *9* (Suppl. 1), S43 (1987).
194   P. Phillips, J.R. Graybill, R. Fetchick and J.F. Dunn: Antimicrob. Agents Chemother. *31*, 647 (1987).
195   P.K. Sharkey, M.G. Rinaldi, J.F. Dunn, T.C. Hardin, R.J. Fetchick and J.R. Graybill: Antimicrob. Agents Chemother. *35*, 707 (1991).
196   G. Cauwenbergh, H. Degreef, J. Heykants, R. Westenbergh, P. Van Rooy and K. Haverans: J. Am. Acad. Dermatol. *18*, 263 (1988).
197   R.M. Tucker, D.W. Denning, L.H. Hanson, M.G. Rinaldi, J.R. Graybill, P.K. Sharkey, D. Pappagianis and D.A. Stevens: Clin. Infect. Dis. *14*, 165 (1992).
198   R.J. Hay, Y.M. Clayton, M.K. Moore and G. Midgely: Brit. J. Dermatol. *119*, 359 (1988).
199   J.T. C. Kwan, P.J.D. Foxall, D.G.C. Davidson, M.R. Bending and A.J. Eisinger: Lancet 2, 282 (1987).
200   D. Trenk, W. Brett, E. Jahnchen and D. Birnbaum: Lancet 2, 1335 (1987).
201   M.R. Kramer, S.E. Marshall, D.W. Denning, A.M. Keogh, R.M. Tucker, J.N. Galgiani, N.J. Lewiston, D.A. Stevens and T. Theodore: Ann. Intern. Med. *113*, 327 (1990).

202   M.K. Sachs, L.M. Blanchard and P.J. Green: Clin. Infect. Dis. *16*, 400 (1993).
203   A. Espinel-Ingroff, S. Shadomy and R.J. Gebhart: Antimicrob. Agents Chemother. *26*, 5 (1984).
204   G. Cauwenbergh and P. De Doncker: Recent Trends in the Discovery, Development and Evaluation of Antifungal Agents, R.A. Fromtling (Ed.). J.R. Prous Science Publishers, S.A., Barcelona. 1987, p. 273.
205   G.P. Bodey: Clin. Infect. Dis. *14* (Suppl. 1), S161 (1992).
206   M.A. Viviani, A.M. Tortorano, M. Langer, M. Almaviva, C. Negri, S. Cristina, S. Scoccia, R. De Maria, R. Fiocchi, P. Ferrazzi, A. Goglio, G. Gavazzeni, G. Faggian, R. Rinaldi and P. Cadrobbi: J. Infect. *18*, 151, (1989).
207   D.W. Denning, R.M. Tucker, L.H. Hanson, J.R. Hamilton and D.A. Stevens: Arch. Int. Med. *149*, 2301 (1989).
208   M.A. Viviani, A.M. Tortorano, A. Pagano, G.M. Vigevani, G. Gubertini, S. Cristina, M.L. Assaisso, F. Suter, C. Farina, B. Minetti, G. Faggian, M. Caretta, N. Di Fabrizio and A. Vaglia: J. Am. Acad. Dermatol. *23*, 587 (1990).
209   D.M. Denning, R.M. Tucker, L.H Hanson and D.A. Stevens: J. Am. Acad. Dermatol. *23*, 602 (1990).
210   G. Cauwenbergh: Mycoses *36*, 221 (1993).
211   R.M. Tucker, D.W. Denning, B. Dupont and D.A. Stevens: Ann. Intern. Med. *112*, 108 (1990).
212   J.R. Graybill, D.A. Stevens, J.N. Galgiani, W.E. Dismukes, G.A. Cloud and the NIAID Mycoses Study Group: Am. J. Med. *89*, 282 (1990).
213   R.M. Tucker, D.W. Denning, E.G. Arathoon, M.G. Rinaldi and D.A. Stevens: J. Am. Acad. Dermatol. *23*, 593 (1990).
214   M. Diaz, R. Puente, L.A. de Hoyos and S. Cruz: Chest *100*, 682 (1991).
215   R. Negroni, O. Palmieri, F. Koren, I.N. Tiraboschi and R.L. Galimberti: Rev. Infect. Dis. *9* (Suppl. 1), S47 (1987).
216   B. Dupont and E. Drouhet: Rev. Infect. Dis. *9* (Suppl. 1), S71 (1987).
217   R. Negroni, A.M. Robles, A. Arechavala and A. Tarboda: Mycoses *32*, 123 (1989).
218   L.J. Wheat, P.A. Connolly-Stringfield, R.L. Baker, M.F. Curfman, M.E. Eads, K.S. Israel, S.A. Norris, D.H. Webb and M.L. Zeckel: Medicine (Baltimore) *69*, 361 (1990).
219   W.E. Dismukes, R.W. Bradsher, Jr., G.C. Sloud, C.A. Kauffman and S.W. Chapman: Am. J. Med. *93*, 489 (1992).
220   L.J. Wheat, R.E. Hafner, M. Wulfsohn, J. Johnson and S. Owens: Program and Abstracts of the 32nd Interscience Conference on Antimicrobial Agents and Chemotherapy. Anaheim, California, October 10–14, 1992. Washington, D.C.: American Society for Microbiology, 1992, p. 312.
221   L.J. Wheat: Clin. Infect. Dis. *14* (Suppl. 1), S91 (1992).
222   L.J. Wheat, R. Hafner, M. Wyulfsohn, P. Spencer, K. Squires, W. Powderly, B. Wong, M. Rinaldi, M. Saag, R. Hamill, R. Murphy, P. Connolly-Stringfield, N. Briggs, S. Owens and the NIAID Clinical Trials and Mycoses Study Group: Ann. Intern. Med. *118*, 610 (1993).
223   D.W. Denning, R.M. Tucker, L.H. Janson and D.A. Stevens: Am. J. Med. *86*, 791 (1989).
224   B. Dupont: J. Am. Acad. Dermatol. *23*, 607 (1990).
225   P. Phillips, G. Bryce, J. Shepard and D. Mintz: Rev. Infect. Dis. *12*, 277 (1990).

226 M.K. Sachs, R.G. Paluzzi, J.H. Moore, Jr., J.S. Framinow and D. Ost: Lancet *335*, 1475 (1990).

227 J.W. Van't Wont, E.J.M. Raven and J.W.M. Van der Meer: J. Infect *20*, 147 (1990).

228 D.W. Denning, J.E. Van Wye, M.J. Lewiston and D.A. Stevens: Chest *100*, 813 (1991).

229 S. Kloss, A. Schuster, J. Schroten, J. Lamprecht and V. Wahn: Eur. J. Pediatr. *150*, 483 (1991).

230 T.S. Jennings and T.C. Hardin: Ann. Pharmacother. *27*, 1206 (1993).

231 A. Restrepo, I. Gomez, J. Robledo, M.M. Patino and L.E. Cano: Rev. Infect. Dis. *9* (Suppl. 1), S51 (1987).

232 A. Restrepo, J. Robledo, J. Gomez, A.M. Tabares and R. Gutierrez: Arch. Dermatol. *122*, 413 (1986).

233 P.K. Sharkey-Mathis, C.A. Kauffman, K.R. Graybill, D.A. Stevens, J.S. Hostetler, G. Cloud, W.E. Dismukes, and the NIAID Mycoses Study Group: Am. J. Med. *95*, 279 (1993).

234 D. Borelli: Rev. Infect. Dis. *9* (Suppl. 1), S57 (1987).

235 P.K. Sharkey, J.R. Graybill, M.G. Rinaldi, D.A. Stevens, R.M. Tucker, J.D. Petrie, P.D. Hoeprich, D.L. Greer, L. Frenkel, G.W. Counts, J. Goodrich, S. Zellner, R.W. Bradsher, C.M. van der Horst, K. Israel, G.A. Pankey and C.P. Barraneo: J. Am. Acad. Dermatol. *23*, 577 (1990).

236 J.W. van't Wout, I. Novakova, C.A.H. Verhagen, W.E. Fibbe, B.E. de Pauw and J.W.M. van der Meer: J. Infect. *22*, 45 (1991).

237 J. de Gans, P. Portegies, G. Tiessens, J. Karel, M.E. Schattenkerk, C.J. van Boxtel, R.J. van Ketel and J. Stam: AIDS *6*, 185 (1992).

238 R. Duchinsky, E. Pleven and C. Heidelberger: J. Am. Chem. Soc. *79*, 4559 (1957).

239 S. Shadomy: Appl. Microbiol. *17*, 871 (1969).

240 P.D. Hoeprich and P.D. Finn: J. Infect. Dis. *125*, 353 (1972).

241 S. Shadomy: Infect. Immun. *2*, 484 (1970).

242 P.L. Steer, M.I. Marks, P.D. Klite and T.C. Eickhoff: Ann. Intern. Med. *76*, 15 (1972).

243 A.G. Vandevelde, A.A. Mauceri and J.E. Johnson III: Ann. Intern. Med. *77*, 43 (1973).

244 S. Shadomy, C.B. Kirchoff and A.E. Ingroff: Antimicrob. Agents Chemother. *3*, 9 (1973).

245 P.D. Hoeprich and A.C. Huston: J. Infect. Dis. *132*, 133 (1975).

246 A. Polak and H.J. Scholer: Chemother. *21*, 113 (1975).

247 J. Schonebeck and S. Ansehn: Sabouraudia *11*, 10 (1973).

248 S. Shadomy, H.J. Shadomy, J.A. McCay and J.P. Utz: Antimicrob. Agents Chemother. *8*, 452 (1969).

249 E.R. Block, A.E. Jennings and J.E. Bennett: Antimicrob. Agents Chemother. *4*, 392 (1973).

250 E. Drouhet, L. Mercier-Soucy and S. Montplaisir: Ann. Microbiol. *126B*, 25 (1975).

251 R.A. Fromtling, G.K. Abruzzo and G.S. Bulmer: Mycopathologica *94*, 27 (1986).

252 J. Schonebeck: Scand. J. Urol. Nephrol. *6* (Suppl. 11) (1972).

253 J. Neuhard and J. Ingraham: J. Bact. *95*, 2431 (1968).

254 M. Grenson: Eur. J. Biochem. *11*, 249 (1969).

255 R. Jund and F. Lacroute: J. Bact. *102*, 607 (1970).

256 S. Normark and J. Schonebeck: Antimicrob. Agents Chemother. *2*, 114 (1972).

257 R.B. Diasio, R.B. Bennett and C.E. Meyers: Biochem. Pharmacol. *27*, 703 (1978).

258 J. Horowitz and E. Chargaff: Nature *184*, 1213 (1959).

259   P. Francis and T.J. Walsh: Clin. Infect. Dis. *15*, 1003 (1992).

260   J.P. Greenstein, C.E. Carter, H.W. Chalkley and F.M. Leuthardt: J. Natl. Cancer Inst. *7*, 9 (1946).

261   J. Kream and E. Chargaff: J. Am. Chem. Soc *74*, 5157 (1952).

262   B.E. Harris, R.B. Diasio, B.W. Manning and T.W Federle: Antimicrob. Agents Chemother. *29*, 44 (1986).

263   J.L. Ingraham and J. Neuhard: J. Biol. Chem. *247*, 6259 (1972).

264   M. Faoli and D. Kerridge: Ann. N.Y. Acad. Sci. *544*, 260 (1988).

265   P.D. Hoeprich, J.L. Ingraham, E. Kleker and M.J. Winship: *130*, 112 (1974).

266   J. Schonebeck, A. Polak, M. Fernex and J.J. Scholer: Chemother. *18*, 321 (1973.

267   A. Polak, E. Eschenhof, M. Fernex and H.J. Scholer: Chemother. *22*, 137 (1976).

268   M.A. Saubolle and P.D. Hoeprich: Program and Abstracts of the 15th Interscience Conference on Antimicrobial Agents and Chemotherapy, 1975.

269   B.A. Koechlin, F. Rubio, S. Palmer, T. Gabriel and R. Duschinsky: Biochem. Pharmac. *15*, 435 (1966).

270   H.J. Scholer: Chemother. *22*, 103 (1976).

271   C.A. Kauffman, J.A. Carleton and P.T. Frame: Antimicrob. Agents Chemother. *9*, 381 (1976).

273   E. Drouhet, P. Babinet, J. Chapusot and K. Kleinknecht: Biomedicine *19*, 408 (1973).

274   E.A. Block and J.E. Bennett: Antimicrob. Agents Chemother. *1*, 176 (1972).

275   D.J. Levinson, D.C. Silcox, J.W. Ripon and S. Thomson: Arthritis Rheum. *17*, 1037 (1974).

276   A.B. Richards, B.R. Jones, J. Withwell and Y. Clayton: Trans. Ophthalm. Soc. *89*, 867 (1969).

277   J.E. Pennington, E.R. Block and H.Y. Reynolds: Antimicrob. Agents Chemother. *6*, 324 (1974).

278   R.E. Cutler, A.D. Blair and M.R. Kelly: Clin. Pharm. Ther. *24*, 333 (1978).

279   D.N. Wade and G. Sudlow: Aust. N.Z. Med. *2*, 153 (1972).

280   J.A. Dawborn, M.D. Page and D.J. Schiavone: Brit. Med. J. *4*, 382 (1973).

281   R.M. Rault, B. Hulme and R.R. Davies: Clin. Nephrol. *3*, 225 (1975).

282   C.A. Kauffman and P.T. Frame: Antimicrob. Agents Chemother. *11*, 244 (1977).

283   S.M. Finegold: Calif. Med. *110*, 455 (1969).

284   T. Korzybski, Z. Kowszyk-Gindifer and W. Kurylowicz: Antibiotics. Origin Nature, and Properties. Washington, D.C.; American Society for Microbiology, 1978, p. 1766.

285   A.E. Oxford, H. Raistrick and R. Simonart: Biochem. J. *33*, 240 (1939).

286   L. Goldman, J. Schwarz, R.H. Preston, A. Beyer and J. Loutzinhiser: J. Am. Med. Assoc. *172*, 532 (1960).

287   F.M. Huber: Antibiotics. Mechanisms of Action (Volume I). D. Gottlieb and P.D. Shaw, editors. New York; Springer Verlag, 1967, p. 181.

288   W.L. Epstein, V.P. Shah and S. Riegelman: Arch. Dermatol. *106*, 344 (1972).

289   R. Aly, C.I. Bayles, R.A. Oakes, D.J. Bibel and H.I. Maibach: Clin. Exp. Dermatol. *19*, 43 (1994).

290   R.M. Atkinson, C. Bedford, K.T. Child and F.G. Tomich: Antibiot. Chemother. *12*, 232 (1962).

291   R.G. Grounse: J. Invest. Dermatol. *37*, 529 (1961).

292   D.W. Anderson: Ann. Allergy *231*, 103 (1965).

293 R.S. Gordee, D.J. Zeckner, L.F. Ellis, A.L. Thakker and L.C. Howard: J. Antibiot. *37*, 1054 (1984).

294 B.W. Dobbeling. B.D. Fine, Jr., M.A. Pfaller, C.T. Sheetz, J.B. Stopkes and R.P. Wenzel: Program and Abstracts of the 30th Interscience Conference on Antimicrobial Agents and Chemotherapy, 1990. Washington, D.C.; American Society for Microbiology, 1990, p. 183.

295 G.S. Hall, C. Myles, K.J. Pratt and J.A. Washington: Antimicrob. Agents Chemother. *32*, 1331 (1988).

296 S.M. Ringel, R.C. Greenough, S. Roemer, D. Connor, A.L. Gutt, B. Blair, G. Kanter and M. von Strandtmann: J. Antibiot. *30*, 371 (1977).

297 S.M. Ringel: Antimicrob. Agents Chemother. *13*, 762 (1978).

298 S. Shadomy, D.M. Dixon, A. Espinal-Ingroff, G.E. Wagner, J.P. Yu and H.J. Shadomy: Antimicrob. Agents Chemother. *14*, 99 (1978).

299 H.B. Levine, S.M. Ringel and J.M. Cobb: Chest *73*, 202 (1978).

300 S. Shadomy, C.J. Utz and S. White: Antimicrob. Agents Chemother. *14*, 95 (1978).

301 S.M. Ringel: Mycopathologica *109*, 75 (1990).

302 R. Cooper, I. Trumees, T. Barrett, M. Patal and J. Schwarz: J. Antibiot. *43*, 897 (1990).

303 J.P. Utz: Recent Trends in the Discovery, Development and Evaluation of Antifungal Agents. R.A. Fromtling (Ed.). J.R. Prous Science Publishers, S.A. (1987) p. 633.

304 V.T. Andriole, J.P. Utz and S.M. Sabesin: Am. Rev. Resp. Dis. *84*, 538 (1961).

305 M.J. Thurmalachar, S.K. Menon and V.V. Bhutt: Hindustan Antibiot. Bull. *3*, 136 (1961).

306 J.P. Utz, P. Witorsch, T.W. Williams, C.W. Emmons, H.J. Shadomy and W. Piggott: Am. Rev. Resp. Dis. *95*, 506 (1967).

307 M.J. Thirumalachar and M.J. Narasimhan, Jr.: Recent Trends in the Discovery, Development and Evaluation of Antifungal Agents. R.A. Fromtling (Ed.). Barcelona; J.R. Prous Science Publishers, S.A., 1987, p. 619.

308 J.E. Bennett, W.E. Dismukes, R.J. Duma, G. Medoff, M.A. Sande, H. Gallis, J. Leonard, B.T. Fields, M. Bradshaw, H. Haywood, Z.A. McGee, T.R. Cate, C.J. Warner and D.W. Alling: New Engl. J. Med. *301*, 126 (1979).

309 A. Polak, H.J. Scholer and M. Wall: Chemother. *28*, 461 (1982).

310 A. Polak: Chemother. *33*, 381 (1987).

311 J.R. Graybill, D.M. Williams, E. Van Cutsem and D.J. Drutz: Rev. Infect. Dis. *2*, 551 (1980).

312 A. Schaffner and P.G. Frick: J. Infect. Dis. *151*, 902 (1985).

313 R. Allendoerfer, A.J. Marquis, M.G. Rinaldi and J.R. Graybill: Antimicrob. Agents Chemother. *35*, 726 (1991).

314 A. Polak: Mycoses *36*, 43 (1993).

Progress in Drug Research, Vol. 44 (E. Jucker, Ed.)
© 1995 Birkhäuser Verlag, Basel (Switzerland)

Newer antifolates in cancer therapy

By Richard M. Schultz

Division of Cancer Research, Lilly Research Laboratories, Indianapolis, IN 46285, USA

> *By opposites, opposites are cured.*
> Hippocreates, *De Flatibus,* vol. i., p. 570

1 Introduction

Folate vitamins are a class of cofactors that serve as one-carbon donors in biochemical reactions. Folate-requiring enzymes provide excellent targets for cancer chemotherapy due to the close relationship of folic acid metabolism to cell replication. Several of these enzymes are essential for important steps in DNA synthesis, including biosynthesis of purines and conversion of deoxyuridine monophosphate (dUMP) to deoxythymidine monophosphate (dTMP) (Figure 1). It is interesting to reflect that of the 18 or so known reactions of folate metabolism, exhaustive research of some 30 years has seemingly produced only folate antimetabolites targeted to block dihydrofolate reductase (DHFR). Over recent years, we now see the emergence of new folate antimetabolites with specificities other than DHFR, such as

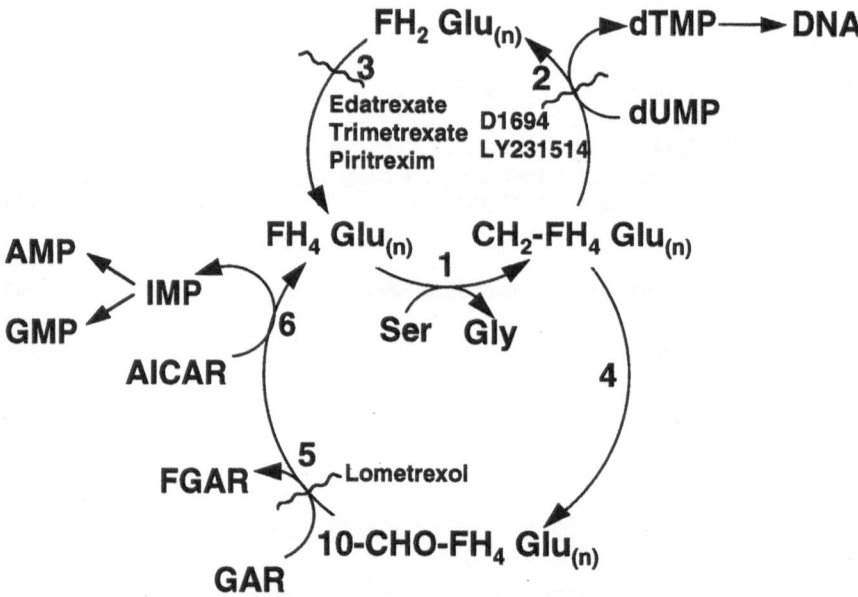

Figure 1.
Inhibition by various antifolates of metabolic cycles involved in purine and pyrimidine synthesis. Enzymes: 1, serine hydroxymethyltransferase; 2, thymidylate synthase; 3, dihydrofolate reductase; 4, C_1-tetrahydrofolate synthase, a trifunctional enzyme involving 10-formyltetrahydrofolate synthetase, 5,10-methenyltetrahydrofolate cyclohydrolase, and 5,10-methylenetetrahydrofolate dehydrogenase; 5, glycinamide ribonucleotide formyl transferase; 6, amino-imidazolecarboxamide ribonucleotide formyl transferase.
Abbreviations: FH_2, dihydrofolate; FH_4, tetrahydrofolate; CH_2-FH_4, 5,10-methylene-tetrahydrofolic acid; 10-CHO-FH_4, 10-formyltetrahydrofolate.

thymidylate synthase (TS) and glycinamide ribonucleotide formyl transferase (GARFT).

The established roles of methotrexate and 5-fluorouracil in cancer therapy
further exemplify how interference with two of these enzymes, DHFR and
TS, can produce meaningful clinical results. Several promising new antifolates have been introduced into clinical trials as anticancer agents over recent
years. These compounds are largely the result of rational drug design based
on current understanding of folate metabolism and transport, exploration of
multiple folate-requiring enzymes, and mechanisms of cellular resistance to
methotrexate. The biology and biochemical pharmacology of six antifolates
farthest along in clinical testing, including edatrexate, trimetrexate, piritrexim, ZN-D1694, LY231514, and lometrexol are discussed in this review (for
structures, see Table 1). These compounds offer exciting opportunities to
expand the role of antifolates in cancer chemotherapy.

2   Historical perspective

Lucy Wills, an English physician working in India in 1931, found that a
diet, largely consisting of wheat, caused pregnant women to develop anemia. This anemia differed from that induced by iron deficiency in that the
red cells were large and hyperchromic. Wills found that this anemia in
Hindu women responded to treatment with yeast extract or liver extract
given by mouth, but was not cured by refined liver extract used for treating
pernicious anemia [1–3]. It is now known that this megaloblastic anemia
was found solely in pregnant women due to their higher requirement for the
"Wills factor", which was needed for cellular proliferation in bone marrow.
This anemia could be produced in monkeys fed restricted diets, and the
resultant leukopenia was termed "nutritional cytopenia" [4].

This anti-anemia factor discovered by Wills was subsequently named folic
acid by Mitchell and coworkers in 1941 [5]. This hematopoietically active
material was isolated from spinach and other "foliage". Angier èt al.
successfully synthesized folic acid in 1945 in the form of pteroylmonoglu-
tamate with a therapeutic activity equal to the natural material [6]. A
research program was started immediately by scientists from Lederle Laboratories and the Calco Chemical Division of American Cyanamid Company
to produce folate analogues for chemotherapeutic testing. Since folic acid
deficiency produced leukopenia, it was proposed that an antagonist of folic
acid could be used to treat leukemia.

Table 1.
Newer antifolates

Structure	Agent	Primary action
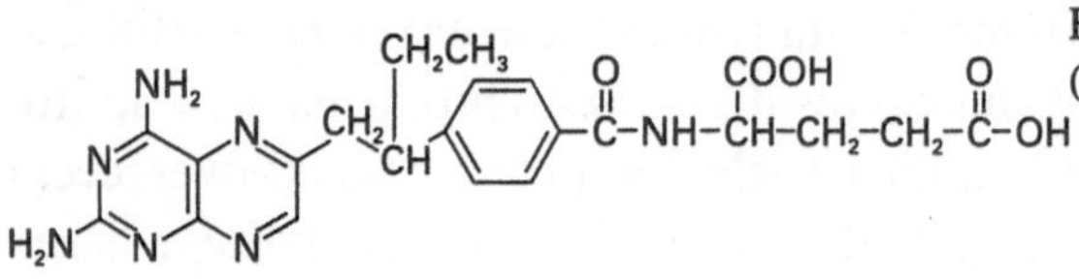 NH₂ ... CH₂CH₃ ... CH₂ CH ... C-NH-CH-CH₂-CH₂-C-OH (COOH) ... H₂N	Edatrexate (10-EdAM)	DHFR inhibition polyglutamates inhibit TS
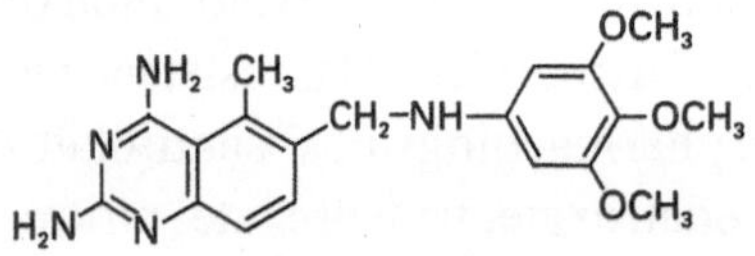 NH₂ CH₃ ... CH₂-NH- ... OCH₃ OCH₃ OCH₃ ... H₂N	Trimetrexate	DHFR inhibition
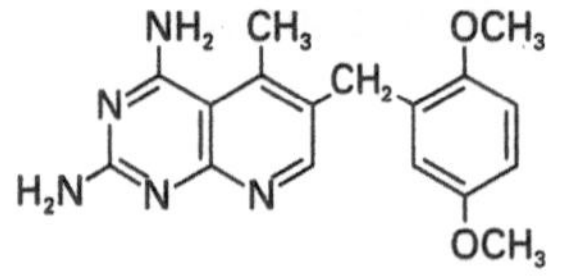 NH₂ CH₃ OCH₃ ... CH₂ ... OCH₃ ... H₂N	Piritrexim (BW 301U)	DHFR inhibition
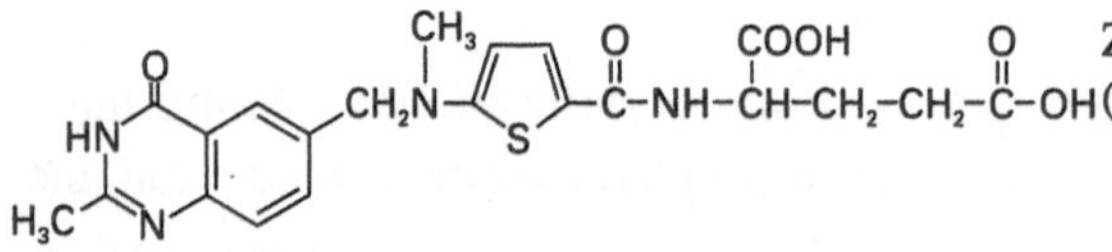 CH₃ ... CH₂N ... S ... C-NH-CH-CH₂-CH₂-C-OH (COOH) ... HN ... H₃C	ZN-D1694 (Tomudex)	TS inhibition
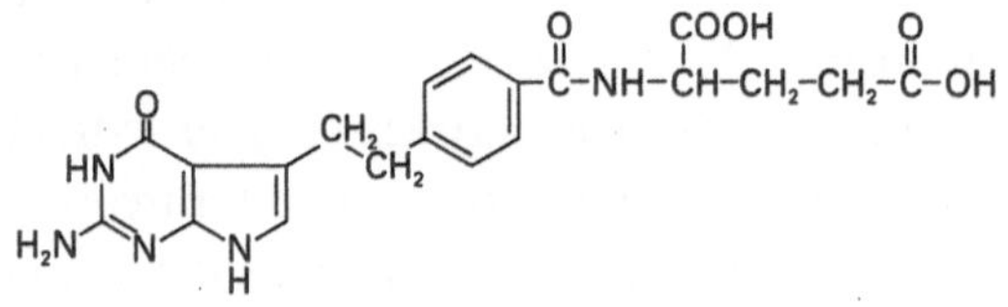 O ... CH₂ CH₂ ... C-NH-CH-CH₂-CH₂-C-OH (COOH) ... HN ... H₂N ... H	LY231514	TS inhibition
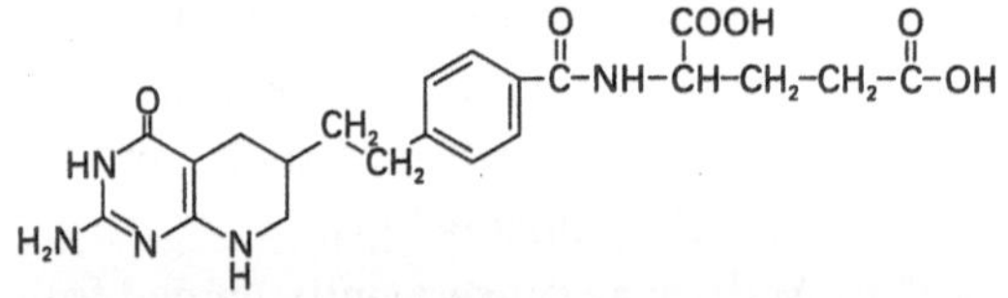 O ... CH₂ CH₂ ... C-NH-CH-CH₂-CH₂-C-OH (COOH) ... HN ... H₂N ... H	Lometrexol (DDATHF; LY264618)	GARFT inhibition

Abbreviations: DHFR, dihydrofolate reductase; TS, thymidylate synthase; GARFT, glycin-amide ribotide formyl transferase.

Lewisohn and colleagues observed in 1945 that folic acid as the triglutamate pteroyltriglutamic acid (teropterin) isolated from bacterial fermentation had antitumor activity against spontaneous mouse mammary tumors [7]. Lewisohn used teropterin for several cancer patients, including George Herman Ruth, who thus became the first and greatest of the major league home run hitters to be associated with folic acid analogues in the therapy of neoplastic diseases [8]. However, the antitumor activity of teropterin in experimental models could not be confirmed by subsequent studies [9].

Antifolate therapy was first shown to have clinical importance in cancer chemotherapy when Farber and associates demonstrated in 1948 that aminopterin treatment could produce temporary remissions in childhood acute lymphocytic leukemia [10]. Aminopterin (4-aminofolic acid) had been synthesized by Seeger et al. in 1947 [11]. 2,4-diamino-10-methyl folic acid (first known as amethopterin and now as methotrexate) was synthesized by Smith and colleagues in 1948 [12]. Methotrexate had reduced potency, but was better tolerated than aminopterin. The most outstanding success in the early clinical testing of methotrexate was treatment of malignant chorionic tumors in women [13]. Complete remissions lasted for over 5 years. Since that time, methotrexate has become the most commonly used antineoplastic antifolate and remains a mainstay in the treatment of several malignant diseases. It is widely used as the treatment of choice for choriocarcinoma and in acute lymphocytic leukemia. It is also included in a variety of combination regimens to treat diffuse lymphomas, osteogenic sarcoma, and lung, head and neck, cervical, ovarian and bladder carcinomas. The antitumor activity of early antifolates has been the subject of several excellent reviews [8, 14–17].

3   Dihydrofolate reductase (DHFR) inhibitors

Dihydrofolic acid   Dihydrofolate reductase   Tetrahydrofolic acid
+ NADPH + H$^+$ $\xrightarrow{\hspace{3cm}}$ + NADP$^+$

Dihydrofolate reductase (DHFR) is the enzyme which catalyzes the reduction of dihydrofolate to tetrahydrofolate, and its importance as a target of cancer chemotherapy has long been recognized [18]. Inhibition of this enzyme initiates a series of intracellular events that culminate in the cessation of *de novo* synthesis of purines and thymidylate. Cell death presumably follows in the wake of nucleotide depletion and, perhaps, due to the genetic injury produced by the misincorporation of the expanded pool of uridine nucleotides into DNA.

Methotrexate is a potent inhibitor of DHFR [19, 20]. The major limitations of methotrexate are its limited tumor spectrum, its acute and chronic toxicities, and the rather frequent development of acquired resistance. These limitations raise the possibility that better analogues, or at least analogues with better antitumor spectrum, could be discovered. In addition, high resolution X-ray crystallography studies of the interaction of dihydro-folate reductase with folate analogs [21] have raised the possibility of computer-assisted drug design of more potent and selective inhibitors.

The movement of methotrexate and other antifolates across cell mem-branes has received a great deal of attention because of the relevance of transport abnormalities to clinical drug resistance. Membrane transport of methotrexate and natural reduced folate compounds, including the rescue agent leucovorin is primarily mediated by the reduced folate carrier (RFC), a high affinity/low capacity influx mechanism [reviewed in ref. 19]. Transport by the RFC involves an energy-dependent, temperature sensitive, and concentrative process that probably depends on the function of specific intramembrane protein(s).

This mechanism is anion dependent and accounts for all methotrexate influx at extracellular drug concentrations up to 50 μM [22].

The formation of intracellular polyglutamates of methotrexate is a critical determinant of its cytotoxicity and tumor selectivity. After transport of methotrexate into the cell, additional glutamic acid moieties are added to the terminal glutamate by the enzyme folylpolyglutamate synthetase (FPGS). These polyglutamate forms appear to be selectively retained within the cell and have an increased affinity for folate-requiring enzymes. Aside from DHFR, methotrexate polyglutamates inhibit thymidylate synthase, AICAR transformylase, and GAR transformylase [23, 24]. In addition, the accumulation of dihydrofolate and 10-formyldihydrofolate that builds as a consequence of DHFR inhibition also directly inhibit folate-requiring en-zymes of thymidylate and purine synthesis [19].

3.1   Edatrexate (10-EdAM; 10-ethyl-10-deazaaminopterin)

Edatrexate is one of several derivatives synthesized by DeGraw and co-workers in which the N^{10}-amine of aminopterin is replaced by a methylene group [25]. It is roughly equivalent to methotrexate as an inhibitor of DHFR [26]. Edatrexate is among the few anticancer agents which exploit differ-ences between tumor cells and normal cells to achieve greater selectivity, and hence, less toxicity. Specifically, it has been shown to have enhanced uptake and polyglutamate formation in tumor cells relative to normal proliferative tissues [27], favoring much greater accumulation of cytotoxic polyglutamates in tumor cells. Sirotnak and coworkers demonstrated that compounds with the greatest ratio for influx K_m of gut epithelial cells to tumor cells are the most effective in prolonging survival in tumor-bearing mice [26, 29]. In addition, edatrexate's polyglutamates appear to have substantial inhibitory activity against thymidylate synthase [28].

Edatrexate was shown to be superior to methotrexate against 4 of 6 murine ascites tumors (L1210, S180, Ehlich, and Tapper) and far superior against 4 of 6 murine solid tumors *in vivo* (S180, Tapper, E0771 mammary adeno-carcinoma, and T241 fibrosarcoma) [26, 29, 30]. It produced 10–30% complete regressions against S180, E0771, and T241 tumors. Both agents demonstrated similar activity against P288 and 1498c leukemias and the Lewis lung tumor, but were inactive against B16 melanoma.

Schmid and associates tested edatrexate against a group of human tumor xenografts in nude mice [26, 31]. They noted that this analog at or near the LD10 dose (2–4.5 mg/kg) given once per day × 5 produced frank regressions in MX-1 mammary carcinoma and LX-1 lung carcinoma. Activity of edatrexate against the CX-1 colon carcinoma was less, but retardation of tumor growth was observed with some minor regressions. In contrast, methotrexate was inactive against all three xenograft models studied. Similarly, only edatrexate was active against two head and neck tumor xenografts, HNX-PI and HNX-LP [32].

Schmid et al. also studied edatrexate in combination with other cytotoxic agents against a number of tumor models [33]. Edatrexate was tested in combination with 5-fluorouracil and/or cyclophosphamide, cisplatin and melphalan. When edatrexate was administered 16 h prior to cyclophosphamide, melphalan, or cisplatin, the therapeutic activity was greatly enhanced, and a substantial number of long-term survivors were seen. Similarly, Sirotnak et al. noted some tumor-free long-term survivors with a combination of edatrexate and cisplatin against a mouse ovarian carcinoma model [34].

Recently, Grant and coworkers reviewed the clinical experience of edatrexate in Phase I and Phase II trials [35]. Antitumor activity has been observed in patients with non-small cell lung cancer, breast cancer, cancer of the head and neck, and non-Hodgkin's lymphoma. The dose-limiting toxicity is mucositis. Other side effects have been mild and include leukopenia, thrombocytopenia, and skin rashes. There is evidence that toxicity resulting from standard doses of edatrexate can be ameliorated with the use of leucovorin rescue. When edatrexate was combined with cyclophosphamide and cisplatin in previously untreated patients with non-small cell lung cancer, a 47% response rate was obtained, but significant stomatitis and myelosuppression limited treatment. However, patients on the same regimen with oral leucovorin (15 mg every 6 hours for 4 doses starting 24 h after edatrexate) experienced less stomatitis without a significant decrease in the response rate [36]. Studies are also underway to determine whether edatrexate is synergistic with alkylating agents, since preclinical studies [33, 34] have predicted such activity. A trial of edatrexate with mitomycin-C and vinblastine in chemotherapy naive patients with non-small cell lung cancer produced a 60% response rate [37].

3.2   Trimetrexate

Trimetrexate (TMQ, JB11) belongs to a group of "nonclassical" antifolates, which also includes piritrexim (part C of this section). They are more lipophilic than methotrexate and lack a terminal glutamic acid residue. Trimetrexate is a potent inhibitor of dihydrofolate reductase derived from bacterial, protozoal, mammalian, and human sources [38, 39]. It was synthesized in an effort to circumvent certain types of resistance associated with classical antifolates. It is taken up by passive diffusion in cells, rather than the active transport mechanism used by naturally-occurring folates and methotrexate, is not polyglutamated, and penetrates areas of the body, such as the lung and brain, which methotrexate enters slowly or not at all [40–42]. In this regard, trimetrexate is effective against several tumor cell lines resistant to methotrexate on the basis of transport, but not against lines resistant because of elevated dihydrofolate reductase [43, 44].

Some experimental data suggests that lipophilic antifols may enter cells by a common but more complex transport process than simple diffusion and that cellular resistance can develop, possibly due to impairment of a specific transport system or alteration in membrane structure [45, 46].

The mechanisms of resistance to trimetrexate have been extensively studied. Trimetrexate is more effective than methotrexate in cells with increased dihydrofolate reductase, presumably because of higher intracellular levels of drug [47]. However, changes in the structure of the target enzyme dihydrofolate reductase due to mutations can also cause trimetrexate resistance [48]. In addition, several reports show that the multidrug-resistance phenotype is a mechanism of resistance to trimetrexate [49–52], probably due to enhanced drug efflux, with partial reversal by verapamil [49] and complete reversal by resperpine [52]. The relative importance of these mechanisms of resistance in clinical practice is not yet clear. Sobrero and colleagues noted that resistance to trimetrexate or methotrexate developed rapidly in cultures of human colon carcinoma cells *in vitro*, and that changing the schedule of administration does not overcome resistance [53].

Several studies compared the antitumor activity of trimetrexate to methotrexate against mouse solid tumors and leukemias. The initial studies showed that trimetrexate has moderate to good activity against L1210 and P388 leukemias, colon 26 and 38, and B16 melanoma, whereas methotrexate is only active against the leukemias [38]. Subsequent reports also demonstrated modest activity against the M5076 ovarian carcinoma [54]. Neither drug is active against the human CX-1 colon, LX-1 lung or MX-1 mammary carcinoma xenografts in nude mice [55, 56].

Trimetrexate has also been tested in combination with other agents. Trimetrexate has demonstrated synergy with carboxypeptidase G_2, a folate-cleaving enzyme that removes glutamic acid from folates, against L1210 leukemia cells *in vivo* [57]. This synergy may be due to folate depletion, leading to decreased levels of the substrate dihydrofolate and intensifying the inhibition of dihydrofolate reductase by trimetrexate [58]. Trimetrexate also has synergistic antitumor activity with 5-fluorouracil, vincristine, 6-thioguanine, doxorubicin, and cyclophosphamide against the P388 leukemia *in vivo* [59]. The combination of cyclophosphamide and trimetrexate was particularly synergistic, produced greater than 4.6 logs tumor cell kill than the optimal regimen with either agent alone. Trimetrexate has also been reported to potentiate etoposide cytotoxicity in L1210 leukemia [60].

Trimetrexate has shown evidence of activity in head and neck [61], non-small cell lung [62, 63], breast [64], prostrate [65],and esophageal [66] cancer. In these studies, relatively mild hematologic toxicity was observed, with rapid recovery, and no cumulative dose effects were noted. Many of the early Phase II trial results with trimetrexate have been summarized [58, 67].

3.3   Piritrexim (BW 301U)

Piritrexim, like trimetrexate, is a nonclassical, lipophilic inhibitor of DHFR that crosses cell membranes rapidly without the need for active transport and is not polyglutamated. It was selected out of over 300 heterocyclic structures based on a series of 6-substituted 2,4-diaminopyrido[2,3-d]-pyridines originally synthesized as potential antimicrobial agents [68–70]. In subsequent years, piritrexim was shown to have significant antitumor activity against Walker 256 carcinoma [71]. Piritrexim had greater affinity for DHFR than metoprine, a previously developed lipophilic antifolate and similar activity as methotrexate (5 nM IC$_{50}$). Unlike metoprine, piritrexim is a relatively weak inhibitor of histamine N-methyltransferase and diamine oxidase. Inhibition of these enzymes had been linked to the CNS toxicity which plagued metoprine in clinical trials [72].

The growth inhibition of leukemia cells in culture induced by most inhibitors of DHFR such as methotrexate and trimetrexate can be fully reversed by a combination of thymidine and hypoxanthine. In contrast, full protection from piritrexim cytotoxicity is afforded only by a combination of hypoxanthine, thymidine, adenosine, and either cytidine or uridine in S180 cells [73, 74]. Furthermore, leucovorin alone is capable of protecting cells from methotrexate and other antifolates, but not from piritrexim. Complete protection can be achieved, however, by the combination of leucovorin and thymidine.

Taylor and coworkers demonstrated the selective toxicity of piritrexim for methotrexate-resistant cells with reduced drug uptake [75]. It has also shown some effectiveness against cell lines that are resistant to methotrexate because of amplification of DHFR [76]. However, selection of cells for resistance to piritrexim has been reported to result in overexpression of DHFR as well as in a non-P-glycoprotein-mediated mechanism that confers cross-resistance to trimetrexate, but not to methotrexate [77, 78].

Piritrexim has *in vivo* antitumor activity against P388 and L1210 leukemias, sarcoma 180, Ehrlich ascites carcinoma, and Walker 256 choriosarcoma [73, 79]. The compound is ineffective against the B16 melanoma [73].

The clinical experience with piritrexim suggests that schedules with prolonged drug exposure time may be optimal for nonclassical antifolates. Since nonclassical antifolates cannot benefit from enhanced cellular retention and concentration associated with polyglutamation, it seems logical that this schedule may overcome the effects of passive efflux of lipid-soluble compounds from cells [80].

Piritrexim has demonstrated activity in Phase II trials against metastatic urothelial cancer [81], advanced squamous head and neck cancer [82], malignant melanoma [83, 84], advanced bladder cancer [85], and non-small cell lung cancer [86]. The prolonged low-dose oral administration of piritrexim appears to have a superior efficacy and toxicity profile [87]. The major toxicities were myelosuppression, stomatitis, and rash in these studies.

4   Thymidylate synthase (TS) inhibitors

N^5, N^{10}-methylene $\xrightarrow{\text{Thymidylate synthase}}$ Dihydrofolic acid + dTMP
tetrahydrofolic acid + dUMP

Thymidylate synthase catalyzes the methylation of deoxyuridine mono-phosphate to thymidine monophosphate in a reaction that requires the reduced folate 5,10-methylene-tetrahydrofolate as a cofactor. The enzyme's crucial role in the synthesis of the only nucleotide required exclusively for DNA synthesis makes it an obvious target for antimetabolite attack. The role of the thymidylate synthesis cycle in anticancer drug development has been the subject of several excellent reviews [88–91]. To date, 5-fluorouracil remains the only oncolytic agent in general use that targets thymidylate synthase.

An alternative approach to the inhibition of thymidylate synthase has been directed toward the synthesis of analogues of the folate cofactor. For example, the antitumor activity of the dihydrofolate reductase inhibitor methotrexate may partially be due to potent inhibition of thymidylate synthase catalytic activity by methotrexate polyglutamates [92, 93]. 5,8-Dideaza-10-propargylfolic acid (CB3717), the first specific inhibitor of thymidylate synthase to advance to clinical trial [94–96], demonstrated activity in ovarian, breast, and liver carcinomas during Phase I trials [97–99]. Its clinical development was discontinued, however, because of associated renal and hepatic toxicity. The kidney toxicity apparently was not related to the antiproliferative properties of the drug, but possibly due to very poor water solubility of the compound at urinary pH with resultant drug precipitation in the renal tubules [100, 101]. The demonstration of clinical activity for this new class of compounds has stimulated extensive research aimed at identifying other folate-based thymidylate synthase inhibitors that may be better clinical candidates.

4.1   ZN-D1694

Efforts to obtain a more water-soluble analogue of CB3717 led to the synthesis of 2-desamino-CB3717 [96, 102]. Despite being 10-fold less potent than CB3717 as an inhibitor of thymidylate synthase, this compound was 6- to 10-fold more potent as an inhibitor of cell growth. Moreover, it lacked the renal and hepatic toxicity seen with CB3717. Subsequent studies demonstrated that the replacement of the C_2-amino group of CB3717 with small lipophilic constituents yielded thymidylate synthase inhibitors which were both more soluble and more cytotoxic than CB3717. These studies led to the selection of D1694 as a second generation quinazoline thymidylate synthase inhibitor [103].

D1694 is a potent inhibitor of TS (K_i 60 nmol/l) and does not cause toxic side effects in the kidney or liver [104]. The synthetic γ-polyglutamates are up to 2 orders of magnitude more potent as inhibitors of TS; e.g., the tetraglutamate has a K_i of 1.0 nM [103, 105]. Although the inhibitory activity of D1694 toward rat liver DHFR was similar to TS ($K_i = 92$ nM), the polyglutamate derivatives did not show enhanced activity.

D1694 inhibited aminoimidazolecarboxamide ribotide formyl transferase (AICARFT) weakly ($K_i = 170$ μM), but the polyglutamates were very potent (e.g., D1964 tetraglu, $K_i = 12$ nM) [106]. GARFT was not inhibited. D1694 was a potent inhibitor of L1210 leukemia cell growth [$IC_{50} = 8$ nM), and growth inhibition was not observed in the presence of thymidine [103], consistent with TS being the locus of action. Thymidine also prevented the antitumor activity of D1694 against L1210 leukemia *in vivo*.

Jackman and colleagues showed that the high cytotoxic potency of D1694 is due to both good cellular uptake via the reduced folate/methotrexate carrier and extensive intracellular polyglutamation [107, 108]. They developed two cell lines where acquired resistance to D1694 was either associated with a defective reduced folate carrier (human ovarian 41 M:R line) or reduced levels of FPGS (L1210:MB3 line). Furthermore, Jackman et al. showed that the L1210:1565 cell line, which has greatly impaired reduced folate/methotrexate transport and thus is resistant to methotrexate, was greater than 100-fold cross-resistant to D1694 [103]. Gibson and associates measured polyglutamate metabolites of D1694 in mouse and human cultured cells [109]. Although cell lines differed in the total level of polyglutamates formed and the pattern of chain length observed, rapid and extensive polyglutamation of D1694 occurred in all cell types examined.

Keyomarsi and coworkers demonstrated that, although D1694 is a potent cytotoxic agent against cultured mammary epithelial cells with TS as its sole locus of action, it also has a novel and major biochemical limitation [110]. Specifically, they noted the accumulation of thymidylate synthase protein, but not its RNA, following treatment of human mammary epithelial cells with D1694. Following D1694 treatment, TS levels in desalted cell extracts increased by up to 40-fold in normal (70N) and 10-fold in human mammary cancer [21PT) cells. Their results suggest that TS is negatively regulated mainly by a feedback of its translational machinery [111, 112], and that D1694 inhibits this specific translational "detainment" resulting in accumulation of this protein. This accumulation and constitutive expression of TS induced by D1694 should increase drug resistance under a clinical setting.

The antitumor activity of D1694 was compared with that of CB3717, 5-fluorouracil, and methotrexate against 10 human tumor xenografts (3 lung, 2 ovarian, 4 colon, and 1 gastric) [113]. Tumor responses were compared by determining the dose required to produce a 15-day growth delay. D1694 produced this response in all tumors at doses below the maximum tolerated dose (MTD) (doses ranged from 1–100 mg/kg/day). By comparison, CB3717 produced this level of effect at its MTD in only 1 tumor (ovarian). 5-FU was active in 4 tumors (small cell lung, ovarian, colon, gastric) at its MTD, and methotrexate was active in 2 tumors (small cell lung, ovarian) at its MTD and 1 tumor (small cell lung) just below its MTD. They concluded that D1694 is superior to the other compounds in these models with respect to both spectrum of antitumor activity and therapeutic margin. In addition, D1694 has been shown to cure the L1210:ICR ascitic tumor in mice at 0.4 mg/kg daily for 5 days [103], and is also active against the murine L5178Y lymphoma thymidine kinase mutants when bolus dosed i.p. [114, 115].

D1694 is currently undergoing phase II testing in a variety of malignancies. In early results, it has shown evidence of activity against advanced colorectal cancer [116], non-small cell lung cancer [117], and advanced pancreatic cancer [118].

4.2   LY231514

LY231514 is a novel pyrrolopyrimidine antifolate that inhibits thymidylate synthase. It has potent cytotoxic activity against CCRF-CEM human leukemia cells (IC_{50} = 7 ng/ml), and thymidine alone is able to substantially reduce this cytotoxicity [119, 120]. In addition, folinic acid antagonized CCRF-CEM growth inhibition in a competitive fashion such that the highest folinic acid concentration used (16 µM) increased the 50% inhibitory activity >100-fold. This is consistent with folinic acid competing with LY231514 for uptake into the cell, intracellular polyglutamation and common enzyme binding sites. When tested against recombinant mouse thymidylate synthase purified from a bacterial expression system, inhibition was competitive (K_i 0.34 µM). Moreover, LY231514 was an extremely efficient substrate for polyglutamation, and these polyglutamates are up to

2-orders of magnitude more potent as inhibitors of TS [K_i 3.4 nM as pentaglutamate] [120].

Jackman and associates have suggested that standard murine models and human tumor xenograft models are not appropriate for the evaluation of pure TS inhibitors [121]. While thymidine levels in the plasma compartment in humans are very low and thus not a problem, substantial levels of thymidine are found in mouse plasma. Unless a tumor model is used which cannot salvage thymidine, only limited antitumor effects have been observed for specific TS inhibitors when drug is administered over a one-week period. LY231514 was active against the thymidine kinase- and hypoxanthine phosphoribosyl transferase-deficient tumor, L5178Y/TK-/HX-, when administered i.p. daily for 8 consecutive days [120]. Complete inhibition of tumor growth was achieved at doses from 12.5 mg/kg to 200 mg/kg, and an excellent therapeutic index was observed. In contrast, CB3717 was completely inactive in this tumor model with daily i.p. administration up to the maximally tolerated dose of 100 mg/kg. Despite the mouse thymidine problem, LY231514 was very effective against the VRC5 and GC3 human colon xenografts in nude mice. Good growth inhibition (>80%) was observed when mice were treated at 25 mg/kg and 50 mg/kg (i.p. daily × 10 beginning 7 days after tumor implantation).

Rinaldi and coworkers described an initial phase I evaluation of LY231514 in patients with advanced solid tumors [122]. Patients with advanced, refractory, solid tumors were given escalating doses of LY231514 intravenously over 10 minutes, weekly for 4 weeks, repeated 42 days. Reversible grade IV neutropenia was the dose-limiting toxicity, and non-hematologic toxicities included mild fatigue, anorexia, and nausea. The maximally-tolerated dose using this schedule was 40 mg/m^2. Alternative phase I schedules are being explored to attempt greater dose intensity prior to phase II testing.

5   Glycinamide ribotide transformylase (GARFT) inhibitors

Glycinamide ribonucleotide (GAR)   GARFT   N-formyl glycinamide
+ N^5,N^{10}-methenyl-tetrahydrofolic acid $\xrightarrow{\hspace{1cm}}$ ribonucleotide +
+ H_2O tetrahydrofolate

Inhibitors of glycinamide ribotide transformylase suppress *de novo* purine synthesis and result in depletion of cellular pools of adenosine triphosphate (ATP) and guanosine triphosphate (GTP). Several investigators have studied whether the cellular effects of GARFT inhibitors are limited to cytosta-sis or extend to cytotoxicity, a question of primary importance to the clinical development of these compounds. Prior studies that concurrent inhibition of purine synthesis by methotrexate tended to prevent the efficiency of "thymineless death" [123] and that purines enhance the cell kill by metho-trexate [124] further complicate this issue. However, studies using trypan blue exclusion, soft agar cloning, and limiting dilution outgrowth for quantitation of cytotoxicity have clearly shown that inhibitors of purine synthesis are cytocidal agents [125–127]. Moreover, Smith et al. reported that substantial (99–99.9%) tumor cell kill can be induced by a pure inhibitor of purine synthesis, but that the rate of commitment to cell death and the extent of cell kill is greater with a pure inhibitor of thymidylate synthesis [127].

5.1   Lometrexol (DDATHF; LY249543)

Lometrexol (5,10-dideaza-5,6,7,8-tetrahydrofolic acid) is the first potent inhibitor of glycinamide ribonucleotide formyl transferase, which mediates the first formyl transfer reaction in purine *de novo* biosynthesis [128–131]. Lometrexol depletes cellular pools of adenosine triphosphate (ATP) and guanosine triphosphate (GTP). It does not cause significant inhibition of dihydrofolate reductase or thymidylate synthase [132, 133].

Lometrexol is a potent inhibitor of L1210 and CCRF-CEM human leukemia cells in culture with 50% inhibition of growth achieved by 10 to 30 nM drug concentrations [129]. The addition of hypoxanthine or aminoimidazole carboxamide to the culture medium is adequate to completely reverse the cytotoxicity of lometrexol up to 1 mM drug concentrations. Lometrexol retains activity against a cell line with a 63-fold increase in DHFR that is resistant to methotrexate, trimetrexate, and edatrexate [134]. Lometrexol is an excellent substrate for folylpolyglutamate synthetase (FPGS); the poly-glutamate forms bind up to 100 times more tightly to GARFT than dose lometrexol itself, and polyglutamation appears to be very important for antitumor activity [131]. Structural analogues of lometrexol that cannot be converted to polyglutamates show little activity *in vitro* [135]. Matherly and colleagues demonstrated that even for tumor cells with severely impaired antifolate transport, the extensive conversion of DDATHF to polyglutamyl forms required for GARFT inhibition preserves high levels of antitumor activity [136, 137]. In addition, markedly decreased cytotoxic activity has been observed for lometrexol against cell lines deficient in FPGS [138,

139]. Pizzorno and associates showed that enhanced target enzyme levels, impaired polyglutamylation, and enhanced pools of natural folates are associated with resistance to lometrexol in CCRF-CEM human leukemia cells [140].

Lometrexol binds to and is apparently transported by the "classical" reduced folate carrier which mediates the uptake of both methotrexate and tetrahydrofolate cofactors in mammalian cells [141–143]. In addition to this transport system, Pizzorno and colleagues noted that lometrexol can be transported in MA104 monkey kidney epithelial cells by a high affinity membrane-associated folate-binding protein (mFBP) [142]. In this regard, it is interesting to note that 90% of human ovarian carcinomas contain overexpressed mFBP [144, 145]. Since lometrexol has a 25–50 fold greater affinity for mFBP than methotrexate [146], it is possible that lometrexol may preferentially be targetted to tumors expressing high levels of mFBP. The role of mFBP in mediating uptake of antifolate in tumor cells has not been well defined. Schultz and coworkers noted a lack of correlation between levels of mFBP and function of mFBP in DDATHF transport in the tumor models that they studied [147].

Lometrexol has demonstrated remarkable antitumor activity against a broad spectrum of murine solid tumors and human tumor xenografts which are refractory towards conventional antifolate (methotrexate) therapy [133, 148]. Diastereomer B of DDATHF (lometrexol) was highly active against the X5563 plasma cell myeloma, AC755 adenocarcinoma, 6C3HED lymphosarcoma, colon 26 carcinoma, B-16 melanoma, Lewis lung carcinoma, and Madison lung carcinoma. It also showed excellent activity against the human colon xenograft (VRC5) and produced complete inhibition of tumor growth at 50 mg/kg/every other day in nude mice. Mice placed on a folate-free diet had reduced drug clearance and suffered a 100-fold increase in toxicity [149, 150]. In these studies, folic acid was able to inhibit toxicity, but not the antitumor activity of lometrexol, suggesting a role for oral folic acid in reducing the toxicity of lometrexol in clinical trials.

During phase I clinical studies, lometrexol showed severe and unexpected hematological and gastrointestinal toxicity in some patients [151–153]. Some antitumor responses have been observed, including a partial response in a patient with malignant fibrous histiocytoma, and a complete response in a patient with squamous cell cancer of the lung. Two approaches are currently under clinical investigation to reduce the risk of toxicity: i) the concomitant administration of oral folic acid and ii) the use of leucovorin as an antidote. Both of these approaches are based on findings in mice, although the mechanism(s) by which folic acid and leucovorin counteract lometrexol toxicity is not well understood. [149, 150]. Young and coworkers demonstrated the improved clinical tolerance of lometrexol with oral folic acid [154]. In their study, a patient with oropharyngeal cancer has had a complete response of 18 months duration, and lesser antitumor effects were seen in 8 additional patients. In another clinical study, toxicity was markedly reduced by oral folic acid administration, and a response (>35 days) was obtained in one breast cancer patient following 2 courses of therapy [155].

6   Mechanisms of resistance

Drug resistance, either primary or acquired, has long been considered the major cause in cancer treatment failure [156]. For example, the initial courses of combination chemotherapy can produce over 80% complete remissions in patients who have "limited" small cell lung cancer. Despite many months of remission and continuous drug treatment, the disease usually recurs and thereafter is quite resistant and patients quickly succumb [157]. Hopes of overcoming drug resistance in cancer chemotherapy have been frustrated by a number of reasons, including lack of new analogs that are non-cross-resistant with the parent compound, current failure of clinical trials aimed at reverting multidrug resistance, and conflicting results reported with alternating non-cross-resistant chemotherapy regimens [53, 158]. Moreover, clinical responses to drug treatments are typically short-lived, demonstrating rapid loss of chemosensitivity of neoplastic cell populations.

Several mechanisms of resistance to methotrexate have been identified from both animal and human tumor cell lines. These include: i) active transport defects [46, 159]; ii) DHFR overproduction due to gene amplification [160]; iii) antifolate-dependent DHFR accumulation [161]; iv) decreased polyglutamation of methotrexate [162]; v) reduced affinity for methotrexate of an altered form of DHFR [163]; and vi) decreased thymidylate synthase activity [164]. While any single mechanism may produce drug resistance, more than one mechanism is frequently found to underlie resistance in model systems and clinical specimens. The relative significance and frequency of each of these mechanisms in the development of clinical resistance has not been adequately studied. However, newer antifolate DHFR inhibitors, such as trimetrexate and piritrexim, have been introduced into clinical study due to their ability to overcome certain mechanisms of methotrexate resistance, including transport mechanisms and polyglutamation. Whether or not these "nonclassical" antifolates will be more efficacious than methotrexate or allow for successful combination therapy with methotrexate has not yet been determined. Assaraf and colleagues showed that a lipid-soluble antifolate such as trimetrexate may well circumvent methotrexate resistance due to impaired transport, but at the same time become ineffective due to the multidrug-resistant phenomenon [51]. Sirotnak described approaches to the circumvention of acquired antifolate resistance at the level of new drug design which incorporated a kinetic analysis of the various biochemical phenotypes and a systematic analysis of their structure-activity relationships [165].

7   Synergistic interactions

Recent experimental evidence demonstrates that two antifolates acting at different enzyme sites in mammalian cells can exhibit synergistic drug interactions [166]. The best combination consisted of relatively low levels of a lipid-soluble inhibitor of DHFR such as trimetrexate and a folate analogue inhibiting purine biosynthesis or *de novo* thymidylate synthesis [167–170]. Galivan et al. demonstrated that the presence of the DHFR inhibitors causes a 10-fold increase in the ratio of the TS inhibitor to its substrate; a condition which would favor the inhibition of the enzyme and potentially account for the synergy observed between this combination [167, 171]. Gaumont and coworkers showed that varying the medium folic acid concentration over the range of 0.5 to 100 µM increasingly blocks the growth inhibitory effects of individual antifolates, but increasingly enhances the synergistic interaction of trimetrexate with either lometrexol or the TS inhibitor, CB3717 [172]. Although most of these synergistic interactions were observed *in vitro*, Ferguson and associates noted the synergy between lometrexol and methotrexate in mice bearing L1210 tumors [173]. Quite complex interactions have been noted in combinations of antifolates which do show synergy. The data on hand suggest that the timing of drug administration, the relative concentrations of the inhibitors, and the folate status of the growth medium play an important role in determining whether synergistic or antagonistic interactions predominate. Some other combinations involving antifolates where synergy have been noted include: CB3717 plus dipyridamole, by inhibiting both thymidine salvage and deoxyuridine efflux [174, 175]; edatrexate plus cisplatin [176]; D1694 plus idoxuridine, a thymidine analogue [177]; lometrexol plus 5-fluorouracil [178]; and various DHFR inhibitors plus 5-fluorouracil [179–181].

A combination of the purine inhibitor lometrexol and the TS inhibitor CB3717 or 2-desamino-CB3717 has been shown to produce primarily antagonistic effects [168, 182, 183]. In one study, protection was associated with a decrease in DNA fragmentation and a drop in intracellular dATP pools [183]. In addition, a source of purines has been noted to potentiate the cytotoxicity of methotrexate [184, 185]. These results support the hypothesis that inhibitory effects on *de novo* purine biosynthesis by inhibitors of dihydrofolate reductase may limit cytotoxicity, and indicate that a rise in dATP pools may be an important signal for apoptosis.

8   Unresolved issues and future directions

The clinical development of several new antifolates with distinctive chemical features, membrane transport characteristics, and target enzymes provides new opportunities to expand the role of this class of agents in cancer chemotherapy. To make the most effective use of these agents, several key research questions need to be addressed. These include:

1) Since membrane transport is the first limiting step in the chemotherapeutic efficacy of folate analogues, a thorough knowledge of each transport system in the antitumor efficacy of newer antifolates needs to be established. For example, human ovarian carcinomas contain elevated levels of type α folate-binding protein. Studies to date have not clarified the role of this folate receptor in transport of antifolates in ovarian cancer [147]. Clearly, differences in transport need to be exploited between normal and malignant tissues.

2) *De novo* and acquired resistance mechanisms to antifolates need to be better characterized and understood, including relative significance and frequency of individual mechanisms in the development of resistance. Results from these studies can then be utilized for the design of better antitumor agents. It is possible, but by no means well established, that nonclassical DHFR inhibitors overcome critical mechanisms of methotrexate resistance, including intracellular transport and polyglutamation. Moreover, these lipophilic compounds suffer from their own resistance patterns, including transport [45, 46] and the multidrug-resistant phenotype [51]. In another example, D1694 appears to increase drug resistance by inducing the accumulation and constitutive expression of TS [110]. It would

be desirable to overcome this major biochemical limitation in the further development of D1694 analogues.

3) Numerous studies suggest that two antifolates acting at different enzyme sites in mammalian cells can exhibit either synergistic or antagonistic drug interactions. The significance of these observations is complicated by the fact that most, if not all glutamate-containing folate analogues are known to inhibit multiple enzymes. For example, methotrexate itself has relatively low affinity for TS, GARFT, and AICARFT, whereas the longer polygluta-mates of MTX have been found to bind more strongly to these enzymes [23, 92, 186], leading to the suggestion that methotrexate, and by implication other classical antifolates [187], should be viewed as prodrugs [24]. However, polyglutamation appears to have a major role in selective antitumor action in certain tumor systems [188–190], arguing against the exclusive use of nonclassical antifolates in cancer therapy. The lack of pure inhibitors prevents the definitive studies necessary to assess enzyme specificities required for synergistic tumor killing. Moreover, the biochemical basis for optimal cytotoxicity by antifolates needs to be defined. Fundamental questions remain to be answered, including the contribution of purine synthesis' inhibition to methotrexate cytotoxicity [191]. Studies to date suggest synergy between relatively low levels of a DHFR inhibitor such as trimetrexate and a folate analogue inhibiting either purine biosynthesis or *de novo* thymidylate synthesis [167–170], but these combinations have not been tested clinically.

4) Techniques need to be developed to enhance the therapeutic effectiveness of antifolates by selectively suppressing systemic toxicity. For example, attempts have been made to modulate the activity of methotrexate at the metabolic level through the use of reversal agents, such as folinic acid (leucovorin), that may be termed either protective or rescue agents depending on the time of administration [192–195]. Similarly, folic acid administration has been shown experimentally to reverse the toxicity, but not the antitumor activity of lometrexol [149, 150]. However, the dose and timing of the reversal agent is critical, since it can also negate the antitumor effects. A careful definition of the folate status of the patient is probably necessary to titrate the dose of the protective agent necessary for achieving optimal therapeutic efficacy.

9 Closing remarks

We have realized considerable advances in the science of rational drug design, since the introduction of methotrexate into clinical cancer chemotherapy in 1949. Methotrexate was brought to clinical trial and found to be effective when little was known about its mechanism of action [196]. Since then, a detailed understanding of the pathways and regulation of folate-dependent enzymes has been developed. Many newer antifolates have been synthesized in attempts to produce agents that have a wider spectrum of activity and less toxicity than methotrexate. The enthusiasm in this area has been sparked by the fairly new recognition of enzymatic targets with potential clinical utility and by new strategies for circumventing some forms of resistance and toxicity. In this brief review, I have highlighted six relatively new antifolates that are undergoing clinical evaluation. The new generation of antifolates holds great promise for improvements in cancer chemotherapy.

References

1   L. Wills: Br. Med. J. *1*, 1059 (1931).
2   L. Wills: Proc. R. Soc. Med. *25*, 1720 (1932).
3   L. Wills: Indian J. Med. Res. 21, 669 (1934).
4   P. L. Day, W. C. Langston and W. J. Darby: Proc. Soc. Exp. Biol. Med. *38*, 860 (1938).
5   H. K. Mitchell, E. E. Snell and R. J. Williams: J. Am. Chem. Soc. *63*, 2284 (1941).
6   R. B. Angier, J. H. Boothe, B. L. Hutchings, J. H. Mowat, J. Semb, E. L Stokstad, Y. Subbarow, C. W. Waller, D. B. Cosulich, M. J. Fahrenback, M. E. Hultquist, E. Kuh, E. H. Northey, D. R. Selgar, J. P. Sickels and J. M. Smith: Science *102*, 227 (1945); Science *103*, 667 (1946).
7   R. Leuchtenberger, C. Leuchtenberger, D. Laszlo and R. Lewisohn: Science *101*, 46 (1945).
8   T. H. Jukes: Cancer Res. *47*, 5528 (1987).
9   D. J. Hutchison and F. A. Schmid: Experimental cancer chemotherapy with folate antagonists. In: Folate Antagonists as Therapeutic Agents: Vol 2. Pharmacology, Experimental and Clinical Therapeutics, eds. F. M. Sirotnak, J. J. Burchall, W. D. Ensminger and J. A. Montgomery. Academic Press, New York 1984, p. 1.
10   S. Farber, L. K. Diamond, R. D. Mercer, R. F. Sylvester and J. A. Wolff: N. Engl. J. Med. *238*, 787 (1948).
11   D. R. Seeger, J. M. Smith and M. E. Hulquist: J. Am. Chem. Soc. *69*, 2567 (1947).
12   J. M. Smith, D. B. Cosulich, M. E. Hultquist and D. R. Seeger: Trans. N. Y. Acad. Sci. *10*, 82 (1948).
13   R. Hertz, J. L. Lewis and M. B. Lipsett: Proc. Am. Assoc. Cancer Res. *3*, 235 (1961).
14   R. C. Jackson: Parmac. Ther. *25*, 61 (1984).

15   B. A. Kamen: Folic acid antagonists. In: Metabolism and Action of Anti-cancer Drugs, eds. G. Powis and R. A. Prough. Taylor and Francis, New York 1987, p. 141.

16   M. G. Nair: Antifolates. In: Cancer Management in Man: Biological Response Modifiers, Chemothrapy, Antibiotics, Hyperthermia and Supporting Measures, ed. P. V. Wooley. Kluwer Academic Publishers, Boston 1989, p. 35.

17   A. Rosowsky: Chemistry and biological activity of antifolates. In: Progress in Medicinal Chemistry, Vol 26, eds. G. P. Ellis and G. B. West. Elsevier Science Publishers, B. V. 1989, p. 1.

18   J. E. Gready: Dihydrofolate reductase: binding of substrates and inhibitors and catalytic mechanism. In: Advances in Pharmacology and Chemotherapy, Vol 17, eds. S. Garattini, A. Goldin, F. Hawking, and I. J. Kopin. Academic Press, New York 1980, p. 37.

19   C. J. Allegra: Antifolates. In: Cancer Chemotherapy: Principles and Practice, eds. B. A. Chabner and J. M. Collins. J. B. Lippincott Co., New York 1990, p. 110.

20   J. Jolivet, K. H. Cowan, G. A. Curt, N. J. Clendeninn, and B. A. Chabner: N. Engl. J. Med. *309*, 1094 (1983).

21   J. H. Freisheim and D. A. Matthews: The comparative bio-chemistry of dihydrofolate reductase. In: Folate antagonists as Therapeutic Agents, eds. F. M. Sirotnak, J. J. Burchall, W. D. Ensminger, and J. A. Montgomery. Academic Press, Orlando 1984, p. 69.

22   G. B. Henderson, J. M. Tsuji, and H. Kumar: Biochem. Pharmacol. *36*, 3007 (1987).

23   J. J. McGuire, E. Mini, P. Hsieh, and J. R. Bertino: Folylpoly-glutamate synthetase: Relation to methotrexate action and as a target for new drug development. In: Development of Target-Oriented Anticancer Drugs, ed. Y.-C. Cheng. Raven Press, New York 1983, p. 97.

24   B. A. Chabner, C. J. Allegra, G. A. Curt, N. J. Clendeninn, J. Baram, S. Koizumi, J. C. Drake, and J. Jolivet: J. Clin. Invest. *76*, 907 (1985).

25   J. I. DeGraw, V. H. Brown, H. Tagawa, R. L. Kisliuk, Y. Gaumont, and F. M. Sirotnak: J. Med. Chem. *25*, 1227 (1982).

26   F. M. Sirotnak, F. A. Schmid, L. L. Samuels, and J. I. DeGraw: NCI Monogr. *5*, 127 (1987).

27   F. M. Sirotnak, J. I. DeGraw, D. M. Moccio, L. L. Samuels, and L. J Goutas: Cancer Chemother. Pharmacol. *12*, 18 (1984).

28   M. G. Nair, N. T. Nanavati, and P. Kumar: J. Med. Chem. *31*, 181 (1988).

29   F. M. Sirotnak, J. I. DeGraw, F. A. Schmid, L. J. Goutas, and D. M. Moccio: Cancer Chemother. Pharmacol. *12*, 26 (1984).

30   F. M. Sirotnak: Cancer Treat. Symposia, 855 (1986).

31   F. A. Schmid, F. M. Sirotnak, G. M. Otter, and J. I. DeGraw: Cancer Treat. Rep. *69*, 551 (1985).

32   D. H. Brown, B. J. M. Braakhuis, and G. A. M. S. van Dongen: Anticancer Res. *9*, 1549 (1989).

33   F. A. Schmid, F. M. Sirotnak, and G. M. Otter: Cancer Treat. Rep. *71*, 727 (1987).

34   F. M. Sirotnak, F. A. Schmid, and J. I. DeGraw: Cancer Res. *49*, 2890 (1989).

35   S. C. Grant, M. G. Kris, C. W. Young, and F. M. Sirotnak: Cancer Investigation *11*, 36 (1993).

36   J. S. Lee, W. K. Murphy, and M. H. Shirinian: Cancer Chemother. Pharmacol. *28*, 199 (1991).

37   M. G. Kris, F. J. Gralla, and L. M. Potanovich: Proc. Am. Soc. Clin. Oncol. 8 (abstract) (1989).

38   J. R. Bertino, W. L. Sawicki, B. A. Moroson, A. R. Cashmore, and E. F. Elslager: Biochem. Pharmacol. 28, 1983 (1979).

39   J. R. Bertino and W. L. Sawicki: Proc. Am. Assoc. Cancer Res. 18, 168 (abstr.) (1977).

40   L. M. Werbel: Design and synthesis of lipophilic antifols as anticancer agents. In: Folate Antagonists as Therapeutic Agents, eds. F. M. Sirotnak, J. J. Burchall, W. D. Ensminger, and J. A. Montgomery. Academic Press, Orlando 1984, p. 261.

41   E. F. Elslager, J. L. Johnson, and L. M. Werbel: J. Med. Chem. 26, 1753 (1983).

42   B. A. Kamen, B. Eibl, A. Cashmore, and J. Bertino: Biochem. Pharmacol. 33, 1697 (1984).

43   K. Scanlon, T. Ohnuma, R. J. Lo, C. A. Nichol, S. Waxman, E. M. Greenspan, and J. F. Holland: Proc. Am Soc. Clin. Oncol. 23, 12 (abstr) (1982).

44   H. Diddens, D. Niethammer, and R. C. Jackson: Cancer Res. 43, 5286 (1983).

45   H. Arkin, T. Ohnuma, Y. Takemura, B. A. Damen, Y. Kano, and J. F. Holland: Proc. Am. Assoc. Cancer Res. 26, 25 (1985).

46   D. W. Fry and R. C. Jackson: Cancer Surv. 5, 47 (1986).

47   J. T. Lin and J. R. Bertino: Cancer Treat. Res. 42, 79 (1989).

48   H. Diddens, D. Niethammer, and R. C. Jackson: Cancer Res. 43: 5286 (1983).

49   W. D. Klohs, R. W. Steinkampf, and J. A. Besserer: Cancer Lett. 31, 253 (1986).

50   H. Arkin, T. Ohnuma, and J. F. Holland: Proc. Am. Assoc. Cancer Res. 27, 269 (1986).

51   Y. G. Assaraf, A. Molina, and R. T. Schimke: J. Natl. Cancer Inst. 81, 290 (1989).

52   W. D. Klohs, R. W. Steinkampf, W. R. Leopold, and D. W. Fry: Proc. Am. Assoc. Cancer Res. 28, 391 (1986).

53   A. Sobrero, C. Aschele, R. Rosso, A. Nicolin, and J. R. Bertino: J. Natl. Cancer Inst. 83, 24 (1991).

54   R. C. Jackson, D. W. Fry, T. J. Boritzki, J. A. Besserer, W. R. Leopold, B. J. Sloan, and E. F. Elslager: Adv. Enz. Reg. 22, 187 (1984).

55   P. J. O'Dwyer, D. D. Shoemaker, J. Plowman, J. Cradock, A. Grillo-Lopez, and B. Leyland-Jones: Invest. New Drugs 3, 71 (1985).

56   J. T. Lin and J. R. Bertino: J. Clin. Oncol. 5, 2032 (1987).

57   A. Romaini, A. F. Sobrero, and T. C. Chou: Cancer Res. 49, 6019 (1989).

58   J. T. Lin and J. R. Bertino: Cancer Invest. 9, 159 (1991).

59   W. R. Leopold, D. D. Dykes, and D. P. Griswold, Jr.: Proc. Am. Assoc. Cancer Res. 27, 253 (1986).

60   D. W. Fry: Proc. Am. Assoc. Cancer Res. 29, 483 (1988).

61   F. Robert: Semin. Oncol. 15 (Suppl.2), 22 (1988).

62   K. Mattson, P. Maasilta, and L. Tammilehto: Semin. Oncol. 15 (Suppl. 2), 32 (1988).

63   J. Maroun: Semin. Oncol. 15 (Suppl. 2), 17 (1988).

64   J. M. Leiby: Sem. Oncol. 15 (Suppl. 2), 27 (1988).

65   T. Curley, C. Engstrom, and H. Scher: Proc. Am Soc. Clin. Oncol. 8, 140 (1989).

66   A. S. Alberts, G. Falkson, and M. Badata: Invest. New Drugs 6, 319 (1988).

67   G. F. Fleming and R. L. Schilsky: Semin. Oncol. 19, 707 (1992).

68   B. S. Hurlbert, K. W. Ledig, B. F. Valenti, and G. H. Hitchings: J. Med. Chem. 11, 703 (1968).

69   B. S. Hurlbert and B. F. Valenti: J. Med. Chem. 11, 708 (1968).

70 B. S. Hurlbert, R. Ferone, T. A. Herrmann, and G. H. Hitchings: J. Med. Chem. *11*, 711 (1968).

71 E. M. Grivsky, S. Lee, C. W. Sigel, D. S. Duch, and C. A. Nichol: J. Med. Chem. *23*, 327 (1980).

72 D. S. Duch, M. P. Edelstein, and C. A. Nichol: Mol. Pharmacol. *18*, 100 (1980).

73 D. S. Duch, M. P. Edelstein, S. W. Bowers, and C. A. Nichol: Cancer Res. *42*, 3987 (1982).

74 D. S. Duch, C. W. Sigel, S. W. Bowers, M. P. Edelstein, J. C. Cavallito, R. G. Foss, and C. A. Nichol: Lipid-soluble inhibitors of dihydrofolate reductase: selection and evaluation of 2,4-diaminopyrimidine BW 301U and related compounds as anticancer agents. In: Current Chemotherapy and Infectious Disease, eds. J. D. Nelson and C. Grassi. The American Society for Microbiology, Washington DC 1980, p. 1597.

75 I. W. Taylow, P. Slowiaczek, M. L. Fiedlander, and M. H. N. Tattersall: Cancer Res. *45*, 978 (1985).

76 W. D. Sedwick, M. Hamrell, and O. E. Brown: Mol. Pharmacol. *22*, 766 (1982).

77 Y. G. Assaraf, A. Molina, and R. T. Schimke: Proc. Am. Assoc. Cancer Res. *30*, A1895 (1989).

78 Y. G. Assaraf, A. Molina, and R. T. Schimke: J. Biol. Chem. *264*, 18326 (1989).

79 J. Laszlo, H. J. Iland, and W. D. Sedwick: Adv. Enzyme Regul. *24*, 357 (1986).

80 E. M. Berman and L. M. Werbel: J. Med. Chem. *34*, 479 (1991).

81 R. deWit, S. B. Kaye, J. T. Roberts, G. Stoter, J. Scott, and J. Verweij: Br. J. Cancer *67*, 388 (1993).

82 W. C. Uen, A. T. Huang, R. Mennel, S. E. Jones, M. B. Spaulding, K. Killion, K. Havlin, P. Keegan, and N. J. Clendeninn: Cancer *69*, 1008 (1992).

83 L. G. Feun, R. Gonzalez, N. Savaraj, J. Hanlon, M. Collier, W. A. Robinson, and N. J. Clendeninn: J. Clin. Oncol. *9*, 464 (1991).

84 L. G. Feun, W. A. Robinson, N. Savaraj, J. Hanlon, M. Collier, and N. J. Clendeninn: Proc. Am. Assoc. Cancer Res. *30*, A1087 (1989).

85 N. J. Clendeninn, N. Savaraj, P. Benedetto, S. Waldman, J. Antunez, E. Donnelly, K. Offenhauser, and L. G. Feun: Proc. Am. Assoc. Cancer Res. *32*, A1110 (1991).

86 M. G. Kris, R. J. Gralla, M. T. Burke, L. D. Berkowitz, L. D. Marks, D. P. Kelsen, and R. T. Heelan: Cancer Treat. Rep. *71*, 763 (1987).

87 N. J. Clendeninn, M. A. Collier, L. G. Feun, and W. A. Robinson: Prolonged low-dose administration of piritrexim: A better way to deliver an antifolate? In: Sixth NCI-EORTC Symposium on New Drugs in Cancer Therapy. Amsterdam, A461 (1989).

88 K. T. Douglas: Medicinal Res. Rev. *7*, 441 (1987).

89 P. V. Danenberg: Biochim. Biophys. Acta *473*, 73 (1977).

90 A. L. Jackman, T. R. Jones, and A. H. Calvert: Thymidylate synthetase inhibitors: experimental and clinical aspects. In: Cancer Treatment and Research, ed. W. L. McGuire. Martinus Nijhoff Publishers, Boston 1985, p. 155.

91 M. Friedkin: Adv. Enzymol. Relat. Areas Mol. Biol. *38*, 235 (1973).

92 C. J. Allegra, B. A. Chabner, J. C. Drake, R. Lutz, D. Rodbard, and J. Jolivet: J. Biol. Chem. *260*, 9720 (1985).

93 W. M. Hryniuk: Cancer Res. *35*, 1085 (1975).

94 K. R. Harrap, A. L. Jackman, D. R. Newell, G. A. Taylor, L. R. Hughes, and A. H. Calvert: Adv. Enzyme Regul. *29*, 161 (1989).

95   T. R. Jones, A. H. Calvert, A. L. Jackman, S. J. Brown, M. Jones, and K. R. Harrap:
      Eur. J. Cancer *17*, 11 (1981).
96   A. L. Jackman, G. A. Taylor, B. M. O'Connor, J. A. Bishop, R. G. Moran, and A. H.
      Calvert: Cancer Res. *50*, 5212 (1990).
97   A. H. Calvert, D. L. Alison, S. J. Harland, B. A. Robinson, A. L. Jackman, T. R. Jones,
      D. R. Newell, Z. H. Siddik, E. Wiltshaw, T. J. McElwain, I. E. Smith, and K. R. Harrap:
      J. Clin. Oncol. *4*, 1245 (1986).
98   S. Vest, E. Bork, and H. H. Hansen: Eur. J. Cancer Clin. Oncol. *24*, 201 (1988).
99   C. Sessa, M. Zucchetti, M. Ginier, Y. Willems, M. D'Incalci, and F. Cavalli: Eur. J.
      Cancer Clin. Oncol. *24*, 769 (1988).
100   D. R. Newell, Z. H. Siddik, A. H. Calvert, A. L. Jackman, D. L. Alison, K. G. McGhee,
      and K. R. Harrap: Proc. Am. Assoc. Cancer Res. *23*, 181 (1982).
101   D. L. Alison, D. R. Newell, C. Sessa, S. J. Harland, L. I. Hart, K. R. Harrap, and A. H.
      Calvert: Cancer Chemother. Pharmacol. *14*, 265 (1985).
102   T. R. Jones, T. J. Thornton, A. Flinn, A. L. Jackman, D. R. Newell, and A. Calvert: J.
      Med. Chem. *32*, 847 (1989).
103   A. L. Jackman, G. A. Taylor, W. Gibson, R. Kimbell, M. Brown, A. H. Calvert, I. R.
      Judson, and L. R. Hughes: Cancer Res. *51*, 5579 (1991).
104   S. Clark and A. Jackman: Proc. Am. Assoc. Cancer Res. *34*, 274 (1993).
105   W. H. Ward, R. Kimbell, and A. L Jackman: Biochem. Pharmacol. *43*, 2029 (1992).
106   R. Ferone, D. Duch, M. Hanlon, J. Humphreys, C. See, S. Singer, and K. Waters: Proc.
      Am. Assoc. Cancer Res. *32*, 326 (1991).
107   A. L. Jackman, M. Brown, L. Kelland, W. Gibson, G. Abel, F. T. Boyle, and 1. Judson:
      Proc. Am. Assoc. Cancer Res. *34*, 326 (1991).
108   A. L. Jackman, W. Gibson, M. Brown, R. Kimbell, and F. T. Boyle: Adv. Exp. Med.
      Biol. *339*, 265 (1993).
109   W. Gibson, G. M. Bisset, P. R. Marsham, L. R. Kelland, I. R. Judson, and A. L. Jackman:
      Biochem. Pharmacol. *45*, 863 (1993).
110   K. Keyomarsi, J. Samet, G. Molnar, and A. B. Pardee: J. Biol. Chem. *268*, 15142
      (1993).
111   E. Chu, D. Voeller, D. M. Koeller, J. C. Drake, C. H. Takimoto, G. F. Maley, F. Maley,
      and C. J. Allegra: Proc. Natl. Acad. Sci. USA *90*, 517 (1993).
112   E. Chu, D. M. Voeller, P. F. Morrison, K. L. Jones, T. Takechi, G. F. Maley, F. Maley,
      and C. J. Allegra: J. Biol. Chem. *269*, 20289 (1994).
113   T. C. Stephens, B. E. Valcaccia, M. L. Sheader, I. R. Hughes, and A. Jackman: Proc.
      Am. Assoc. Cancer Res. *32*, 328 (1991).
114   T. C. Stephens, J. A. Calvete, D. Janes, S. E. Waterman, B. E. Valcaccia, L. R. Hughes,
      and A. H. Calvert: Proc. Am. Assoc. Cancer Res. *31*, 342 (1990).
115   T. C. Stephens, M. N. Smith, S. E. Waterman, M. L. McCloskey, A. L. Jackman, and
      F. T. Boyle: Use of the murine L5178Y Iymphoma thymidine kinase mutants for in
      vitro and in vivo antitumour efficacy: evaluation of novel thymidylate synthase
      inhibitors. In: Chemistry and Biology of Pteridines and Folates, ed. J. E. Ayling.
      Plenum Press, New York 1993, p. 589.
116   J. Zalcberg, E. Francois, E. Van Cutsem, J. H. Schornagel, A. Adenis, M. Green, H.
      Starkhammer, A. Hanrahan, and P. Ellis: Proc. Amer. Soc. Clin. Oncol. *13*, 199 (1994).
117   R. Heaven, K. Bowen, D. Rinaldi, F. Robert, T. Jenkins, J. Eckardt, S. Fields, J. Hardy,

S. Patton, G. Kennealey, D. VonHoff, and H. Burris: Proc. Amer. Soc. Clin. Oncol. *13*, 355 (1994).

118   R. Pazdur, E. S. Casper, N. J. Meropol, C. Fuchs, and G. T. Kennealey: Proc. Amer. Soc. Clin. Oncol. *13*, 207 (1994).

119   G. B. Grindey, C. Shih, C. J. Barnett, H. L Pearce, J. A. Engelhardt, G. C. Todd, S. M. Rinzel, J. F. Worzalla, L S. Gossett, T. P. Everson, T. M. Wilson, M. E. Kobierski, M. A. Winter, J. R. Bewley, D. Kuhnt, E. C. Taylor, and R. G. Moran: Proc. Amer. Assoc. Cancer Res. *33*, 411 (1992).

120   E. C. Taylor, D. Kuhnt, C. Shih, S. M. Rinzel, G. B. Grindey, J. Barredo, M. Jannatipour, and R. G. Moran: J. Med. Chem. *35*, 4450 (1992)

121   A. L. Jackman, G. A. Taylor, A. H. Calvert, and K. R. Harrap: Biochem. Pharmacol. *33*, 3269 (1984).

122   D. A. Rinaldi, H. A. Burris, F. A. Dorr, J. Nelson, S. M. Fields, J. G. Kuhn, J. R. Eckardt, P. Lu, J. R. Woodworth, S. W. Corso, and D. D. Von Hoff: Proc. Am. Soc. Clin. Oncol. *13*, 159 (1994).

123   J. Borsa and G. F. Whitmore: Cancer Res. *29*, 737 (1969).

124   C. R. Fairchild, J. Maybaum, and J. A. Straw: Cancer Chemother. Pharmacol. *22*, 26 (1988).

125   J. B. J. Kwok and M. H. N. Tattersall: Biochem. Pharmacol. *42*, 507 (1991).

126   G. K. Smith, D. S. Duch, I. K. Dev, and S. H. Kaufmann: Cancer Res. *52*, 4895 (1992).

127   S. G. Smith, N. L. Lehman, and R. G. Moran: Cancer Res. *53*, 5697 (1993)

128   G. P. Beardsley, E. C. Taylor, C. Shih, G. A. Poore, G. B. Grindey, and R. G. Moran: Proc. Amer. Assoc. Cancer Res. *27*, 259 (1986).

129   R. G. Moran, E. C. Taylor, and G. P. Beardsley: Proc. Amer. Assoc. Cancer Res. *26*, 231 (1985).

130   G. P. Beardsley, B. A. Moroson, E. C. Taylor, and R. G. Moran: J. Biol. Chem. *264*, 328 (1989).

131   S. W. Baldwin, A. Tse, L. S. Gossett, E. C. Taylor, A. Rosowsky, C. Shih, and R. G. Moran: Biochemistry *30*, 1997 (1991).

132   E. C. Taylor, P. J. Harrington, S. R. Fletcher, G. P. Beardsley, and R. G. Moran: J. Med. Chem. *28*, 914 (1985).

133   G. P. Beardsley, E. C. Taylor, G. B. Grindey, and R. G. Moran: Deaza derivatives of tetrahydrofolic acid, a new class of folate Antimetabolites. In: Chemistry and Biology of Pteridines, eds. B. A Cooper and V. M. Whitehead. Walter de Gruyter, Berlin 1986, p. 953.

134   B. F. A. M. van der Laan, G. Jansen, and I. Kathmann: Eur. J. Cancer *27*, 1274 (1991).

135   M. G. Nair, A. Abraham, and R. L. Kisliuk: Proc. Amer. Assoc. Cancer Res. *32*, 324 (1991).

136   L. H. Matherly, S. M. Angeles, and J. J. McGuire: Biochem. Pharmacol. *46*, 2185 (1993).

137   L. H. Matherly and S. M. Angeles: Adv. Exp. Med. Biol. *338*, 783 (1993)

138   G. Pizzorno, J. A. Sokoloski, and A. R. Cashmore: Mol. Pharmacol. *39*, 85 (1990).

139   O. Russello, B. A. Moroson, and A. R. Cashmore: Proc. Amer. Assoc. Cancer. Res. *32*, 324 (1991).

140   G. Pizzorno, A. R. Cashmore, B. A. Moroson, A. D. Cross, C. Shih, and G. P. Beardsley: Proc. Amer. Assoc. Cancer Res. *30*, 480 (1989).

141 D. H. Boschelli, S. Webber, J. M. Whiteley, A. L. Oronsky, and S. S. Kerwar: Arch. Biochem. Biophys. *265*, 43 (1988).

142 G. Pizzorno, A. R. Cashmore, B. A. Moroson, A. D. Cross, A. K. Smith, M. Marling-Cason, B. A. Kamen, and G. P. Beardsley: J. Biol. Chem. *268*, 1017 (1993).

143 F. M. Sirotnak, G. M. Otter, J. R. Piper, and J. I. DeGraw: Biochem. Pharmacol. *37*, 4775 (1988).

144 S. Mioti, S. Canevari, S. Menard, D. Mezzanzanica, G. Porro, S. M. Pupa, M. Regazzoni, E. Tagliabue, and M. I. Colnaghi: Int. J. Cancer *39*, 297 (1987).

145 L. R. Coney, A. Tomassetti, L. Carayannopoulos, V. Frasca, B. A. Kamen, M. I. Colnaghi, and V. R. Zurawski: Cancer Res. *51*, 6125 (1991).

146 S. D. Weitman, A. G. Weinberg, L. R. Coney, V. R. Zurawski, D. S. Jennings, and B. A. Kamen: Cancer Res. *52*, 6708 (1992).

147 R. M. Schultz, S. L. Andis, S. B. Gates, K. A. Shackelford, L. G. Mendelsohn, C. Shih, and G. B. Grindey: Proc. Amer. Assoc. Cancer Res. *35* (1994); Oncology Res., submitted, 1994.

148 C. Shih, G. B. Grindey, P. J. Houghton, and J. A. Houghton: Proc. Amer. Assoc. Cancer Res. *29*, 283 (1988).

149 G. B. Grindey, T. Alati, and C. Shih: Proc. Amer. Assoc. Cancer Res. *32*, 324 (1991).

150 T. Alati, C. Shih, R. C. Pohland, R. J. Lantz, and G. B. Grindey: Proc. Amer. Assoc. Cancer Res. *33*, 407 (1992).

151 C. Sessa, L. Gumbrell, S. Hatty, H. Kern, and F. Cavalli: Ann. Oncol. *1* (suppl.), 5 (1990).

152 F. Muggia, T. Martin, M. Ray, C. G. Leichman, S. Grunberg, and I. Gill: Proc. Amer. Soc. Clin. Oncol. *9*, 74 (1990).

153 M. Ray, F. Muggia, C. G. Leichman, L. Leichman, R. Moran, and R. Dyke: Ann. Oncol. *3* (Suppl. 1), 137 (1992).

154 C. W. Young, V. E. Currie, J. F. Muindi, L. B. Saltz, K. M. W. Pisters, A. J. Esposito, and R. W. Dyke: Proc. Amer. Assoc. Cancer Res. *33*, 406 (1992).

155 S. R. Wedge, S. Laohavinij, G. A. Taylor, D. R. Newell, C. J. Charlton, M. Proctor, F. Chapman, D. Simmons, A. Oakey, L. Gumbrell, and A. H. Calvert: Proc. Amer. Assoc. Cancer Res. *34*, 274 (1993).

156 V. T. DeVita, Jr.: Principles of chemotherapy. In: Cancer, Principles and Practive of Oncology, eds. V. T. DeVita, Jr., S. Hellman, and S. A. Rosenberg. Lippincott, Philadelphia 1989, p. 276.

157 J. Laszlo, H. J. Iland, and W. D. Sedwick: Adv. Enz. Regul. *24*, 357 (1986).

158 G. Morstyn, G. P. Schechter, and D. C. Ihde: Cancer Treat. Rep. *68*, 1439 (1984).

159 G. A. Fischer: Biochem. Pharmacol. *11*, 1233 (1962).

160 F. W. Alt, R. E. Kellems, J. R. Bertino, and R. T. Schimke: J. Biol. Chem. *253*, 1357 (1978).

161 M. R. Hamrell, J. Laszlo, and W. D. Sedwick: Mol. Pharmacol. *19*, 491 (1981).

162 K. H. Cowan and J. Jolivet: Clin. Res. *31*, 508a (1983).

163 W. F. Flintoff and K. Essani: Biochemistry *19*, 4321 (1980).

164 D. Ayusawa, H. Koyama, and T. Seno: Cancer Res. *41*, 1497 (1981).

165 F. M. Sirotnak: NCI Monogr. *5*, 27 (1987).

166 J. Galivan: Biochemical mechanisms of the synergistic interaction of antifolates acting on different enzymes of folate metabolic pathways. In: Synergism and Antagonism in

Chemotherapy, eds.T.-C. Chou and D. C. Rideout. Academic press, Inc., New York 1991, p. 339.

167 J. Galivan, M. S. Rhee, T. B. Johnson, R. Dilwith, M. G. Nair, M. Bunni, and D. G. Priest: J. Biol. Chem. *264*, 10685 (1989).

168 J. Galivan, Z. Nimec, M. Rhee, D. Boschelli, A. L. Oronsky, and S. S. Kerwar: Cancer Res. *48*, 2421 (1988).

169 J. Galivan, A. Nimec, and M. Rhee: Cancer Res. *47*, 5256 (1987).

170 J. Thorndike, Y. Gaumont, J. Powers, R. L. Kisliuk, and J. R. Piper: Proc. Amer. Assoc. Cancer Res. *29*, 285 (1988).

171 J. Galivan, M. S. Rhee, T. B. Johnson, M. G. Nair, and D. Priest: Proc. Amer. Assoc. Cancer Res. *29*, 284 (1988).

172 Y. Gaumont, R. L. Kisliuk, J. C. Parsons, and W. R. Greco: Cancer Res. *52*, 2228 (1992).

173 K. Ferguson, D. Boschelli, P. Hoffman, A. Oronsky, J. Whiteley, S. Webber, J. Galivan, J. Freisheim, J. Hynes, and S. S. Kerwar: Cancer Chemother. Pharmacol. *25*, 173 (1989).

174 N. J. Curtin and A. L. Harris: Biochem. Pharmacol. *37*, 2113 (1988).

175 N. J. Curtin, D. R. Newell, and A. L. Harris: Biochem. Pharmacol. *38*, 3281 (1989).

176 T.-C. Chou, Q.-H. Tan, and F. M. Sirotnak: Cancer Chemother. Pharmacol. *31*, 259 (1993).

177 J. Pressacco, D. W. Hedley, and C. Erlichman: Cancer Res. *54*, 3772 (1994)

178 G. Pizzorno, S. J. Davis, D. J. Hartigan, and O. Russello: Biochem. Pharmacol. *47*, 1981 (1994).

179 W. L. Elliott, C. T. Howard, D. J. Dykes, and W. R. Leopold: Cancer Res. *49*, 5586 (1989).

180 J. R. Bertino, E. Mini, and D. J. Fernandes: Sem. Oncol. *10* (suppl. 2), 2 (1983).

181 E. Mini, M. Coronnello, S. Carotti, A. Gerli, A. Pesciullesi, B. A. Moroson, T. Mazzsel, P. Periti, and J. R. Bertino: J. Chemother. *2*, 17 (1990).

182 R. L. Kisliuk, Y. Gaumont, J. F. Powers, J. Thorndike, M. G. Nair, and J. R. Piper: Synergistic growth inhibition by combinations of antifolate. In: Folic Acid Metablism in Health and Disease, eds. M. F. Picciano, E. L. R. Stokstad, and J. F. Gregory. Liss, New York 1990, p. 79.

183 J. B. J. Kwok and M. H. N. Tattersall: Biochem. Pharmacol. *42*, 507 (1991).

184 J. Borsa and G. F. Whitmore: Cancer Res. *29*, 737 (1969).

185 C. R. Fairchild, J. Maybaum, and J. A. Straw: Cancer Chemother. Pharmacol. *22*, 26 (1988).

186 C. J. Allegra, J. C. Drake, J. Jolivet, and B. A. Chabner: Proc. Natl. Acad. Sci. USA *82*, 4881, 1985.

187 A. Rosowsky, J. Galivan, G. P. Beardsley, H. Bader, B. M. O'Connor, O. Russello, B. A. Moroson, M. T. DeYarman, S. S. Kerwar, and J. H. Freisheim: Cancer Res. *52*, 2148 (1992).

188 D. W. Fry, L. A. Anderson, M. Borst, and I. D. Goldman: Cancer Res. *43*, 1087 (1983).

189 I. Fabre, G. Fabre, and I. D. Goldman: Cancer Res. *44*, 3190 (1984).

190 B. G. Rumberger, J. R. Barrueco, and F. M. Sirotnak: Cancer Res. *50*, 4639 (1990).

191 R. C. Jackson: NCI Monogr. *5*, 9 (1987).

192 J. R. Bertino: Semin. Oncol. *4*, 203 (1977).

193 H. M. Pinedo, D. S. Zaharko, and J. M. Bull: Cancer Res. *36*, 4418 (1976).

194   A. Leyva, H. Nederbragt, J. Lankelma, and H. M. Pinedo: Cancer Treat. Rep. *65* (Suppl. 1), 45 (1981).
195   K. R. Harrap: Biochem. Soc. Trans. *4*, 856 (1976).
196   J. H. Burchenal, D. A. Karnofsky, and C. M. Southam: Am. J. Med. *7*, 420 (1949)

Progress in Drug Research, Vol. 44 (E. Jucker, Ed.)
© 1995 Birkhäuser Verlag, Basel (Switzerland)

Non-steroidal menses-regulating agents:
The present status[1]

By P. K. Mehrotra*, Sanjay Batra** and A. P. Bhaduri**

* Division of Endocrinology, and ** Division of Medicinal Chemistry, Central Drug
Research Institute, Lucknow 226001, India

---

1   CDRI Communication No. 5340.

1   Introduction

The desire to dissociate pregnancy from the act of coitus has led to the development of various contraceptive techniques. With the exception of condoms, contraceptive methods are mainly concerned with females. The reason is not because they are directly affected by unwanted pregnancies but because our present knowledge of the female reproductive system offers ways of interfering with the female cycle at more than one stage. Two distinct methods of fertility control have received acceptance: the intra-uterine device (IUD) and the steroidal pill. The use of IUD has been described as a "contraception divorced from coitus" [1]; oral contraception entails the intake of more than 250 tablets per female per year. Fertility control involves healthy subjects; however, the use of chemical agents for almost all the days of the female cycle is bound to cause physiological insults. In order to achieve the highest degree of user safety, stringent requirements for oral contraceptives have been described [2]. For example, an oral contraceptive should:

(i)   express an absolute specificity of action preferably by intercepting a discrete mechanism,
(ii)   cause a predictably low level of menstrual bleeding and possess a potential for regulating the timing of onset,
(iii)   possess 100% efficacy with a potential to be used at any time in the cycle,
(iv)   be devoid of life-threatening side effects,
(v)   be appropriate for use over many years, and at any stage from menarche to menopause,
(vi)   be reversible without resorting to any therapeutic measures,
(vii)   not compromise with the reproductive potential of the user,
(viii) maintain the endogenous levels of sex steroids within the safe and prophylactic window,
(ix)   be able to contribute to potential health care with respect to reproductive oncology, menstrual days, function, osteoporosis, well being and longevity.

It is beyond the purview of this article to initiate discussions on the merits and demerits of individual contraceptive pills in the light of these requirements but it is perhaps appropriate and essential to discuss the logistics of the use of contraceptive pills. The two main considerations which govern the logistics are: (1) the number of pills required per month to protect a female subject from unwanted pregnancies and (2) the cost involved to attain this objective. The step from a sequential steroidal pill to a once-a-week non-steroidal pill has been achieved [3], but is it adequate and does it not provoke the development of a "once-a-month pill"? Even if this envisaged pill is made available, what would it offer as distinct advantages over the existing pills and what should its desired profile of biological activity be? Besides these concerns, the envisaged once-a-month pill is a challenge to medicinal chemists and may provoke regulatory agencies to lay down special parameters for clinical studies. The emerging concept for the development of menses regulators, therefore, requires detailed analysis. Carl Djerassi [4] recommended the use of a "once-a-month pill" because it can be self-administered and is more suitable for short-term use without causing long-term side effects. This pill is intended for both pregnant and non-pregnant women and the onset of menses assures the users of their planned protection. The menses inducers, therefore, aim at agents for short-term use, the ideal situation being the use of one tablet per month. The opinion in favour of such tablet(s) has also come recently from the Human Reproduction Programme of the World Health Organisation [5].

In principle, a single tablet with a longer half-life in biophase may (depending on the day of administration) either interfere with the process of implantation, or may lead to the detachment of the embryo during the early stages of implantation, selectively interacting with trophoblast and/or utero-trophoblast junction and eliciting its contragestational activity. It is, therefore, important to understand the sequence of events in endometrium and blastocyst during the implantation and peri-implantation stages. Without going into the details of the biology of implantation, we shall discuss the changes which may be relevant for menses induction.

2 Preparation for implantation

The most pressing requirement for the implantation of the embryo in the wall of the uterus is the critical "synchrony" between the uterus and the embryo. This stage is described by events which make the endometrium "receptive" and embryos attain the expanded blastocyst stage. The driving forces for endometrial receptivity are the levels of endogenous hormones, mainly estrogen and progesterone, which fluctuate from the pre-sensitive to the sensitive stage of the uterus. Since the uterine receptivity is a transitory phase, the blastocyst has to implant during this period, otherwise the uterus may change to the "refractory stage" [6–8]. In spite of these critical requirements, the implantation process is not an isolated event; it represents a complex sequence of events which has to be understood from morphological, physiological and biochemical perspectives.

Morphologically, the attachment of embryos to the uterine epithelium happens in two phases, apposition and adhesion [9]. Apposition is the progressive intimacy of contact between trophoblast and uterine epithelium. During this phase interdigitation of microvilli and an intimate association between the membranes of blastocyst and endometrium occur. The adhesion in rodents begins on the antimesometrial side of the uterus [10–12], while in some higher species the "trophoblastic knobs" lying over the embryonic cell mass occupy the mesometrial area [13, 14].

The exact biochemical or molecular basis of apposition, clasping and attachment of the embryo has not been worked out but the available information does indicate the involvement of progesterone and estrogen [15–17]. Endocrine-dependent absorption of fluid from the lumen by way of irregular (large) cytoplasmic projections termed as "pinopods" and estrogen-induced mild edema of the endometrium are almost accepted events [18–20].

In order to understand the molecular basis of adhesion of the trophoblast, one has searched for cell surface glycoconjugates and extracellular cell adhesion molecules on the surface of peri-implantation blastocyst and uterine epithelium. The changes in the constitution of glycocalyx of the apical surface of uterine epithelial cells during this period have been extensively studied [21]. There is a loss of anionic sites and reduction in the thickness of uterine glycocalyx at the time of implantation in mouse [22, 23], rat [24, 25], rabbit [26] and primates [27], and the uterine epithelium develops the capacity to bind certain lectins indicating changes in carbohydrate residues of cell surface glycoconjugates [28–32]. Extensive biochemical analysis has revealed uterine production of specific classes of glycoconjugates, including hyaluronate [33], lactosaminoglycans and galactosyl-transferases [24, 34–40] and heparansulphate proteoglycans and their binding proteins [41–45]. It is noteworthy that molecules of extracellular matrix such as laminin, collagen and fibronectin involved in cell adhesion mechanisms are conspicuously absent from the apical surface of uterine epithelium.

Changes in surface molecules of trophoblasts have also been observed at the time of embryo attachment. Immunocytochemical evidences [46–48] reveal that laminin is present as early as the two-cell stage and is found in areas of contact between the cells at the 8- to 16-cell stage of the embryo. Immunohistochemical methods have indicated the presence of cell adhesion molecules CAM 120/80, uvomorulin [51, 52] and cadhedrin [53] in mouse embryos as early as the two-cell stage. The cell adhesion molecule CAM-105 has been reported to be expressed on the surface of the early blastocyst and it is believed that it plays a dominant role in embryo-uterine interaction during implantation [54]. It is known that cell-cell adhesion requires interactions between galactosyltransferase and multivalent lactosaminoglycans [55]. The presence of galactosyltransferase and lactosaminoglycans in the 4- to 8-cell stage of the mouse embryo indicates the role of these cell adhesion systems in implantation. A specific heparansulfate/chondroitin sulfate containing membrane proteoglycan has been detected on the surface of embryos from the 4-cell to early blastocyst stage [56].

The available evidence from immunological studies indicates that appearance of individual glycoconjugate on the apical surface of the uterine epithelium induces a highly specific ligand-receptor recognition mechanism for the attachment of the embryo to the uterine surface [22, 23, 31, 40].

Attachment of the blastocyst on the uterus is followed by the penetration of the trophoblast into the uterine epithelium. This process of penetration varies from species to species and can be broadly classified into three groups, namely intrusive, displacement and fusion penetrations. In intrusive penetration, the embryos are highly invasive and the species involved in this process are guinea pig [57–59] and rhesus monkey [60]. Rat [61] and mouse [62] display the mechanism of displacement penetration, and as the apposition proceeds, the first sign of decidualization appears in the adjacent stroma following the death or detachment of epithelial cells which occur either singly or in groups. The mechanism responsible for the death and detachment of epithelial cells is, however, not known. The rabbit [57, 63–65] furnishes the example for fusion penetration. The apical membrane of the epithelial cells fuses with the trophoblastic knobs which slowly change to syncitium to look like pegs, and there may be more than one peg per trophoblastic knob.

3   Peri-implantation secretory changes

Analysis of the peri-implantation secretory products and their relevance in the physiology of reproduction would enable to identify the possible biochemical target sites for developing menses inducers. Attention has, therefore, been focussed on secretory proteins, endometrial cytokines, histamine and prostaglandin release and finally on the influence of uterine environment on the blastocyst development. Unlike pituitary, prolactin in human endometrium is not stored as secretory granules, and the mechanism responsible for the regulation of endometrial secretions and release is not the same as observed with pituitary [66–68]. The endometrial prolactin possibly facilitates electrolyte exchange across the chorioamnion where the existence of appropriate receptors has been demonstrated [69, 70]. Another secretory protein of human endometrium is 29 KD α_1-globulin (α_1-PEG) which is found in pre-decidual cells but appears after implantation. This protein is considered to be the main insulin-like growth factor-1 (IGF-1) binding protein [71–75]. Besides α_1-PEG, the presence of another dimeric protein, α_2-PEG, and its function as transporting protein is documented [69, 76–79].

The major secretory protein in mouse is lactotransferin, and its production is markedly increased to estrogen stimuli [80]. Uteroferrin is a progesterone-induced iron-binding glycoprotein secreted by the pig endometrium after implantation [81]. Uteroglobin is the pregnancy-specific secretory protein of the rabbit endometrium which is capable of binding with progesterone, inhibits trypsin activity and blocks the antigenicity of the blastocyst and sperm (*in vitro*) [82–89]. Diamine oxidase has been detected in proliferative and secretory human endometrium and significantly increases during the first trimester of pregnancy [90]. It is also reported to be present in uteri of pregnant hamsters and rats [91–94]. Interest for this enzyme arose because of its association with the changes in accumulation, synthesis and degradation of putrescine, spermidine and spermine in the early placenta [76].

Cell proliferation, differentiation, reorganization and recruitment of cells from the bone marrow during embryo implantation and decidualization have prompted to look for endometrial cytokines. The role of IL-6 in the regulation of local changes within the human uterus at the time of implantation is significant. Human trophoblast cells have receptors for IL-6, and in response to this cytokine as well as gonadotropin-releasing hormone, the release of hCG occurs [95]. The role of interferon in peri-implantation events has also been investigated. In humans the epithelial receptors for interferon-γ remain constant but the localized variations in hormone-dependent expression of histocompatibility complex HLA-DR molecules occur [96]. The interferon-γ is produced by the activated T cells within the endometrium and these have estrogen receptors [97].

4   *In vitro* studies on implantation-related events

The understanding of the events related to implantation is not restricted to *in vivo* studies alone since efforts have also been made to understand these events with the help of *in vitro* studies [99–102]. It would be, therefore, pertinent to overview the results obtained from these studies. Mouse uterine tissue strips obtained after days 5–7 of pregnancy have been used to culture the blastocyst [103]. Attempts have also been made to use monolayers of uterine cells in culture dishes on which blastocysts are seeded [104, 105]. The uterine cells have been reported to permit the spreading of trophoblasts covering the blastocyst, and this process has been described as implantation *in vitro* [106]. The method, however, had been a subject of debate since the type of cells used was not identified as pure epithelial or stromal or mixed [107]. Adhesiveness of the blastocyst to the living epithelial cells in suspension could not be demonstrated even after placing them together for several days [108]. However, this could be made possible only when the epithelial cells were allowed to form aggregates which in turn developed sheets of epithelium rolling into vesicles having an original luminal surface exposed [109]. The invasive nature and contact inhibiting ability of trophoblasts have been studied in detail. Glass et al. reported the non-adhesive nature of trophoblasts to other cells [110, 111] but not with the non-living objects like glass or petriplate since they adhere to these surfaces [112, 113]. In an alternate method trophoblasts are allowed to grow on the cell matrix containing heparan sulphate proteoglycan [114–116] or hydrated gels [117, 118]. This not only promotes adhesion but helps in differentiation of these cells *in vitro*. Although the attachment and outgrowth of trophoblast on extra-cellular matrix correspond with *in vivo* developmental changes, there is a lack of progressive interaction between the embryo and the endometrium [119–121]. In another modified *in vitro* method [122], blastocysts are grown on membrane filters coated with Engelbreth Holm Swarm cells (EHS) laden with uterine epithelial cells [123]. However, this culture system did not progress well either. In yet another improved method, mouse trophoblast and uterine endometrial stromal cells of same gestation age are cultured together in hanging droplets. The aim of this is to examine their interaction during culture, an analogous situation these cells face *in vivo* during attachment and further development. It has been reported that embryonic and maternal cells maintain their growth and proliferation longer (for 120 h) in this method [124].

These *in vitro* studies unquestionably represent bold attempts to understand trophoblast-uterine cell interactions under *in vitro* conditions but they have failed to identify any cell-specific biochemical marker which could help in the design of menses inducers.

5   Screening methods for identifying menses inducers

5.1   *In vitro* assay

Since the early eighties *in vitro* assays using mostly 4–8-cell-embryos or early-stage blastocysts have been reported. For example, cadmium chloride, teratogenic to embryo [125–127], arrested trophoblastic outgrowth and reduced the number of giant cell formation when injected in culture medium containing rat blastocyst [128]. *In vitro* effect of an anti-estrogen (CI-628) in culture has been assayed to examine its effect on the embryo for implantation. The drug drastically reduced the implantation rate from 83% to 13% [129]. The same compound is also reported to prevent expansion of mouse blastocyst *in vitro* [130]. A similar assay of another anti-estrogen 'Nafoxidine' has also been reported [131, 132]. Pre-implantation monkey embryo has also been used for in vitro assay to evaluate the effect of RU-486, an antiprogestational agent. At 10^{-7} M concentration it was not found detrimental to the survival of the embryo [133].

Since the pregnancy interceptive agents or the menses regulators may also influence the development of either trophoblasts or the maternal cells (epithelial and stromal) at the embryo attachment site, another *in vitro* assay method using trophoblast cells of hamster and mouse isolated from a preplacental organelle, the ectoplacental cone, has been developed [124, 134]. In this assay growth, proliferation and giant cell formation are considered as markers for determining the efficacy of pregnancy interceptive agents.

5.2   *In vivo* assay

The animals used in an *in vivo* pregnancy interceptive assay, among the rodent species, are rat, hamster, mouse and guinea pig, and among higher animal species, including infrahuman primates, are beagle bitch, rhesus monkey and baboon.

The multiple-day treatment in lower animals varies from 3–8 or 4–8 days of pregnancy in hamster [134, 135] and mouse [136], to 5–10 and 6–10 days of pregnancy in guinea pig and rat [137, 138]. In the case of single administration, the optimal day of pregnancy is day 4 in hamster [139], day 5 in mouse [140] and day 7 in rat [141]. The treated animals are laparotomized 5–6 days after the completion of treatment, when using the multiple-day schedule [142], and 8–10 days after when on the single administration schedule, and are examined for live/dead fetuses, resorption sites or pregnancy scars [143]. The efficacy is determined by counting the number of animals showing partial to complete effect out of a total number of animals treated with the test substance [144].

The multiple-day schedule in the case of beagle bitch runs from days 18–24 of pregnancy and in single day administration it is day 20 of pregnancy [145]. The effect of the test substance is determined on days 35–45 of pregnancy. However, in rhesus monkey and baboon the multiple-day schedule goes from days 16–21 and days 35–44 of pregnancy, respectively. The effect is analyzed two months after the treatment in both species [146, 147].

6   Possible biochemical target sites for developing menses inducers

The search for menses inducers is still at an exploratory stage. The mechanism by which these inducers may intercept pregnancy is linked to the time/period of their administration. A pill after coitus which is capable of intercepting pregnancy till menses is induced, is one possibility; the administration of a pill 5–6 days before the expected date of menses and capable of inducing menstruation, whether or not pregnancy has occurred, represents the second possibility. The pill after coitus may help to identify biochemical target sites different from the ones identified for the pill 5–6 days before menses. Pregnancy interceptive agents developed on the basis of the first possibility require a significantly long half-life in the biophase and the mechanism of interception would probably be concerned with the prevention of implantation. Subjects who do not want an abortion of the fetus may be happy with such interceptive agents. Menses inducers developed on the basis of the second possibility need not exhibit a long half-life but their possible site of action is likely to be the uteroplacental junction and, therefore, may not appeal to those who dislike abortion. The likely biochemical target sites involved in both possibilities are:

a)   Prevention of endometrial preparations for the blastocyst attachment,
b)   Alteration of the physicochemical environment of the uterus to prevent implantation,
c)   Interference with the functions of the utero-placental junction for facilitating detachment/resorption of the implanted blastocyst.

Prevention of blastocyst attachment to the uterus, in principle, is possible either by changing the carbohydrate chemistry of the cell surface glycoconjugates or by interfering with the biosynthesis of these glycoconjugates. Unfortunately, these approaches are conceptual and no definite experimental evidence exists for providing a molecular basis for the development of menses inducers. Alteration of the physicochemical environment of the uterus may be evoked directly or indirectly. While it is possible to believe that an interceptive agent would selectively prevent the penetration of the trophoblast, it is also possible that alteration in secretory proteins or immunological disturbances may help to achieve the desired objective. The interference with pregnancy-specific proteins has been demonstrated [148, 149] but the desired modulation of the immune apparatus exclusively at the uterus has yet to be demonstrated. For example, in rabbit, uteroglobin, a pregnancy-specific endometrial protein, is believed to sequester progesterone. Since this protein has a specific binding affinity towards progesterone any compound which can compete with progesterone for the binding sites will exhibit antiprogestational activity. It was found that non-steroidal compounds such as diaryl ketones (I) are able to elicit such a biological response and compounds structurally related to these can even bring changes in the conformation of pregnancy-specific proteins [149]. The largest amount of experimental work in the search for menses inducers relates to the interference with the physiology of the utero-placental junction.

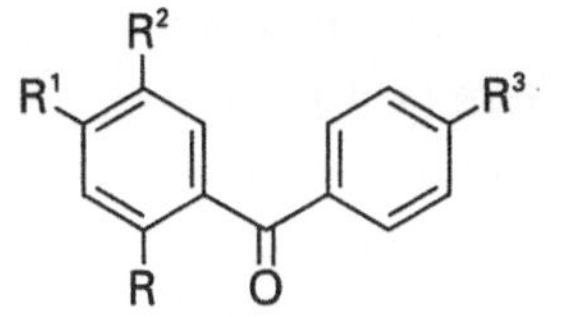

I R = OH, Me
R^1 = OMe
R^2 = H, Me
R^3 = H, Me, OMe

The search for menses inducers

Post-implantation contragestational agents are both steroidal and non-steroidal in nature. Progesterone is the most essential hormone required for successful initiation and maintenance of pregnancy. Agents exhibiting a antagonistic property towards progesterone may also elicit a menses-inducing property. The antiprogestational compound may cause disturbance in the hypothalamus-pituitary-gonadal-adrenal axis or may directly interfere with progesterone receptors at the uteroplacental junction. The post-implantation contragestational progesterone antagonists of importance are:

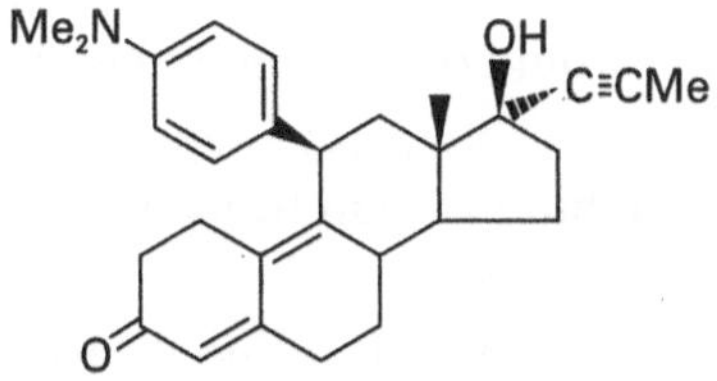

RU-486 (Mifepristone)

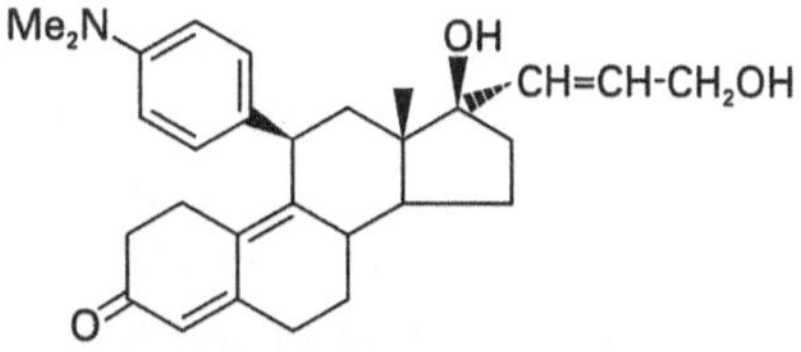

ZK-734 (Lilopristone)

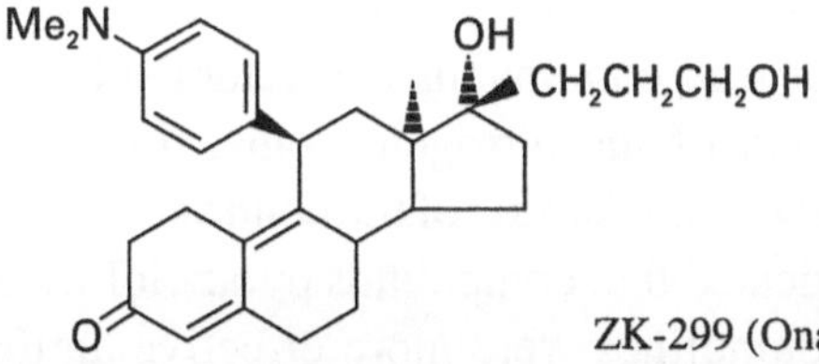

ZK-299 (Onapristone)

RU-486 discovered during the search for antiglucocorticoid activity, is being marked as the post-coital pill. In cases of established pregnancy, a single dose of 600 mg of RU-486, followed by 1 mg of gemprost (a prostaglandin) induces abortion in 97.4% cases [5]. The mechanism of RU-486 has already been discussed in detail elsewhere [150].

The search for non-steroidal contraceptive agents commenced in the mid-seventies when workers from Lepetit Research Laboratories first reported [151] the antifertility action of 2-(3-methoxyphenyl)-5H-triazolo-[5,1-α]-isoindole (L-10492] and 2-(3-methoxyphenyl)-5,6-dihydro-triazolo[5,1-α]isoquinoline (L 10503).

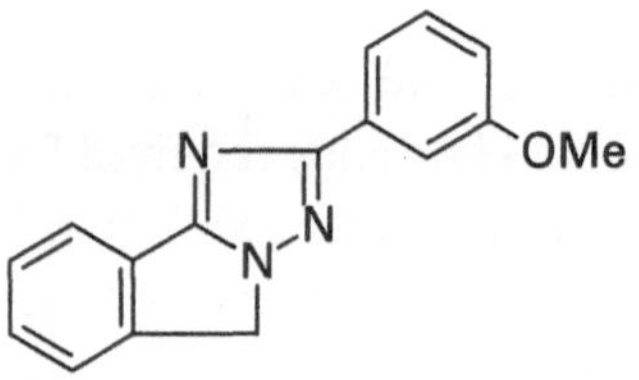

L 10492 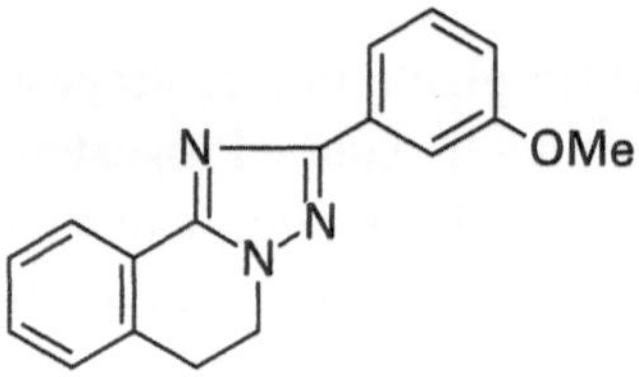   L 10503

This group of workers was exploring the possibility of developing compounds which may inhibit prostaglandin (PG) metabolism, thereby leading to an elevated level of PG [152]. This situation would be detrimental to the placental physiology and may thus help in intercepting pregnancy. The initial results inspired them to undertake an ambitious plan to synthesize and evaluate the contragestational efficacy of nitrogen heterocycles. The heterocycles which attracted their attention are described in Fig. 1 [153–157].

The compounds belonging to the pyrazolo[5,1-a]isoindole (IX) pyrazolo[5,1-a]isoquinoline (VI) triazolo[5,1-a]isoindoles (XII), triazolo[5,1-a]isoquinoline (XIV) and their open chain analogs (XIII and XV) exhibited promising pregnancy interceptive activity. Studies were directed towards optimizing the biological activity of lead compounds and establishing the influence of the number and position of the nitrogen atoms; this led to syntheses of analogs of these heterocycles. Analysis of the contragestational efficacy of various heterocycles indicated that compounds pyrazolo[5,1-a]-indoles and the pyrazolo[5,1-a]isoquinolines were more effective antifertility agents.

The most potent compound was obtained when a double bond was introduced between positions 5 and 6 in pyrazolo [5,1-a]isoquinoline [158]. The presence of a phenyl group in pyrazolo [5,1-a]isoquinoline (XVI) was found to be essential for the activity since its replacement with a methyl group

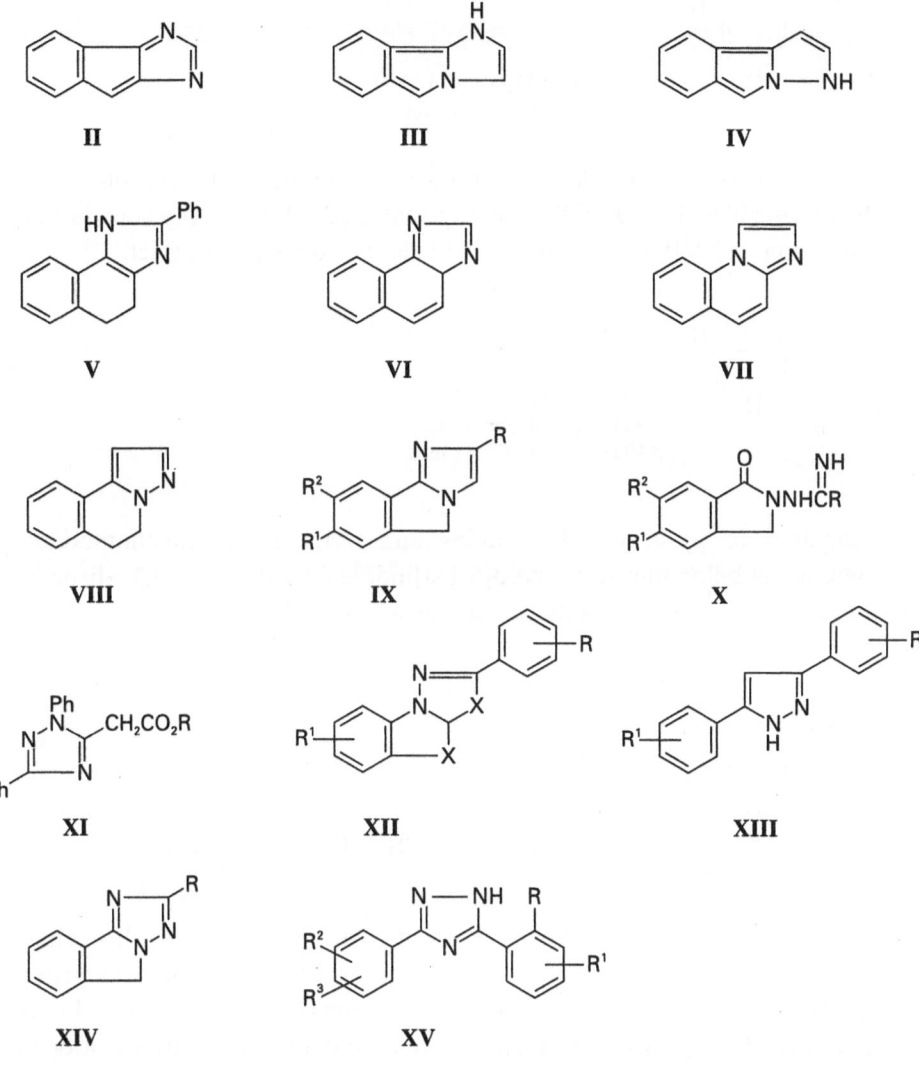

Fig. 1

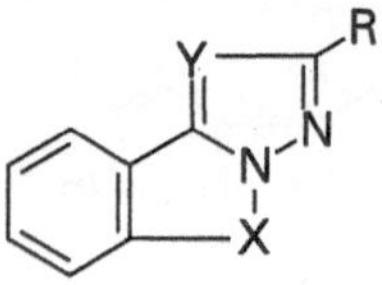

X = CH, CH$_2$–CH$_2$, CH = CH
Y = CH, C–CH$_2$OH, C–CO$_2$H
R = Me, substituted phenyl

(XVII) led to complete loss of antifertility activity. Substitution in the phenyl ring also decreased the contragestational efficacy. Any substitution at position 4 (XVIII) of the pyrazole nucleus had a similar effect.

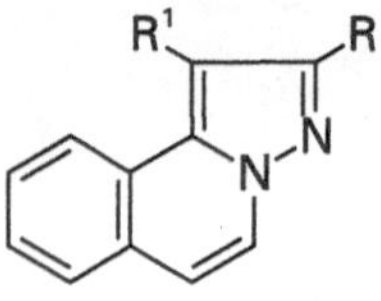

XVI   R = Ph, R^1 = H
XVII R = Me, R^1 = H
XVIII R = Ph, R^1 = Me

Compared to pyrazolo[5,1-a]indoles and pyrazolo[5,1-a]isoquinolines, compounds belonging to triazolo[5,1-a]indoles and triazolo[5,1-a]isoquinolines (XIX) exhibited better contragestational efficacy.

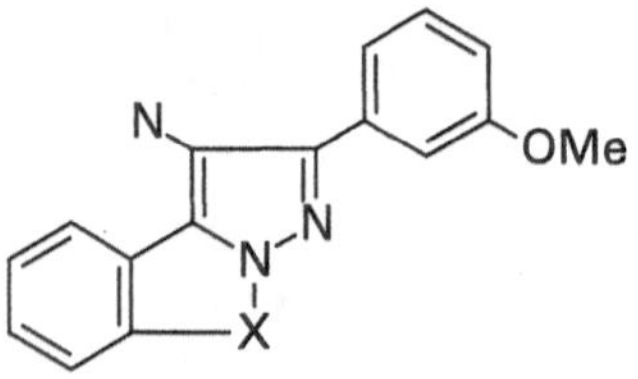

XIX   X = CH$_2$, CH$_2$–CH$_2$, CH = CH

In this class of compounds a phenyl ring at position 3 of the triazole nucleus is an essential feature for activity. The presence of a meta-methoxy group significantly increased the potency of triazoles (XIX). However, lower solubility of tricyclics even in an oily vehicle led to the synthesis of open chain analogs (XX and XXI) of pyrazolo[5,1-a]isoquinolines and triazolo[5,1-a]isoquinolines.

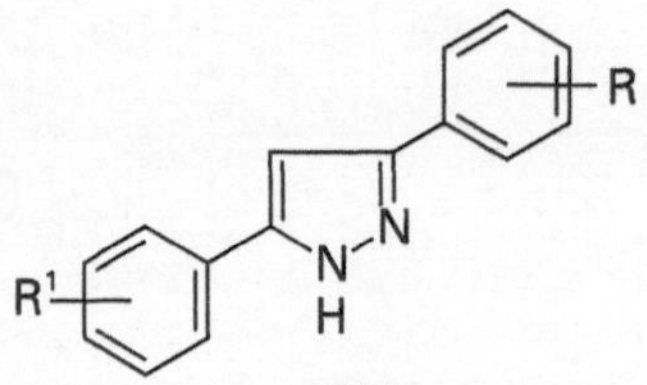

XX

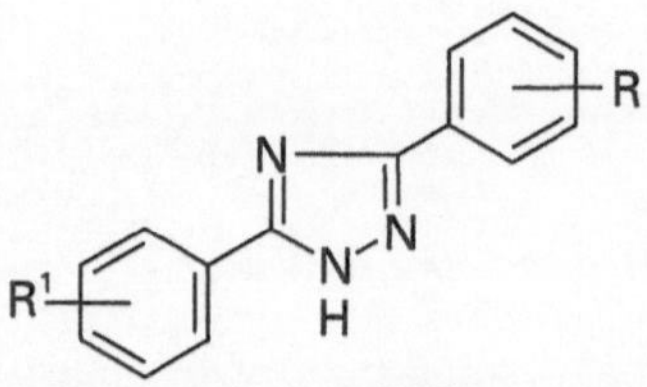

XXI

During the course of this study it was found that the contragestational effect of open-chain pyrazoles were the same as compared to their corresponding tricyclic derivatives but the structural modifications in triazoles produced more active compounds than triazolo[5,1-a]isoquinolines and they exhibited better solubility in oily vehicles [159]. It was observed that in this class of compounds substituents such as methyl, ethyl and hydroxymethyl at the ortho position of the phenyl ring attached to the position 3 of the triazole ring evoked better contragestational activity. The potency was maximum for the ethyl group but decreased with the elongation or branching of the alkyl chain. Another methyl group at the ortho position of this ethyl group evoked a marked increase in biological response. In the other phenyl ring attached to position 5 of the triazole, the presence of a meta-alkoxy group is an essential requirement for biological activity. The number of carbon atoms in this alkoxy group do not influence the activity since analogs with methoxy and ethoxy groups were equipotent. Although the presence of a para-methoxy group in the phenyl ring made the derivative 3-fold less potent than its corresponding meta-methoxy analog, a comparable activity to the most potent compound of this series was obtained with 3,4-dimethoxy or 3,4-methylenedioxy derivatives. The potent compounds selected for detailed study were DL 111-IT and DL 204-IT.

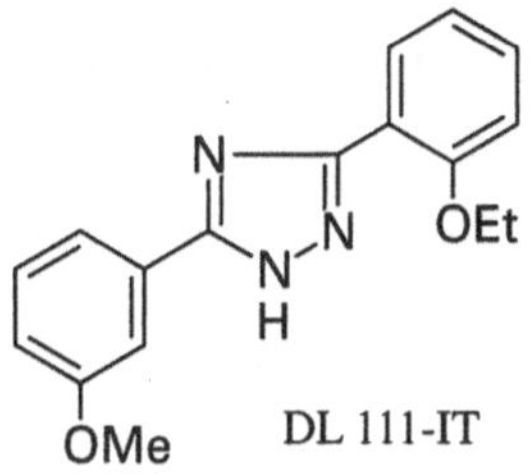

DL 111-IT 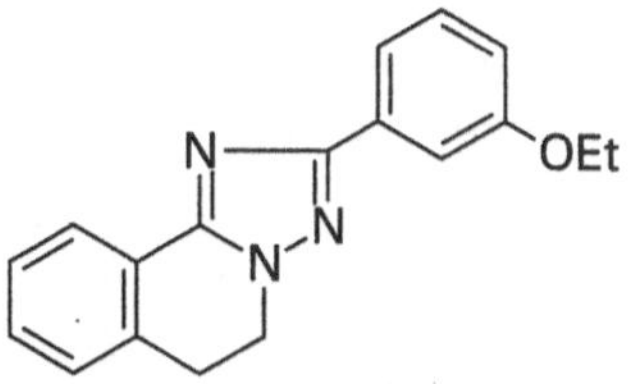   DL 204-IT

The highlights of the detailed studies [143] carried out with these compounds are:

i)   The compounds did not exhibit any implantation-preventing efficacy and the time at which these compounds elicited maximum biological response was the early post-implantation period. The contragestational activity decreased as the pregnancy progressed.

ii) Standard biochemical assays revealed these compounds to be devoid of estrogenic, anti-estrogenic, progestational, antiprogestational, androgenic or anti-androgenic activity even at higher dose than the contraceptive doses.

iii)   The compounds did not disturb the hypothalamo-pituitary-gonadal-adrenal axis.

iv)   No antagonistic action of progesterone on contragestational activity of these compounds was observed.

v)   No interference with prostaglandins, no alteration in the placental hemodynamics and no cytotoxicity of these compounds were recorded.

vi)   The compounds caused selective degradation of decidual cells, increased the number of progesterone receptors and decreased the ornithine decarboxylase (ODC) activity in the blastocyst. It was suggested that these compounds interfere with the chain of events by which progesterone regulates the mitotic activity of decidual and trophoblast cells necessary for the placenta to achieve morphological and functional maturity [143].

The significant contributions from Galliani et al., however, did not reveal the fate of isomeric 4H-1,2,4-triazoles as pregnancy-interceptive agents. It was not clear whether replacement of one nitrogen atom with another ' heteroatom in triazoles would lead to altered contragestational activity. In order to answer these questions, the pregnancy-interceptive activity of triazoles, oxadiazoles and thiadiazoles was evaluated [160, 161]. The results in table 1 reveal that the isomeric 4H-triazoles were less active than 1H-triazoles; oxadiazoles were less potent than triazoles and thiadiazoles were inactive.

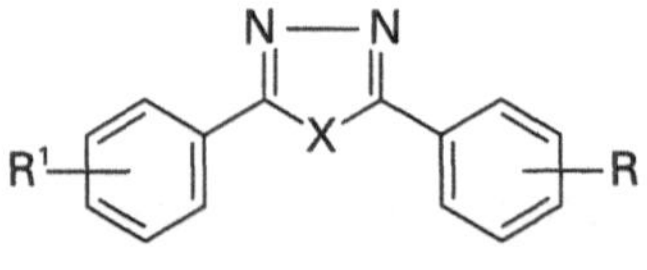

XXII X = NH
XXIII X = O
XXIV X = S

The contragestational activity of other heterocycles such as furans (XXV), isoxazoles (XXVI) and isoxazolones (XVII, XVIII) revealed potential of 5(2H)-isoxazolone derivatives (XXVIII) (Table I) [162, 163]. However, the isomeric 5(4H)-isoxazolones (XXVII) were inactive. These results indicated the need of the nitrogen atom(s) in a five-membered heterocyclic system to evoke pregnancy-interceptive activity.
Contragestational efficacy of six-membered heterocycles with one or more nitrogen atoms such as 1,4-dihydropyridine (XXIX) and pyridazine deriva-

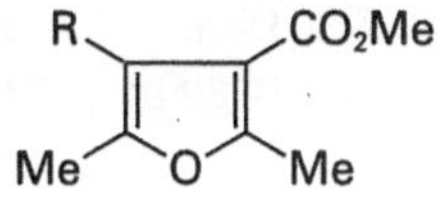

XXV

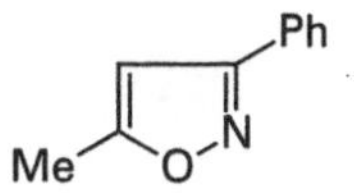

XXVI

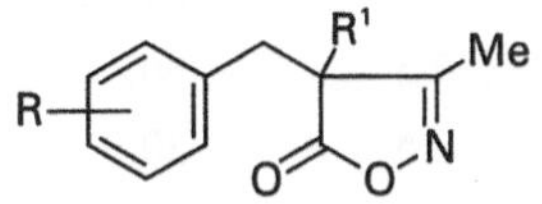

XXVII

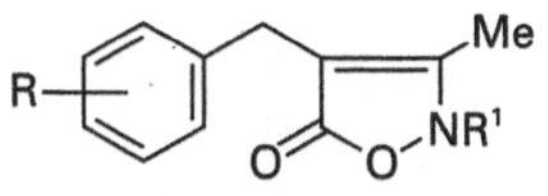

XXVIII

Table 1.
Five-membered heterocycles exhibiting pregnancy-terminating activity in hamsters

Structure		Dose (mg/kg)	Fetal resorption (% of animals)

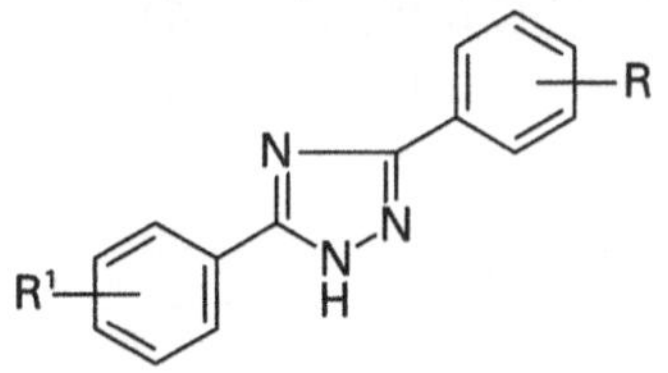

	R	R^1		
1.	2-Me	3-OMe	2.5	60
2.	2-Et	3-OMe	5.0	100
3.	3-Me	3,4-(OMe)$_2$	2.5	100
4.	2,5-Me$_2$	3-OMe	2.5	60
5.	4-Me	3-OMe	2.5	60

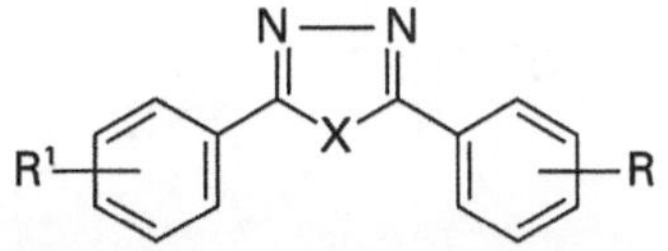

	R	R^1	X		
6.	2-Et	3-OMe	NH	2.5	80
7.	3-Me	3-Me	NH	2.5	50
8.	2-Me	3-Me	NH	2.5	60
9.	3,4-(OMe)$_2$	3,4-(OMe)$_2$	NH	5.0	50
10.	2-Me	2-Me	O	5.0	50

Structure			Dose (mg/kg)	Fetal resorption (% of animals)
11.	3-Me	3-Me	O	2.5	70
12.	4-Me	4-Me	O	7.5	88
13.	4-Me	2-OH	O	7.5	50
14.	H	H	S	7.5	50
14a. 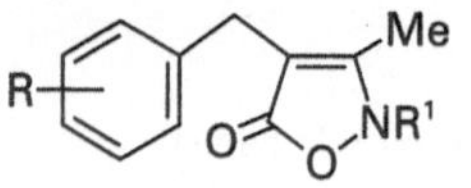	3,4-(OMe)$_2$	3,4-(OMe)$_2$	S	5.0	80

	R	R^1		
15.	Naphtyl	H	10.0	70
16.	H	Me	10.0	80
17.	H	Et	10.0	60
18.	4-Me	Et	10.0	60
19.	3,4-(OMe)$_2$	Et	10.0	100
20.	3,4-OCH$_2$O	COMe	10.0	60
21.	4-OMe	COMe	10.0	75
22.	4-OMe	CO$_2$Me	10.0	100
23.	3,4-(OMe)$_2$	CO$_2$Me	10.0	100
24.	H	CH$_2$CH$_2$CO$_2$Et	10.0	80

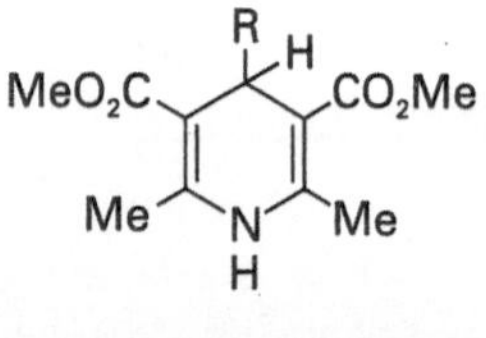

XXIX

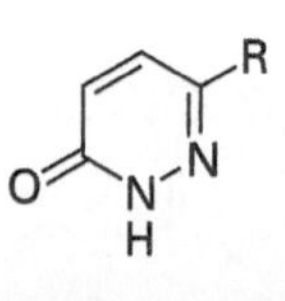

XXX

tives (XXX) has been evaluated [142, 162]. Of these only dihydropyridine derivatives evoked a potent contragestational effect (Table 2). A variety of linearly annealed heterocycles such as dihydroquinoline (XXXI) and imidazolo[1,2-a]pyridine (XXXII) [137, 164] have also been evaluated as pregnancy interceptive agents. The most potent compounds amongst these were 3-amino-6,7-dimethoxy[3,4-d]quinoline (XXXIII) which was found

to be effective both in rodent and primate models [134], and 3-hydroxy-
furo[2,3-a]furo[2,3-b]quinoline-2-carboxamide (XXXIV).

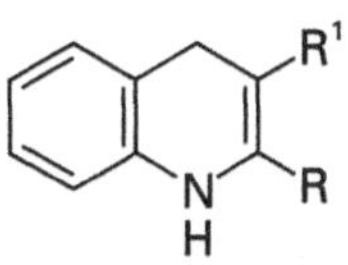

XXXI

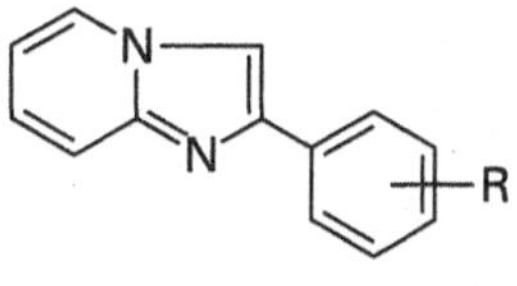

XXXII

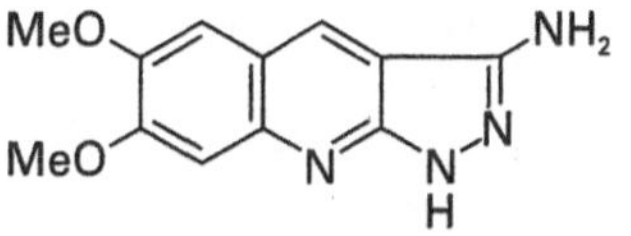

XXXIII

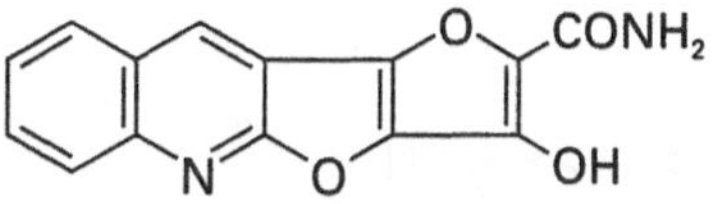

XXXIV

Table 2.
Six-membered and other heterocycles exhibiting pregnancy-terminating activity in hamsters

Structures	Dose (mg/kg)	Fetal resorption (% of animals)
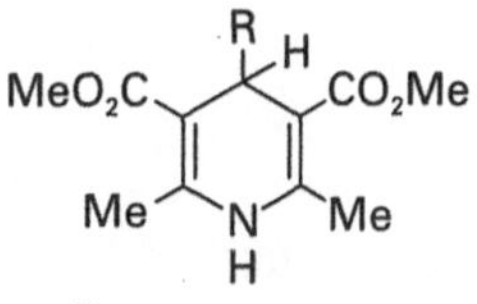 R		
1. 4-Acetamido phenyl	10.0	83
2. 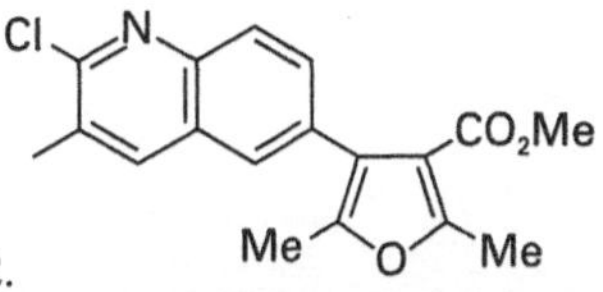	10.0	100
3. 3-Nitro-4-chlorophenyl-	10.0	60
4. 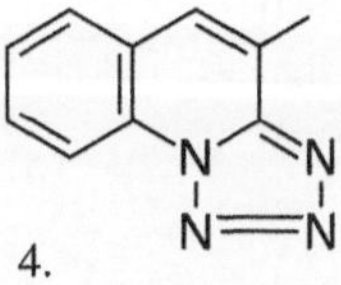	10.0	66

Structures	Dose (mg/kg)	Fetal resorption (% of animals)
5. (3-methyl-2-chloroquinoline)	10.0	100
6. (H H OHOH / OHOHH H —CH₂OH)	10.0	100
7. (3-CN, 2-SMe dihydroquinoline)	10.0	80
8. (3-CN, 2-oxo dihydroquinoline)	10.0	100

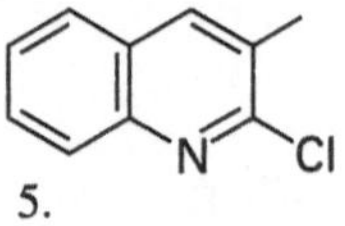

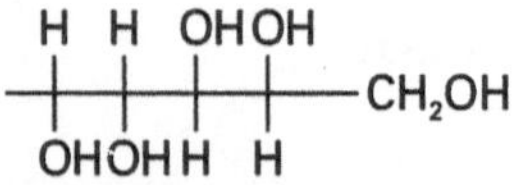

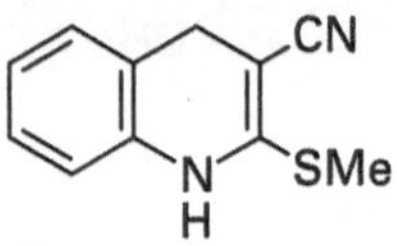

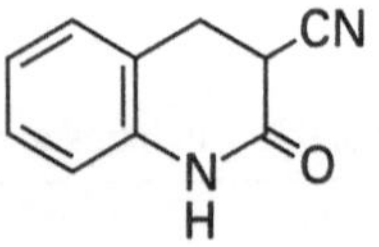

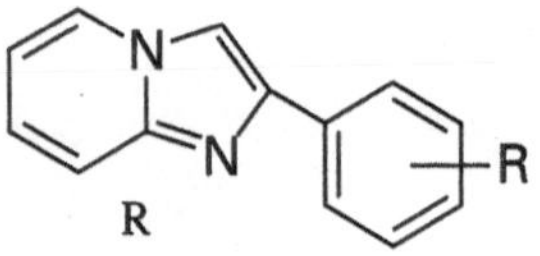

$$\text{6.} \quad \overset{\text{H H OH OH}}{\underset{\text{OH OH H H}}{|\,|\,|\,|}}\text{—CH}_2\text{OH}$$

Structures	R	R¹	Dose (mg/kg)	Fetal resorption (% of animals)
9.	3-OH		3.5	100
10.	4-Cl		10.0	75
11.	OMe	Me	7.5	50
12.	OMe	NH₂	10.0	100
13.	H	Ph	10.0	50
14. 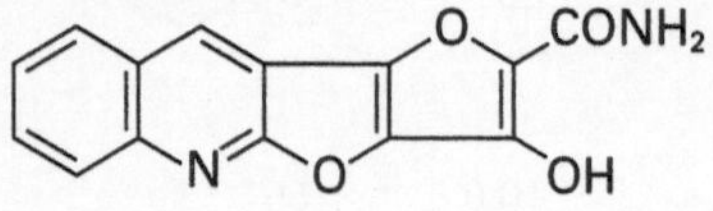	H	N = CMe₂	10.0	80
16.			15.0	100

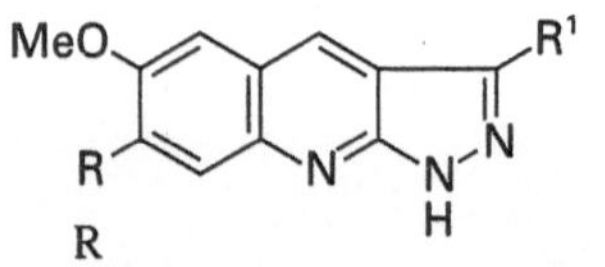

8   Conclusion

An orally effective once-a-month pill as menses inducer is going to be the future choice for avoiding unwanted pregnancies. It is difficult to envisage the chemical nature of the first candidate compound which would exhibit unquestionable clinical efficacy since the prospects for both steroidal and non-steroidal compounds are evenly weighed. Immediate research inputs required for successful development of menses inducers are: identification of biochemical markers which, besides facilitating *in vitro* screening of pregnancy interceptive activity, would also guarantee a correlation of *in vitro* and *in vivo* contragestational efficacy of test compounds. The second input relates to the identification of pharmacophores which after oral administration would direct the test compounds to the uterus in concentrations adequate to intercept pregnancy. The search for exact biochemical target site(s) affected by compounds exhibiting a contragestational effect in experimental animals represents the third input.

Identification of the "hit compound" for the desired biological activity, amongst compounds representing molecular diversity may become possible with this help of combinatorial technology [165]. Since interception of pregnancy is possible by intervening the immunological status of the uterus, a combinatorial approach to discovering a new class of menses inducers should be possible after ascertaining the correct bioassay system. The present century is likely to end with exciting developments in this area, and the early part of the next century may see the dawn of the development of a once-a-month pill.

References

1   C. Djerassi: Science *169*, 941 (1970).
2   D. W. Lincoln: Br. Med. Bull. *49* (1), 224 (1993).
3   V. P. Kamboj, S. Ray and B. N. Dhawan: Drugs of Today *28* (4), 227 (1992). .
4   C. Djerassi: Science *245*, 356 (1989).
5   M. F. Fathalla. In: Challanges in reproductive health research, p. 75. Eds. J. Khanna, P. F. A. Vanlook and P. D. Griffin, W.H.O. Geneva (1994).
6   A. Psychoyos: Ciba Foundation study group on egg implantation, p 4. Churchill, London (1966).
7   A. Psychoyos: Vitamins Horm. *31*, 201 (1973).
8   A. Psychoyos: J. Reprod. Fertil. *25* Suppl., 17 (1976).
9   S. R. Glasser and S. A. McCormack: Endocrinology *104*, 1112 (1979).

180　　　　P.K. Mehrotra, Sanjay Batra and A.P. Bhaduri

10　　R. L. Gardner, V. E. Papaioannou and S. C. Barton: J. Embryol. Exp. Morphol. *30*, 561
　　　(1973).
11　　S. Tachi, C. Tachi and H. R. Lindner: J. Reprod. Fertil. *21*, 37 (1970).
12　　T. A. Parkening: J. Anat. *122*, 211 (1976).
13　　M. Knoth and J. F. Larsen: Acta Obstet. Gynec. Scand. *51*, 385 (1972).
14　　J. F. Larsen: Prog. Reprod. Biol. *7*, 284 (1980).
15　　L. Martin, C. A. Finn and J. Carter: J. Reprod. Fertil. *21*, 461 (1970).
16　　K. Hedlund and O. Nilsson: J. Reprod. Fertil. *26*, 267 (1971).
17　　R. M. Pollard and C. A. Finn: J. Endocrinol. *55*, 293 (1972).
18　　A. C. Enders and D. M. Nelson: Am. J. Anat. *138*, 277 (1973).
19　　F. Leroy, J. VanHoeck and C. Bogaert: J. Reprod. Fertil. *47*, 59 (1976).
20　　M. B. Parr and E. L. Parr: Biol. Reprod. *11*, 220 (1974).
21　　A. C. Enders and S. Schlafke: Anat. Rec. *180*, 31 (1974).
22　　D. J. Chavez and T. L. Anderson: Biol. Reprod. *32*, 1135 (1985).
23　　D. J. Chavez, in: Trophoblast Invasion and Endometrium Receptivity: Novel Aspects
　　　of the Cell Biology of Embryo Implantation. Trophoblast Res *4*, p. 259. Eds. H. Denker
　　　and J. D. Aplin (1990).
24　　K. Hewitt, A. E. Beer and F. Grinnel: Biol. Reprod. *21*, 691 (1979).
25　　A. C. Enders, S. Schlafke and A. O. Welsh: Am. J. Anat. *159*, 59 (1980).
26　　T. L. Anderson and L. H. Hoffman: Am. J. Anat. *171*, 321 (1984).
27　　T. L. Anderson, J. A. Simon and G. D. Hodgen, in: Trophoblast Invasion and En-
　　　dometrium Receptivity: Novel Aspects of the Cell Biology of Embryo Implantation.'
　　　Trophoblast Res. *4*, p 273. Eds. H. Denker and J. D. Aplin. (1990).
28　　S. A. Lampelo, A. P. Ricketts and D. W. Bullock: J. Reprod Fertil. *75*, 475 (1985).
29　　B. P. Nalbach and H. W. Denker: Eur. J. Cell Biol. *4* (Suppl), 13 (1983).
30　　A. Bukers, N. J. Friedrich, B. P. Nalbach and H. W. Denker, in: Trophoblast Invasion
　　　and Endometrial Receptivity: Novel Aspects of the Cell Biology of Embryo Implan-
　　　tation. Trophoblast Res. *4*, p 285. Eds. H. Denker and J. D. Aplin (1990).
31　　T. L. Anderson, G. E. Olson and L. H. Hoffman: Biol. Reprod. *34*, 701 (1986).
32　　L. H. Hoffman, V. P. Winfrey, T. L. Anderson and G. E. Olson, in: Trophoblast Invasion
　　　and Endometrial Receptivity: Novel Aspects of Cell Biology of Embryo Implantation.
　　　Trophoblast Res. *4*, p 243. Eds. H. Denker and J. D. Aplin (1990).
33　　D. D. Carson, A. Dutt and J. P. Tang: Dev. Biol. *120*, 228 (1987).
34　　J. D. Nelson, J. J. Jato-Rodriguez and S. Mookerjee: Arch. Biochem. Biophys. *169*,
　　　181 (1975).
35　　A. Dutt, J. Tang and D. D. Carson: Dev. Biol. *119*, 27 (1987).
36　　A. Dutt, J. Tang and D. D. Carson: J. Biol. Chem. *263*, 2270 (1988).
37　　A. Dutt and D. D. Carson: J. Biol. Chem. *265*, 430 (1990).
38　　B. S. Babiarz and H. J. Hathaway: Biol. Reprod. *39*, 699 (1988).
39　　S. J. Timber, S. Lindenberg and A. Lundblad: J. Reprod. Immunol. *22*, 297 (1988).
40　　S. J. Timber and S. Lindenberg: J. Reprod. Fertil. *89*, 13 (1990).
41　　H. Munakata, M. Isemura and Z. Yosizawa: Int. J. Biochem. *17*, 1077 (1985).
42　　J. Tang, J. Julian, S. R. Glasser and D. D. Carson: J. Biol. Chem. *262*, 12832 (1987).
43　　J. E. Morris, S. W. Potter and G. Gaza-Bulseco: Endocrinology *122*, 242 (1988).
44　　J. E. Morris, S. W. Potter and G. Gaza-Bulseco: J. Biol. Chem. *263*, 4712 (1988).
45　　O. Wilson, A. L. Jacobs, S. Stewart and D. D. Carson: J. Cell. Physiol. *143*, 60 (1990).
46　　M. Dziadek and R. Timpl: Dev. Biol. *111*, 372 (1985).

47   I. Leivo, A. Vaheri, R. Timpl and J. Wartiovaara: Dev. Biol. *76*, 100 (1980).

48   T. Wu, Y. Wan and A. E. Chung: Dev. Biol. *100*, 496 (1983).

49   J. Richa, C. H. Damsky, C. A. Buck, B. B. Knowles and D. Solter: Dev. Biol. *108*, 513 (1985).

50   I. Damjanov, A. Damjanov and C. H. Damsky: Dev. Biol. *116*, 194 (1986).

51   D. Vestweber, A. Gossler, K. Boller and R. Kemler: Dev. Biol. *124*, 451 (1987).

52   D. Vestweber and R. Kemler: Exp. Cell Res. *152*, 169 (1984).

53   C. Noro-Yoshida, N. Suzuki and N. Takeichi: Dev. Biol. *101*, 19 (1984).

54   P. C. Svalander, P. Odin, B. O. Nilsson and B. O'brink: Development *100*, 653 (1987).

55   B. D. Shur: Mol. Cell Biochem. *61*, 143 (1984).

56   A. E. Sutherland, R. D. Sanderson, M. Mayes, M. Seibert, P. G. Calarco, M. R. Bernfield and C. H. Damsky: Development *113*, 339 (1991).

57   A. C. Enders and S. Schlafke: Am. J. Anat. *125*, (1969).

58   A. C. Enders and S. Schlafke, in: Pre-implantation stages of Pregnancy: CIBA Foundation Symposium. Little, Brown: Boston, p. 29, Eds. G. E. W. Wolstenholme and M. O'Connor (1965).

59   E. L. Parr: Biol. Reprod. *8*, 531 (1973).

60   A. C. Enders, A. G. Hendrickx and S. Schlafke: Am. J. Anat. *167*, 275 (1983).

61   A. C. Enders and S. Schlafke: Am. J. Anat. *120*, 185 (1967).

62   C. A. Finn and A. M. Lawn: J. Reprod. Fertil. *15*, 333 (1968).

63   A. C. Enders and S. Schlafke: Am. J. Anat. *132*, 219 (1971).

64   W. Steert: J. Anat. *107*, 315 (1970).

65   W. Steert: J. Anat. *110*, 445 (1971).

66   A. Golander, J. Barrett, T. Hurley, S. Barry and S. Handwerger: Endocrinology *49*, 787 (1979).

67   S. Handwerger, S. Barry and P. M. Conn: Mol. Cell. Endocrinol. *37*, 83 (1984).

68   S. Handwerger, I. Hamman, A. Costello and E. Markoff: Mol. Cell. Endocrinol. *50*, 99 (1987).

69   J. D. Aplin, in: Biology of Uterus, p. 89. Eds. R. M. Wynn and W. P. Jollie, Plenum Medical Book Company, New York (1989).

70   A. C. Herington, J. Graham and D. L. Healy: J. Clin. Endocrinol. Metab. *51*, 1466 (1980).

71   S. C. Bell, S. Patel, M. W. Hales, P. H. Kirwan and J. O. Drife: J. Reprod. Fertil. *74*, 261 (1985).

72   S. C. Bell, M. W. Hales, S. Patel, P. H. Kirwan and J. O. Drife: Br. J. Obstet. Gynaecol. *92*, 793 (1985).

73   S. C. Bell, S. Patel, P. H. Kirwan and J. O. Drife: J. Reprod. Fertil. *77*, 221 (1986).

74   S. C. Bell, M. W. Hales, S. Patel, P. H. Kirwan, J. O. Drife and A. Milford-Ward: Br. J. Obstet. Gynaecol. *93*, 909 (1980).

75   G. T. Waites, R. A. Walker and S. C. Bell; J. Reprod. Fertil. *36* (Suppl.), 182 (1988).

76   S. C. Bell: J. Reprod. Fertil. *36* (Suppl.), 109 (1988).

77   S. C. Bell, J. W. Keyte and G. T. Waites: J. Clin. Endocrinol. Metab. *65*, 1067 (1987).

78   S. C. Bell and F. Dore-Green: J. Reprod. Immunol. *11*, 13 (1987).

79   S. C. Bell and S. Smith, in: Contemporary Obstetrics and Gynecology, Vol. 1 Part 2, p. 273. Eds G. V. P. Chamberlin, Butterworths, London (1988).

80   B. T. Pentecost and C. T. Teng: J. Biol. Chem. *262*, 10134 (1987).

81   T. T. Chen, F. W. Bazer, J. J. Cetorelli, W. E. Pollard and R. M. Roberts: J. Biol. Chem. *248*, 6560 (1973).
82   H. M. Beier: Biochim. Biophys. Acta *160*, 289 (1968).
83   H. M. Beier: J. Reprod. Fertil. *25* (Suppl.), 53 (1976).
84   D. W. Bullock and K. M. Conell: Biol. Reprod. *9*, 125 (1973).
85   J. C. Daniel: J. Reprod. Fertil. *25* (Suppl.), 71 (1976).
86   M. Beato and H. M. Beier: J. Reprod. Fertil. *53*, 305 (1978).
87   T. Tancredi, P. A. Temussi and M. Beato: Eur. J. Biochem. *122*, 101 (1982).
88   A. B. Mukherjee, R. E. Ulane and A. K. Agrawal: Am. J. Reprod. Immunol. *2*, 135 (1982).
89   D. C. Mukherjee, A. K. Agrawal, R. Marjunath and A. B. Mukherjee: Science *219*, 989 (1983).
90   C. F. Holinka and E. Gurpide: Am. J. Obstet. Gynecol. *150*, 359 (1984).
91   C. H. Spilman, K. K. Bergstrom and D. C. Beuving: Prostaglandins *20*, 1061 (1980).
92   S. K. Guha and J. Janne: Biochim. Biophys. Acta *437*, 244 (1976).
93   D. V. Maudsley and Y. Kobayashi: Biochem Pharmacol. *26*, 121 (1977).
94   B. Bacus and K. S. Kim: Comp. Gen. Pharmacol. 1, 196 (1970).
95   E. Nishino, N. Matsuzaki, K. Masuhiro, T. Kameda, T. Taniguchi, T. Takagi, F. Saji and O. Tanizawa: J. Clin. Endocrinol. Metab. *71*, 436 (1990).
96   S. S. Tabibzadeh: Endoc. Rev. *12*, 272 (1990).
97   S. S. Tabibzadeh, G. Pondichery and R. G. Satyaswaroop: Am. J. Clin. Pathol. *91*, 656 (1989).
98   T. W. Glenister: Proc. Roy. Soc., London (Biol) *154*, 428 (1961).
99   T. W. Glenister: Int. J. Fertil. *11*, 412 (1966).
100 T. W. Glenister, in: Fertility and Sterility, p 385. Eds. B. Westin and N. Wiquist, Ser. 133, Excerpta Medica Fedn, Amsterdam (1967).
101 M. Shiotani, Y. Noda and T. Meri: Biol. Reprod. *49*, 794 (1994).
102 P. S. Grant: J. Embryol. Exp. Morphol. *29*, 617 (1973).
103 P. S. Grant, I. Ljungkvist and O. Nilsson: J. Embryol. Exp. Morphol. *34*, 299 (1975).
104 D. S. Salomon and M. I. Sherman: Exp. Cell Res. *90*, 261 (1975).
105 M. I. Sherman and L. W. Wudl, in: Cell Surface in Animal Embryogenesis and Development, p 81. Eds. G. Porte and G. L. Nicolson, Elsevier, North Holland, Amsterdam (1976).
106 M. I. Sherman, in: Methods in Mammalian Reproduction, p 81. Ed. J. C. Daniel Jr. Academic Press, New York (1978).
107 A. C. Enders, D. J. Chavez and S. Schlafke, in: Cellular and Molecular Aspects of Implantation, p 365. Eds. S. R. Glasser and D. W. Bullock, Plenum Press, New York (1981).
108 J. E. Morris and S. W. Potter, in: Trophoblast Invasion and Endometrial Receptivity: Novel Aspects of the Cell Biology of Embryo Implantation. Trophoblast Research *4*, p 51. Eds. H. W. Denker and J. D. Aplin, Plenum Press, New York (1990).
109 R. H. Glass, A. I. Spindler and R. A. Pederson: J. Reprod. Fertil. *59*, 403 (1980).
110 D. J. Chavez and J. VanBlerkom, in: Cellular and Molecular Aspects of Implantation, p. 457. Eds. S. R. Glasser and D. W. Bullock, Plenum Press, New York (1981).
111 R. H. Glass, A. I. Spindler and R. A. Pedersen: J. Exp. Zool. *208*, 327 (1979).
112 R. H. Glass, J. Aggeler, A. I. Spindler, R. A. Pedersen and Z. Web: J. Cell Biol. *96*, 1108 (1983).

113 B. G. Boving, in: The Biology of the Blastocyst, p. 423. Ed. R. J. Blandau, Univ. of Chicago Press, Chicago (1971).

114 A. Heifetz, W. J. Lennarz, B. Libbus and Y. C. Hsu: Dev. Biol. *80*, 398 (1980).

115 J. P. Tang, J. Julian, S. R. Glasser and D. D. Carson: J. Biol. Chem. *262*, 12832 (1987).

116 M. C. Farach, J. P. Tang, G. L. Decker and D. D. Carson: Dev. Biol. *123*, 401 (1987).

117 W. Karst and H. J. Merker: Cell Differen. *22*, 211 (1988).

118 S. Strickland, E. Reich and M. I. Sherman: Cell *9*, 231 (1976).

119 E. J. Jenkinson and R. F. Searle: Exp. Zool. *210*, 69–80 (1979).

120 R. Shalgi and M. I. Sherman: J. Exp. Zool. *210*, 69 (1979).

121 S. R. Glasser, J. A. Julian, G. L. Decker, J. P. Tang and D. D. Carson: J. Cell Biol. *107*, 2409 (1988).

122 S. R. Glasser, J. A. Julian, J. Mulholland, S. Mani, D. D. Carson and A. D. Jacobs, in: Early Embryo Development and Paracrine Relationships, p 153. Ed. R. L. Alan, Inc. (1990).

123 R. Shukla: Ph.D. Thesis, Division of Endocrinology, Central Drug Research Institute, Lucknow, India (1990).

124 R. Shukla, P. K. Mehrotra, A. Dwivedi and V. P. Kamboj: Contraception *45*, 605 (1992).

125 N. W. Klein, M. A. Volger, C. L. Chalot and L. J. Pierro: Teratology *21*, 199 (1980).

126 I. R. Record, I. E. Drosti, S. J. Manuel and R. A. Buckley: Life Sciences *31* (24), 2735 (1982).

127 C. W. Warner, T. W. Sadler, S. A. Tulis and M. C. Smith: Teratology *30* (1), 47 (1984).

128 H. S. Yu and S. T. H. Chan: Pharmacol. Toxicol. *60*, 129 (1987).

129 B. M. Bhatt and D. W. Bullock: J. Reprod. Fertil. *39*, 65 (1974).

130 J. Sengupta, S. K. Dey and Z. Dickmann: Steroids *29*, 363 (1977).

131 S. K. Roy, J. Sengupta and S. K. Manchanda: Acta Endocrinol. *96*, 546 (1981).

132 S. K. Roy, J. Sengupta, B. C. Paria and S. K. Manchanda: Acta Endocrinol. *99*, 129 (1982).

133 J. P. Wolf, D. R. Danforth, A. Ulmann, E. E. Beaulieu and G. D. Holgen: Contraception *41*, 185 (1989).

134 P. K. Mehrotra, R. Shukla, A. Dwivedi, R. P. Srivastava, N. Bhat, M. Seth, A. P. Bhaduri and V. P. Kamboj: Contraception *43* (5), 507 (1991).

135 N. Bhat, P. K. Mehrotra, A. P. Bhaduri and V. P. Kamboj: Ind. J. Med. Res. *86*, 256 (1987).

136 A. Galliani, L. Assandri, F. Gallico, C. Luzzani, A. Oldani, A. Omodei-Salé, A. Soffientini and G. Lancini: Contraception *23*, 163 (1981).

137 M. M. Singh, P. K. Mehrotra, A. Agnihotri, R. P. Srivastava, M. Seth, A. P. Bhaduri and V. P. Kamboj: Contraception *36*, 239 (1987).

138 H. J. Zhou, R. Y. Fang, B. Z. Yang and Y. P. Zhang: Contraception *43*, 287 (1991).

139 A. Assandri, E. Perazi, P. Martinelli, P. Fervani, A. Ripamonti, G. Tuan and G. Galliani: Arzneim-Forsch. *31*, 2104 (1981).

140 P. K. Mehrotra, N. Bhat, A. P. Bhaduri and V. P. Kamboj: Ind. J. Med. Res. *83*, 614 (1986).

141 G. Galliani, A. Assandri, D. Barone and L. Gallico: IRCS Med. Sci. *12*, 433 (1984).

142 A. Mukherjee, M. S. H. Akhtar, V. L. Sharma, M. Seth, A. P. Bhaduri, A. Agnihotri, P. K. Mehrotra and V. P. Kamboj: J. Med. Chem. *32*, 2297 (1989).

143 G. Galliani, F. Luzzani, G. Colombo, A. Conz, A. Mistrello, D. Barone, G. Lancini and A. Assandri: Contraception *33*, 263 (1986).

144 G. Galliani, L. Gallico, C. Costaneo and A. Assandri: Arzneim-Forsch. *31*, 972 (1980).

145 G. Galliani, C. Caramel and A. Assandri: J. Small Anim. Pract. *25*, 211 (1984).

146 L. J. Lerner, R. Heywood, J. M. Hall, M. Alison and M. S. Grant: Fertil. Steril. *28*, 290 (1977).

147 G. Galliani, A. Assandri, L. J. Lerner, A. Omodei-Salé, G. Lancini, P. E. Nock and A. M. Grant: Contraception *26*, 165 (1982).

148 S. K. Saxena, M. Seth, A. P. Bhaduri and M. K. Sahib: J. Steroid Biochem. *18*, 303 (1983).

149 S. K. Saxena, M. K. Sahib, S. Kumar, M. Seth and A. P. Bhaduri: Ind. J. Biochem. and Biophy. *21*, 139 (1984).

150 I. M. Spitz and C. W. Bardin: Contraception *48*, 403 (1993).

151 L. J. Lerner, G. Galliani, M. C. Mosca and A. Omodei-Salé. Fed. Proc. *34*, 338 (1975).

152 L. J. Lerner, G. Galliani, P. Carminati and M. C. Mosca: Nature *256*, 130 (1975).

153 A. Omodei-Salé, P. Consonni and L. J. Lerner: U.S. Patent 4,007,276, Chem. Abstr. *83*, 206286v (1975).

154 A. Omodei-Salé, P. Consonni and L. J. Lerner: U.S. Patent 4075, 341, Chem. Abstr. *89*, 24316w (1978).

155 A. Omodei-Salé, P. Consonni, G. Galliani and L. J. Lerner: Ger. Offen. 2,819,372, Chem. Abstr. *90*, 72206c (1979).

156 A. Omodei-Salé, E. Toja, G. Galliani and L. J. Lerner: Ger. Offen. 2, 551,868, Chem. Abstr. *85*, 192731p (1976).

157 G. Winters, G. Odasso, G. Galliani and L. J. Lerner: U.S. Patent, 4,024,149, Chem. Abstr. *85*, 94369g (1976).

158 E. Toja, A. Omodei-Salé, C. Cattaneo and G. Galliani: Eur. J. Med. Chem. *17* (3), 223 (1982).

159 A. Omodei-Salé, P. Consonni and G. Galliani: J. Med. Chem. *26*, 1187 (1983).

160 Neelima, P. K. Mehrotra, A. P. Bhaduri and V. P. Kamboj: Ind. J. Med. Res. *86*, 256 (1987).

161 Neelima: Ph.D. Thesis, Division of Medicinal Chemistry, Central Drug Research Institute, Lucknow, India (1983).

162 M. S. H. Akhtar: Ph.D. Thesis, Division of Medicinal Chemistry, Central Drug Research Institute, Lucknow, India (1987).

163 S. Batra: Ph.D. Thesis, Division of Medicinal Chemistry, Central Drug Research Institute, Lucknow, India (1992).

164 S. P. Vishnoi: Ph.D. Thesis, Division of Medicinal Chemistry, Central Drug Research Institute, Lucknow, India (1993).

165 M. A. Gallop, R. W. Barrett, W. J. Dower, S. P. A. Fodor and E. M. Gordan: J. Med. Chem. *37* (9), 1233 (1994).

Progress in Drug Research, Vol. 44 (E. Jucker, Ed.)
© 1995 Birkhäuser Verlag, Basel (Switzerland)

Developments in anticonvulsants[1]

By Anil K. Saxena and Mridula Saxena

Division of Medicinal Chemistry, Central Drug Research Institute, Lucknow 226 001, India

---

1   CDRI Communication No. 5349

1   Introduction

Epilepsy is one of the oldest of common human ailments and is mentioned in ancient writings such as the Babylonian Code of Hammurabi 2080 BC and in the Hebrew scriptures. Its clinical description was given by Hippocrates in his monograph (ca. 400 BC) on the disease [1]. In earlier times the paroxysmal, uncontrollable behaviour of epileptics was thought to be due to their possession by evil spirits or demons and hence the disease was known as the "sacred disease" in some cultures. Such superstitious beliefs were gradually discarded with the advancement in medical sciences, firstly in diagnosis of epilepsy and a better understanding of its cause and of various types of seizures and secondly in the development of antiepileptic drugs. These advancements have led to the availability of effective medication for epilepsy patients. The agents used in the treatment of different types of epilepsy are termed as anticonvulsants.

In spite of the progress made in this area, approximately 1 to 2 million people in the United States of America and 20 to 40 million people worldwide suffer from epileptic seizures [2]. The present method of treatment is of benefit to only 60–70% of patients. About 25% still continue to suffer from uncontrollable seizures and medication toxicity [3–6]. The disease is more common in children below the age of 7 years [7]. Different medical aspects of epilepsy have been reviewed in recent years [8–11]. The present article outlines different aspects of epilepsy with emphasis on the development of anticonvulsants.

1.1   Types of epileptic seizures

Epilepsy is a collective designation for sudden and transient disorders of the central nervous systems comprising episodes (seizures) of abnormal phenomena of motor (convulsion), sensory, autonomic or psychic origin. The attributory cause of epilepsy can be identified in some patients but in a large number of them, it is difficult to assign a cause. However, it is certain that epilepsy is a "symptom complex", a result of an underlying brain lesion, which in some patients may be due to a genetic abnormality and in others to some other reasons. The causes of epilepsy in infants, children and in adults have been discussed by Porter [9] and are summarized below (Table 1).

Table 1
Causes of seizures in infants, children and adults in order of probable incidence

Infants and children	Adults
No definite cause determined	No definite cause determined
Birth and neonatal injuries	–
Vascular insults (other than above)	Vascular lesions
Head injuries	Head trauma
Congenital or metabolic disorders	–
–	Drug or alcohol abuse
Neoplasia	Neoplasia
–	Infection
Heredity	Heredity

The basic reason for seizures is the abnormal and excessive discharge of the nerve tissue. Seizures can be divided into two broad types: (i) partial and (ii) generalized. Partial seizures can be recorded on an electroencephalograph (EEG)and are further divided into three classes: (a) simple partial; (b) complex partial; and (c) simple partial, secondarily generalized. Simple partial seizure is also termed cortical epilepsy or Jacksonian seizure. In this type of seizure the patient remains conscious and the convulsions are confined to a single limb or group of muscles. In some cases other symptoms are seen as a consequence of localized organic brain lesions which promote rapid discharge in local neurons and may spread to the cortical regions leading to progressive muscular contractions. In another variety of partial seizure called psychomotor seizure, the symptoms may include amnesia, attack of abnormal rage, sudden anxiety and a momentarily incoherent speech. Complex partial seizures are associated with impairment of consciousness and usually involve the bilateral hemisphere. A partial seizure may become secondarily generalized, i.e. it may progress to a generalized tonic-clonic seizure. A generalized seizure involves all parts of the brain and there is no evidence of localized onset. Generalized seizures include: (a) generalized tonic-clonic seizure (grand mal), (b) absence seizure (petit mal), (c) myoclonic seizure, (d) atonic seizure, (e) clonic seizure, and (f) tonic seizure. Characteristics of different types of seizures are summarized in Table 2.

Table 2
Classification, possible progression and characteristics of epileptic seizures

Type of seizure	Progression	Characteristics
1. Partial seizure (focal, local seizure)		
A) Simple partial seizure	SP	Localized convulsions confined to single limb or muscle group without the loss of consciousness, specified and localized sensory disturbances, and other limited signs and symptoms like motor, somatosensory, autonomic and psychic symptoms depending upon the cortical area involved in producing the abnormal discharge.
B) Complex partial seizure (with SP onset)	SP → CP CP	Loss of consciousness or decreased ability to respond normally to exogenous stimuli, with a wide variety of clinical symptoms such as automatism (lip smacking, fumbling, walking) or associated with symptoms described for simple partial seizures, associated with bizarre generalized EEG activity during seizure but with evidence of anterior temporal lobe focal abnormalities even in the interseizure period in many cases.
C) Partial seizure (secondarily generalized)		
2. Generalized seizure (convulsive or nonconvulsive)		Bilaterally symmetrical and without local onset.
A) Partial seizure (secondarily generalized)	SP → GTC	No evidence of localized onset reflects maximal involvement, general convulsions, chewing motion usually a sequence of
– Generalized tonic	CP → GTC	maximal tonic spasms of whole body musculature followed by synchronous clonic
– Clonic seizure (Grand mal)	SP → CP → GTC	jerking and prolonged depression of all central functions.
B1) Absence seizure		Brief motionless decrease in responsiveness, with automation, with mild clonic motion (usually eyelids), increased (arching of back) or decreased (head nodding) postural tone, some times with no motor activity.
B2) Atypical absence seizure		Associated with more heterogeneous EEG along with slower onset and cessation than is usual for absence seizure.

Type of seizure	Progression	Characteristics
C) Myoclonic seizure		Burst of neuronal discharge for a fraction of a second occurs throughout CNS leading to isolated clonic jerks associated with multiple spikes in EEG.
D) Clonic seizure		Loss of consciousness and of memory, the ictal EEG contains well-known generalized rhythmic clonic contractions of cell muscles and marked autonomic manifestations.
E) Tonic seizure		Loss of consciousness, opisthotonus and marked autonomic manifestations.
F) Atonic seizure		Sudden loss of postural tone, with sagging of head or falling.

No evidence is available for the localized onset of a generalized seizure, only the generalized tonic-clonic seizure shows maximal neuronal involvement [17]. The extreme neuronal discharge originating from the mesencephalic portion of the reticular activating system spreads throughout the central nervous system including the cortex, lower portion of brain, spinal cord and leads to tonic convulsions, followed by clonic convulsions. Absence seizure is associated with brief abrupt loss of consciousness with high voltage, bilaterally synchronous, 3-per-second spike and wave pattern in the EEG, increase or decrease in postural tone, mild clonic motion and automatic behaviour [18]. Stereotyped generalized tonic-clonic seizures have been best described by Gastaut and Broughtor [19]. Myoclonic seizures are extraordinarily heterogeneous and are believed to be a fragment of another type of seizure [20, 21]. Atonic seizures are characterized by sudden loss of postural tone. Tonic seizure in many cases may be the fragment of a generalized tonic-clonic seizure. 2.5–5.0 percent of the population suffer from nonepileptic seizures termed as "febrile seizures" [22].

1.2   Nature and mechanism of seizures

The basic etiology of seizures is not clearly understood. The concept of epilepsy is based on the John Hughlings Jackson hypotheses, according to which seizures are caused by occasional, sudden, excessive, rapid and local discharge of gray matter [23]. The result is a generalized convulsion due to invasion of normal brain tissue by the seizure activity initiated in the abnormal focus. The EEG demonstrates that the seizures are associated with abnormal and sometimes massive electrical discharge in the brain. It helps as a tool in the differential diagnosis of epilepsies. Many aspects of epilepsy including the neuronal mechanism underlying the EEG have been explained in the monograph [24]. The different biochemical aspects of epileptic seizures still remain unknown. The proposed hypotheses explaining the electrical discharge lack information about the chemical events underlying the convulsive reactivity of the brain. Various workers have investigated the biochemical aspects of convulsive events [25–27]. Computer modelling of neuronal networks (the properties determined from *in vitro* studies of hippocampal slices) indicates that synchronous and sustained discharge from neurons can be enhanced due to the sensitivity of the excitatory receptors or from decreased efficacy of the inhibitory system [28, 29]. Studies in animals of abnormal neuronal activity in the epileptic focus indicate that the characteristic of neuron showing such activity is burst firing. This recruitment of normal neurons into abnormal activity provides the transition from interictal to ictal activity in EEG records [30]. It has also been demonstrated by Panfield and Jasper that seizures arise in a focus and then propagate to involve additional circuits in the brain [31]. This phenomenon has also been studied in single neurons in man by Wyler and Ward [32]. Singh and Huot [33] have described the neurochemical modifications that occur before, during and after an epileptic seizure. According to them, the pre-ictal changes comprise hypoglycemia, pyridoxine deficiency, and changes in Ca^{++} and Mg^{++} ions. The intra-ictal neurochemical modifications are the result of increased cerebral metabolism, muscular convulsions and apnea. They include changes in metabolism of neurotransmitters, e.g. acetylcholine, catecholamines, serotonin, GABA and glycine [33]. Advances in neurosurgery enable removal of the epileptogenic focus which results in cessation of seizures [34]. Based on the spikes generated by the dendrites of the neuron in EEG, Ward put forward the hypothesis that physiological malfunction in epilepsy occurs at the dendrite level. According to the hypothesis mechanical disruption of dendritic membrane causes depolarization leading to the autonomous activity that characterizes epileptic neurons. These epileptic neuronal dendrites because of their electrical excitability due to relatively nonenveloping structures [34] cause excitable alteration of the adjacent neurons. Among the different mechanisms proposed for epileptogenesis, denervation hypersensitivity of ACTH is one because the epileptogenic cortex is characterized by impairment of acetylcholine binding, metabolic loss of glutamic acid and failure to maintain potassium ion concentration [25]. Though mechanisms implicating excessive acetylcholine have been proposed as contributing factors, it seems unlikely that impaired acetylcholine metabolism is solely responsible for epilepsy, because the selective blockade of cholinergic transmission with an acetylcholine antagonist is not sufficient to bring about complete anticonvulsant action unless the convulsions are specifically due to activation of cholinergic neurons.

Neuronal events at the cellular level relating to epileptic discharges studied in different animal models *in vivo* and hippocampal slice *in vitro* show that the burst discharge is associated with an abnormally large and prolonged depolarizing potential, known as paroxysmal depolarizing shift (PDS). This PDS is an abnormal, excitatory post-synaptic potential and it triggers the action potentials which are very frequent in appearance and in which current is carried by Ca^{++} ions rather than Na^{++} ions. The neurons showing burst discharge during PDS stimulate the normal neurons to a burst of excessive excitatory input. However, this does not lead to recruitment during the interictal period but recruitment takes place in ictal phase. The recruitment process which may be modified according to the activity within the inhibitory system is discussed under the following headings:

(a) Inhibitory synaptic processes and their pharmacological manipulation.
(b) Excitatory transmission and their pharmacological manipulation.
(c) Membrane properties favouring or restricting repetitive firing and their pharmacological manipulation.

1.2.1   Inhibitory synaptic processes and their pharmacological manipulation

GABA, a central neurohormonal inhibitory modulator [35], plays an important role in the etiology and control of epilepsy [33] by mediating the inhibition processes of epilepsy. It is synthesized in the brain by the decarboxylation of glutamic acid by the enzyme glutamic acid decarboxylase which is specifically localized to GABA-ergic neurons. Using the antibodies formed against glutamic acid decarboxylase and glutaraldehyde-GABA-protein complex, the structures of inhibitory interneurons and their connections have been elucidated [36]. These interneurons are excited either by the sustained afferent input to the cortical region or by recurrent collateral pathways from the pyramidal tract or extra-pyramidal neurons or by an excessively sustained local discharge giving rise to excessive output. The GABA-ergic system prevents the excessive syn-chronized discharge or the recruitment of neurons of other cortical regions by hyperpolarization of resting membrane potential of the neurons. This GABA-mediated inhibition is evident from the fact that compounds which block GABA synthesis by inhibiting glutamic acid decarboxylase are potent convulsants when given systemically or locally in the cortex or hippocampus [37, 38]. Thus decrease in GABA concentration leads to convulsive manifestations and enhancement of GABA-mediated inhibi-tion, while its increase produces anticonvulsant effects [39, 40]. Though GABA can be directly administered, it produces significant cardiovascular effects before manifesting anticonvulsant effects due to its poor blood-brain barrier penetration. GABA-mediated inhibition is enhanced by (i) GABA agonists (Muscimol, THIP, Baclofen, Progabide) [41, 42], (ii) GABA uptake inhibitors (Nipecotic acid, Isoguvacine, THPO) [43–45], (iii) GABA transaminase inhibitors (ethanolamine-O-sulphate, γ-ace-tylenic GABA, γ-vinyl GABA, gabaculine and β-difluoromethyl-β-alan-ine) [46], and (iv) compounds acting on allosteric sites (benzodiazepine, triazolopyridazines, anticonvulsant β-carbolines) [38].

The nonspecific regulation of CNS excitation due to GABA has been demonstrated by the studies of Curtis and Watkins [47, 48], in which iontophoretical application of GABA to the external surface membrane of spinal motor neurons, interneurons and Renshaw cells did not produce any change in the resting potential in intracellular recordings, but depressed or blocked the excitatory and inhibitory postsynaptic potentials. The presy-naptic inhibition by picrotoxin, a CNS stimulant, is blocked by GABA, suggesting that the latter has an important role as a neurohormonal trans-mitter or modulator [49]. Adrenal cortical steroids and ACTH can trigger a spontaneous epileptic seizure because of their ability to decrease GABA concentration in brain and to increase brain excitability [50].

The anticonvulsants hydroxylamine and aminooxyacetic acid [51, 52], and the CNS stimulants caffeine and centedrin [51] increase GABA concentra-tion in brain. The anticonvulsant action of the former two has been attributed to the inhibition of the GABA-ketoglutaric transaminase system which appears to be the rate-limiting step of GABA catabolism through succinate and entry to the Krebs TCA cycle. On the other hand glutamic acid γ-hydrazide, an inhibitor of GABA transaminase, causes an increase in GABA concentration in brain but its anticonvulsant action is unable to completely counteract insulin and phenylenetetrazole-induced convulsions in mice [53].

1.2.2   Excitatory synaptic transmission and its pharmacological manipulation

The total range of excitatory neurotransmitter substances in brain has not yet been identified. But it has been established that dicarboxylic amino acids, various peptides and acetylcholine act as neurotransmitters. Aspartate, glutamate and other excitatory amino acids are known to initiate focal discharge when they are applied directly to cortex and deep brain tissue [54]. These compounds and their sulphonic and sulphinic analogs act on the membrane receptor site by depolarizing the resting membrane (dendritic and somatic) and initiating the action potential at the axon hillock, to open channels for Na^{++}, Ca^{++} and K^+ ions. The spread of focal seizure activity from one area of brain to another is due to excitatory transmission caused by compounds acting on excitatory amino acid receptors. The focal seizure activity is initiated by the release of glutamate from the cortical surface. The exact metabolic pathways and rate-limiting steps involved in the synthesis of the enzymes glutamate, aspartate etc. are not known. So the approaches based on inhibition of their synthesis have not been successful in finding anticonvulsant compounds. However, weak anticonvulsant activity has been shown by glutaminase inhibitors [55]. The mechanisms controlling the synaptic release of excitatory neurotransmitters involve autoreceptors responding to glutamate or its analogues and other receptors like $GABA_A$ receptors linked to benzodiazepine receptor site, adenosine receptors, and $GABA_B$ receptors. It has been possible to demonstrate a decrease in the evoked release of excitatory amino acid in brain slice and other *in vitro* preparations in the presence of benzodiazepines, baclofen and adenosine [56–58].

Membrane receptors responsible for the postsynaptic excitatory action of dicarboxylic amino acid have been classified into four subtypes depending on the nature of the agonist present [59], viz. N-methyl-D-aspartate preferring receptor, quisqualate preferring receptor, α-kinate preferring receptor and glutamate-receptor. The postsynaptic excitatory action can be blocked by analogues that compete with the neurotransmitter at the receptor site. The NMDA receptor operates ionic channels with specific current voltage properties of conductance, leading to a paroxysmal depolarizing shift and burst-firing [60].

Several glutamate analogues have been tested as potential antagonists at postsynaptic receptor sites. 2-Amino-7-phosphonoheptanoic acid and CPP (3-(±)-2-carboxypiperazine-4-yl)propyl-1-phosphonate) are highly potent and selective NMDA receptor antagonists and are potent anticonvulsants when administered intracerebroventricularly in mice. These analogues penetrate the blood brain barrier poorly. However, some of them show anticonvulsant activity when given systemically to mice, rats and baboons, e.g. 2-amino-7-phosphonoheptanoic acid is active at a dose of 0.3–1.0 mg/kg, i.p. or i.v. in rodents and primates [46]. γ-D-Glutamylaminomethylsulphonate and piperazine derivatives like 1-(p-bromobenzoyl)-2,3-piperazine dicarboxylate (BBPP) have shown antagonistic action at kainate or quisqualate receptors in preference to NMDA receptors. These compounds show anticonvulsant activity when given intracerebroventricularly in rodents. However, it is difficult to ascertain how much of the anticonvulsant action can be attributed to kainate or quisqualate receptors and how much to the NMDA receptor. Nevertheless, the impairment of excitatory transmission by the use of selective amino acid receptor antagonists may lead to highly selective anticonvulsant action without impairing neurological functions, and thus this approach provides a means for the control of epilepsy.

1.2.3   Membrane stabilization and ionic transport

The importance of membrane stabilization and ionic transport is due to the fact that alteration in neuronal membrane ion conductance can (i) reduce the burst-firing tendency of neurons, (ii) change the properties of the membrane and neurons by modifying their passive and electrical features, and (iii) alter the active transport of ions across the membrane leading to changes in resting and action potentials. Thus drugs having direct action on neuronal membrane ion conductance can act directly on abnormal epileptic neurons in focus and thus prevent the spread of seizure activity. Drugs having primary action on ionic properties of membranes may have secondary action on inhibitory and excitatory neurotransmission, but for understanding molecular mechanism of their action, it is essential to consider their interaction with membrane components responsible for ionic permeability of the membrane. The effects of the anticonvulsant phenytoin on the active transport of sodium, potassium and calcium in neuronal and non-neuronal preparations *in vitro*, have been described by Glaser et al. [61]. The electrophysiological studies of Macdonald et al. [62] support the view that the anticonvulsant action of a drug is due to its membrane stabilizing effect.

1.2.4   Mechanism of anticonvulsant action

A knowledge of the mechanism of action of anticonvulsant drugs provided a rational approach to the design of the new anticonvulsant. In view of the fact that most clinically used anticonvulsant drugs act by more than one mechanism, the mechanism of action of important anticonvulsants will be discussed along with their SAR in subsequent sections.

2   History of anticonvulsant drug development

The history of anticonvulsants dates back to the mid-1800s, when inorganic bromides were used as sedatives. Locock in 1857 first introduced potassium bromide for the treatment of catamenial seizures [63] and it soon replaced all the previous drugs as these failed to control seizures in many patients. It continued to be used for a long period of 50 years until severe side-effects like skin eruptions and psychosis were reported. The first synthetic anticonvulsant drug, phenobarbital, was marketed by Winthrop in 1912. It possessed good sedative and hypnotic action, reduced the frequency of seizures with less toxic effects than potassium bromide [64]. Approximately 50 analogues of phenobarbital were synthesized and marketed in the first 35 years of this century. Among them mephobarbital exhibited the best antiepileptic activity in man [65, 66]. It was marketed in 1935 in the United States. Its efficacy was similar to that of phenobarbital but it produced less sedation [67, 68].

The discoveries of both potassium bromide and phenobarbital were serendipitous. The first experimental model for testing anticonvulsant activity in which seizures were evoked in dogs by direct faradic stimulation of the motor cortex, was used in 1882 [69]. Later, many naturally occurring substances like strychnine, picrotoxin and synthetic compounds like pentylenetetrazole were also used to produce convulsant effects in experimental models [70, 71].

Preclinical evaluation of anticonvulsant drugs started in 1937 with the work of Putnam and Merritt [72, 73] who devised methods of preclinical testing for anticonvulsant activity in experimentally induced convulsions in laboratory animals. They discovered the anticonvulsant property of phenytoin (diphenylhydantoin) while screening compounds synthesized by Park Davis & Co. against electrically induced seizures in cats. Phenytoin was found to be well tolerated by laboratory animals and was effective in clinical trials. It was marketed in the United States in 1938 and was exempted from formal requirements of the Federal Food and Drug Act of 1906 due to the absence of sedative action and dramatic control of seizures when given in combination with barbiturate therapy [74]. Discovery of phenytoin proved that sedation is not important for anticonvulsant action. The reproducibility and accuracy of the techniques developed by Putnam and Merritt prompted researchers to search for safer and more effective antiepileptic drugs. A large number of phenytoin analogues was synthesized and tested. In 1944 Richards and Everett [75] reported trimethadione as a potent analgesic drug [76], which later proved to be the first anti-absence drug to prevent penty-lenetetrazole-induced threshold seizures in rodents. These seizures were also prevented by phenobarbital, but not by phenytoin. The results were confirmed by Goodman and coworkers [77, 78] who concluded that the intensity of the convulsive stimulus is very important in evaluating anticon-vulsant properties and that is the reason why phenytoin and phenobarbital modify the pattern of maximal electroshock seizures [78, 79] while trimethadione does not. These conclusions demonstrate that there is a quantitative difference in the anticonvulsant action of these drugs against threshold and maximal seizures.

The relevance of these findings to the testing of drugs was supported by two facts. The widespread use of electroshock therapy for the treatment of mental disorders provided an opportunity for the observation of artificially' induced seizures in humans. A similar pattern of seizures was observed by Kalinowsky and Kennedy [80] in experimental animals undergoing the same stimulation. They reported the induction of major and minor seizures by pentylenetetrazole and electroshock and the ability of phenobarbital and phenytoin to increase the voltage required to elicit the maximal seizure. These findings were later confirmed by Strauss and Landis [81] and ex-plained the similarity of response to seizure-provoked stimulus in rodents and in the human nervous system.

Petit mal, myoclonic and akinetic seizures were treated with trimethadione in 50 patients who did not respond to other treatments. It was observed that petit mal attacks decreased or stopped but grand mal attacks were not controlled and were even exacerbated in 10 patients [82]. This unique action of trimethadione was also confirmed by the testing of a larger series of compounds [83, 84]. The striking differences in the effects of trimethadione and phenytoin [77, 78] can be seen from their effects on seizures in man and in experimental maximal and threshold seizure models. Trimethadione was marketed in 1946 and became the drug of choice for absence seizure. Investigations from 1945 to 1950 failed to find a seizure model in which all the drugs were active. However, profiles of anticonvulsant activity were uncovered which correlated well with clinical efficacy and specific-ity [85]. Among 65 phenylsuccinimides investigated for anticonvulsant activity against pentylenetetrazole-induced seizures, phensuximide and methsuximide were found to be the most potent by Chen et al. [86] and were approved for the treatment of absence seizures in 1953 and 1957 respectively. Later, ethosuximide was introduced for the same purpose in 1960 [87].

Clinical experience with phensuximide raised doubts about its efficacy which were substantiated by Porter at al. [88]. Methsuximide, on the other hand, was found occasionally effective in generalized tonic-clonic, complex partial as well as in absence seizures. A comparative study of ethosuximide, phensuximide and methsuximide revealed the first to be as effective as methsuximide against subcutaneous pentylenetetrazole seizures, but less potent against maximal electroshock [89].

During 1938 to 1960 two analogues of phenytoin (mephenytoin and ethotoin), two of phenobarbital (metharbital and primidone) and an analogue of trimethadione (paramethadione) were marketed. Each of these analogues had a spectrum of activity similar to that of the parent compound. The use of these drugs has been reviewed by Woodbury et al. [90]. Three other drugs, phenylate, benzchloropropamide and aminoglutethimide were also marketed for epilepsy during the same period. However, the first two were withdrawn in 1960 due to side-effects like hepatic necrosis in phenylates and chronic toxicity of benzchloropropamide in animals [91, 92]. Later, in 1966, aminoglutethimide was also withdrawn because of high incidence of goitre [93, 94].

There followed a period of marked decline in the development of antiepileptic drugs, from 1961 to 1973, because the remarkable improvements shown by many patients convinced the drug industry and many clinicians that existing drugs were adequate for the therapy of epilepsies, and that these drugs used alone or in combination could achieve maximum control of specific seizure disorders. It was highly unlikely that any new drug would capture the market sufficiently to justify the cost of its development which had become substantially higher after the passage of the Kefauver-Harris amendments in 1962 to the Federal Food, Drug and Cosmetic Act of 1938 [95]. These amendments required more stringent proof of efficacy of a new drug which was not possible in the case of antiepileptic drugs due to the limited number of patients for controlled clinical trials and non-availability of patients with well-defined uncontrolled seizures. A dramatic improvement of increased seizures made patients reluctant to participate in such trials. In addition, the use of multidrug therapy made it difficult to design controlled clinical trials that could establish the efficacy of a new drug.

There was a lack of rigorous methodology to measure the clinical response, and medical and ethical guidelines for accepting patients [96]. In 1967 a survey (by an Advisory Committee of Epilepsies (1967) of the U.S. General Public Health Service) of the pharmaceutical industry [97] revealed that no new antiepileptic drugs had been introduced because of the prohibitive cost of development or lack of marketing permission due to inadequate proof of efficacy. Besides, academic researchers accorded low priority to the synthesis of new anticonvulsants as they did not have ready access to pharmacological screening. Furthermore, the discovery of tranquillizers and sedative hypnotics which brought substantial financial returns diverted the attention of the pharmaceutical industry from anticonvulsants to other central nervous system drugs. During this period only diazepam was marketed as a new adjunctive drug for status epilepsies.

2.1   Status of antiepileptic drug therapy in 1970

The armamentarium of drugs available for epilepsy till 1970 consisted of 13 basic drugs, all of which had been marketed before the efficacy requirements under the Kefauver-Harris amendments of 1962 came into force [95]. Their efficacy evaluation had been done by means of retrospective studies, postmarketing uncontrolled trials and case reports. Numerous reports of toxic effects after chronic administration were a matter of concern. Clinical experience of the decade preceding 1970 revealed many shortcomings in both efficacy and safety of available drugs. While many patients did benefit from the drugs, in some poorly defined or improperly diagnosed seizures neither single drugs nor combination therapy could provide satisfactory control. However, some acceptable controlled trials were reported in the literature [98]. The seizure-free period achieved by many patients was at the cost of significant toxic effects observed not only in CNS but also in connective tissues, bone, haematopoietic and some other systems. The toxicity pattern of one drug could not be used to predict those of others. Sedation was an undesirable side-effect of a number of antiepileptic drugs, specially on long-term use. Inaccurate diagnosis of seizure disorders resulted in the wrong choice of agents. Sometimes in spite of proper selection of agent, failure of treatment occurred due to improper administration. In view of the above there was a pressing need in 1970 to develop better drugs for the treatment of epileptic seizures.

2.2   Renewed interest in antiepileptic drugs

A rational selection of therapeutic agents is very important for successful treatment of epilepsy patients. Many attempts were made to overcome the inadequacies of existing methods. Attention was focussed on the definition and diagnosis of seizure disorders. In 1968, the Epilepsy Branch of the National Institute of Neurology and Communicative Disorders and other investigators initiated efforts to improve and validate the classification of seizures and seizure disorders [99]. The Epilepsy Branch in collaboration with others conducted controlled clinical trials of seven drugs, namely albutoin, carbamazepine, clonazepam, clorazepate dipotassium, mexiletine, sulthiame and valproic acid to establish proof of their efficacy as required. The introduction of controlled clinical trials not only decreased the cost of development of anticonvulsants but also led to the improvement in the methodology of quantitative analysis of blood levels of antiepileptic drugs and extended the use of accurate blood drug levels to therapeutic practice [100–105]. The new drug applications for carbamazepine, clonazepam and valproic acid were eventually approved and they were marketed in 1974, 1975 and 1978, respectively. Clorazepate was approved as an adjunctive drug in 1981. Albutoin, mexiletine and sulthiame were unsuccessful in these trials.

3   Anticonvulsant screening

The systemic anticonvulsant screening and preclinical evaluation of anticonvulsant drugs is important in providing clues to their therapeutic properties and clinical efficacy. The test model used for evaluation of anticonvulsant activity should be clinically predictive and capable of distinguishing anticonvulsants from other centrally active compounds. Unfortunately, testing of a number of clinically active drugs in a variety of experimental animal models failed to discover a single test which fulfills the above requirements, and even the specificity of the low frequency electroshock test has been doubted [106]. Millichap has tried to correlate laboratory and clinical evaluation data of anticonvulsants [107]. Suppression of seizure discharge in EEG has shown good correlation with the control of commonly observed clinical symptoms; anticonvulsants that control grand mal tonic seizure are effective against maximal electroshock tonic seizure in mice and rat, but activity against pentylenetetrazole-induced seizure is neither essential for nor always predictive of efficacy against petit mal [107]. The importance of the intensity of the convulsive stimulus in evaluation of anticonvulsant activity was known as far back as 1938 [72, 73]. This fact has been confirmed and it has been demonstrated that the specificity of experimental models of epilepsy is primarily due to the intensity rather than the nature of the stimulus used or the kind of seizure induced [108]. In the absence of an ideal single test model, a wide variety of animal models are used to screen potential antiepileptic drugs [109–117]. Development of models of epilepsy have recently been reviewed [118, 119]. The set of different tests used in a phased manner for detection and measurement of anticonvulsant activity in anticonvulsant drug development programme (ADD programme) [109,110] is outlined in Figure 1.

Two strains each of adult male CF No. 1 albino mice (18–25 g) and adult male Sprague-Dawley albino rats (100–150 g) of the same sex, age and weight are used to minimize the effects of biological variation [120]. These animals are used as experimental animals because they are very docile and mortality is rare during maximal electroshock seizure [121]. Animals are maintained and handled according to HEW publication (NIH) No. 7423 "Guide for the care and use of laboratory animals" [122]. After any transit of animals, the animals are allowed to rest for 24 hrs before the experiment is carried out. The rest is required to compensate for food, water and stress due to transit because in such transit the starvation due to stress or food refusal may increase the intensity of MES [123]. The following five tests are used routinely for detection, measurement and evaluation of anticonvulsant activity, viz. (i) maximal electroshock seizure (MES) test, (ii) subcutaneous pentylenetetrazole seizure threshold test (scMet) (iii) subcutaneous bicuculline seizure threshold test (scBic), (iv) subcutaneous picrotoxin seizure threshold test (scPic), and (v) subcutaneous strychnine seizure pattern test (scStr). After the active compounds have been identified by these tests, they are characterized and differentiated on the basis of their mechanism of action as elucidated by receptor-binding studies.

3.1   Maximal electroshock seizure (MES) test

This test, discovered by Merrit and Putnam [124], is used to detect compounds that prevent the spread of seizure. Such compounds may or may not increase the minimal seizure threshold and may be active against partial

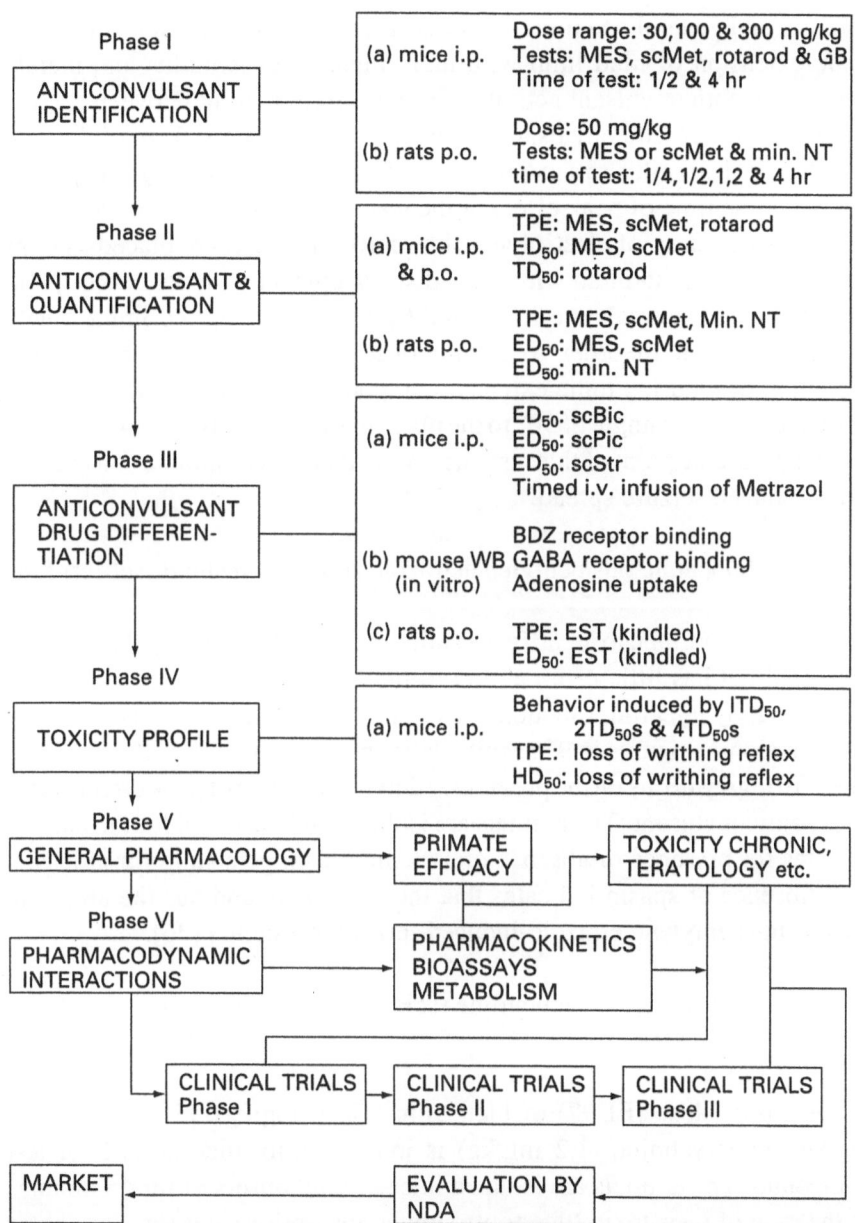

Fig. 1
Schema of the ADD programme
(GB = general behavior, NT = neurotoxicity, HD = hypnotic dose).

seizures and generalized tonic-clonic seizures. The test is characterized by tonic extension of hind limb with high intensity of stimulus and merely detects the anticonvulsant activity without differentiating between seizure spread and other anticonvulsant activities. In the standard form of the test, the electrical stimulus (50 mA in mice, 150 mA in rats; 60 Hz) is given for 0.2 sec at the time of peak effect of the test compound, and two electrodes primed with a drop of electrolyte solution (0.9% NaCl) are placed as clips on the ears or as platinum wire rings/discs in contact with the cornea [110, 125, 126]. The animals are restrained by hand and released immediately after stimulation in order to permit observation of the entire seizure. Abolition of hind leg tonic extensor component (hind-leg tonic extension does not exceed an angle of 90° to the plane of the body) after drug treatment was taken as end-point of this test, indicating that the compound can prevent MES-induced seizure spread.

3.2   Subcutaneous pentylenetetrazole seizure threshold (scMet) test

This test is performed to identify the anticonvulsant that elevates the minimal threshold but has little or no ability to prevent seizure spread. The test is carried out by injecting subcutaneously the convulsant dose (ED 97) (dose causing clonic seizures in 97% animals) of pentylenetetrazole (85 mg/kg in mice; 70 mg/kg in rats) at the previously determined time of peak effect (TPE) of the anticonvulsant. The animals are isolated and observed for the next 30 minutes for presence or absence of a clonic spasm persisting for at least 5 sec. Absence of spasm indicates that the test compound has the ability to elevate the pentylenetetrazole-induced seizure threshold [126].

3.3   Subcutaneous bicuculline (scBic), picrotoxin (scPic), strychnine (scStr) tests

A convulsant dose (ED97) of bicuculline (2.70 mg/kg), picrotoxin (3.15 mg/kg), or strychnine (1.2 mg/kg) is injected into mice at TPE of test compound. The animals are isolated in cages and observed for 45 minutes in the case of picrotoxin (due to its slower absorption) and for 30 minutes in the case of the other two compounds. Absence of clonic seizure in scBic and scPic tests showed the ability of a test compound to elevate the respective seizure threshold. In scStr-treated animals, abolition of hind limb extensor component indicates the ability of the compound to prevent seizure spread [110, 126].

3.4   Receptor binding studies

Crude synaptic membrane (mouse whole brain) preparations made according to the method of Euna and Synder [127] are used for receptor-binding studies. [^{3}H] Flunitrazepam receptor-binding studies are performed according to Braestrup and Squires [128]. GABA receptor-binding studies are done by centrifugation assay [129]. The membrane preparation (1 ml) containing [^{3}H] flunitrazepam (1–10 nM) or [^{3}H] GABA (50 nM), the test compound (0.01–100 μM) and sufficient tris buffer are incubated at 0 to 2°C. The amount of the test compound bound is determined by scintillation counting of the membranes isolated by filtration ([^{3}H] flunitrazepam) or centrifugation ([^{3}H] GABA). Nonspecific binding is determined in the presence of clonazepam (2 μM) or GABA (2 μM). The displacing potency of the compound is estimated as K_i (affinity constant for inhibitor) and IC_{50} (inhibitory concentration that displaces 50% of radiolabelled ligand from membranes).

3.5   Adenosine uptake

[^{3}H] Adenosine uptake is determined by the method of Phillis et al. [130]. Freshly prepared whole brain synaptosomes [131] are incubated in phosphate buffered balanced salt solution with [^{3}H] adenosine at 37°C for 40 sec in the presence of 0.1–100 μM of test compound. The assay is terminated by filtration through Whatman GF/B filters. Nonspecific binding is determined by incubation of [^{3}H] adenosine with boiled synaptosomes.

3.6   Genetically determined seizure models

The genetically epilepsy-prone rat is an important and much utilized model of genetically determined epilepsy and it has been reviewed recently [132]. Epileptic Gerbils appear to predict the anticonvulsant efficacy of GABAmimetic drugs better than other available models [133]. Various genetically determined syndromes of epilepsy in many species have been studied. Important ones are a recessive syndrome in hens where the provocation for seizure is by photic stimulation [134], and a large number of genetically determined syndromes in mice [135, 136]. The most extensively studied syndrome is sound-induced seizures in inbred strains of mice [137–139] and in Wistar and Sprague-Dawley strains of rats [140]. Though all classes of anticonvulsants are effective in sound-induced seizure, the more active compounds are those which antagonize benzodiazepine and EAA receptors and in the later case particularly the NMDA receptor.

3.7   Photosensitive epilepsy in *Papio papio*

This type of epilepsy was discovered in 1966 and has been extensively studied by neuropharmacologists and neurophysiologists [141–145]. This genetically determined syndrome of photically-induced myoclonus and epilepsy is shown by baboons. The triggered myoclonus of the eyelids, face, neck, trunk and limb are scored before and after i.v. or oral administration of the test anticonvulsant drug. This not only provides an accurate picture of dose-response relationship and time course of action but also of the relation between anticonvulsant effect and plasma levels of the drug and its metabolites. Established anticonvulsants like benzodiazepines, carbolines, EAA antagonists etc. are effective in this model and show a spectrum of activity that corresponds to myoclonic syndromes and primary generalized seizures in man [42, 146–148].

3.8   Focal seizures models

There is no optimal model for identifying drugs active against focal (partial) epilepsy. Focal seizure models are based on the use of epileptogenic agents to create a neocortical focus or to provoke limbic seizure either by their direct action by induction of focal pathology or by electrical kindling. A model of focal motor seizure in monkeys induced by alumina cream which has the advantage of close correspondence to partial seizures in man has been used extensively [149–151]. The other important test system is based on kindling [152–154]. It is highly reproducible and anticonvulsants active against complex partial seizures and tonic-clonic seizures are effective in this model. The relevance of kindling to human epileptogenesis has been discussed by Schmutz [155]. It has been found that NMDA receptors are involved in kindling [156, 157] and that competitive and non-competitive NMDA antagonists suppress kindling [158, 159]. These compounds also show antiepileptic action in a variety of animal seizure models [160, 161]. Among them MK-801 has shown limited anticonvulsant efficacy in the clinic [162].

The preclinical assessment of anticonvulsants is based on the median effective dose (protective index $PI = ID_{50}/ED_{50}$), where TD_{50} is the median toxic dose for neurotoxicity in mice (i.p. or p.o.). Neurotoxicity is measured by rotarod, positional sense, Gait and Stance, muscle tone and writhing tests [85, 163–165]. The detection and quantification of anticonvulsant activity is done in a phased manner according to Fig.1.

4   Development of anticonvulsants

4.1   Barbiturates

The barbiturates (5-alkyl and/or aryl derivatives of barbituric acid) have been used clinically for over eight decades as CNS depressants and anti-convulsants [166, 167]. However, some barbiturates may cause CNS exci-tation and subsequently induce seizures or convulsions [168, 169].

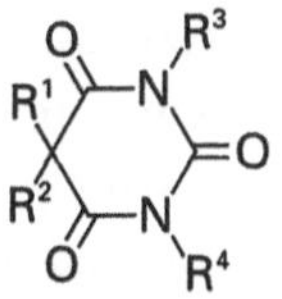

I	$R^1 = Ph, R^2 = Et, R^3 = R^4 = H$
II	$R^1 = Ph, R^2 = Et, R^3 = Me, R^4 = H$
III	$R^1 = R^2 = Et, R^3 = R^4 = H$
IV	$R^1 = R^2 = Et, R^3 = R^4 = H$
V	$R^1 = Ph, R^2 = Et, R^3 = R^4 = CH_2O$ alkyl
VI	$R^1 = Ph, R^2 = Et, R^3 = R^4 = CH_2OMe$
VII	$R^1 = R^2 = Et, R^3 = R^4 = CH_2OMe$
VIII	$R^1 = R^2 = Et, R^3 = R^4 = CH_2OCOMe$
IX	$R^1 = Ph, R^2 = Et, R^3 = CH_2OMe, R^4 = Me$

X $R^1 = Ph, R^2 = Et, R^3 = -CH_2-N$⟨ ⟩$O$, $R^4 = H$

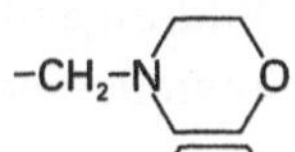

XI $R^1 = Ph, R^2 = Et, R^3 = -CH_2-N$⟨ ⟩ , $R^4 = H$

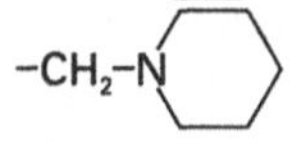

XII $R^1 = Ph, R^2 = Et, R^3 = R^4 = Me$
XIII $R^1 = Ph, R^2 = Et, R^3 = R^4 = Et$
XIV $R^1 = Ph, R^2 = Et, R^3 = R^4 = CH_2-Ph$

The anticonvulsant barbiturates include the first effective organic anticon-vulsant drug, phenobarbital (I), introduced in 1912 and still very widely used. Similar to other barbiturates, it is a powerful sedative but, unlike almost all other barbiturates, it has a selective anticonvulsant action because it shows maximal anti-seizure activity at a dose lower than that which is markedly sedative or hypnotic. It is effective in most animal seizure models viz. partial seizures and generalized tonic-clonic seizures (grand mal epilepsy). It is able to protect against both electroshock and pentylenetetrazole-induced seizures [170–172] and to suppress amygdaloid-kindled seizures [173]. It protects against PTZ seizures at a dose of 10 mg/kg p.o. in mice, and at about twice this dose it prevents electroshock seizures [174]. The hypnotic dose (HD$_{50}$) is 100 mg/kg and the dose for motor toxicity in the rotarod ataxia test (TD$_{50}$) is 70 mg/kg. Since phenobarbital is being used since 1912, it has not been scrutinized under the current regulatory procedure for new drug marketing. The oral daily dose for adults is 1–5 mg/kg (60–250 mg), but since the average plasma half-life is 100 hours it takes weeks to obtain a steady state. So a double dose is required for the initial 4 days to obtain quickly an effective concentration of drug in the plasma. The usual dose for children is 3–6 mg/kg in two divided doses; subsequent doses are monitored as per requirement for control of seizures or as limited by toxicity. It has slow oral absorption and its peak concentration in plasma occurs several hours after single dose. It is bound to plasma proteins and also to other tissues, including brain, to the extent of 40–60%. The volume of distribution is 0.5 l/kg. Its pKa is 7.3 up to 25% of the dose excreted by renal excretion and the remainder is inactivated by hepatic microsomal enzymes. The major metabolite is the p-hydroxyphenyl derivative which is inactive and is excreted in the urine partly as glucuronide. The other major metabolite is the N-glucoside derivative of I. The plasma half-life of phenobarbital in adults is 100 hr; it is longer in neonates and shorter and variable in children. Though it is used for generalized tonic-clonic and partial seizures in both children and adults and for most neonatal seizures, its reputation has come down in recent years because it has shown sedative and behavioural side-effects [175]. It produces irritability and hyperactivity in children and adversely affects general intelligence, perceptual motor and memory function and behaviour [176–178]. In a long-term double-blind study on children with febrile seizure, Farwell et al. reported that phenobarbital caused a significant (8.4 point) depression in cognitive performance as measured in an intelligence test, without providing any prophylaxis against the development of seizures [179]. No significant antiproliferative or cytotoxic effects are shown by phenobarbital in in vitro assays [180], but it is significantly cytotoxic at 1 mM concentration to a primary culture of cerebral cortex neuronal cells [181].

The other barbiturates marketed for epilepsy are N-methylphenobarbital (mephobarbital, II) and N-methylbarbital (metharbital, III) [182]. Mephobarbital (MEBARAL) gets N-demethylated in the hepatic endoplasmic reticulum and so its long-term action is attributed to the accumulation of phenobarbital. Hence it is similar to phenobarbital in pharmacological action, toxicity and clinical utility. However, its oral absorption is incomplete and its dose is approximately twice that of phenobarbital. Metharbital is metabolized to barbital (IV) and shows greater sedative and less antiepileptic activity than phenobarbital [183].

Among a series of 1,3-bis(alkoxymethyl)-5,5-disubstituted barbituric acids tested against MES and PTZ-induced seizures in mice, the 1,3-bis(alkoxymethyl)phenobarbitals (V), including 1,3-bis(dimethoxymethyl)phenobarbital (DMMP, VI), were very effective against both types of seizures while the corresponding analogues of barbital, including VII, were only active against PTZ-induced seizures. None of these compounds showed hypnotic activity [184]. DMMP (etrobarb) exerts its action mainly through its dealkylated metabolite N-monomethoxymethyl phenobarbital. Unlike phenobarbital it is more active in the MES test in mice ($ED_{50} = 14$ mg/kg p.o.) than in the PTZ-induced seizure test ($ED_{50} = 47$ mg/kg) [174]. In clinical studies in man eterobarb showed good antiepileptic activity with less sedation and hypnotic activity than phenobarbital [185, 186]. It was also effective in a variety of seizures in children and induced less severe hyperactivity than phenobarbital [187]. The replacement of the alkoxy group by acyloxy in compounds of type V did not result in any change in the profile of activity, as these compounds were also active against MES and PTZ-induced seizures in mice and were not hypnotic in mice. However, the 1,3-bis(acetoxymethyl)5,5-diethylbarbituric acid (VIII) in which the alkoxy group in VII is replaced by an acetoxy group, showed activity against electroshock seizure unlike VII which was active against PTZ-induced seizures [188]. Substitution at N-1 and N-3 also influenced the effectiveness against MES and PTZ-induced seizures. The 1-methyl-3-methoxymethyl phenobarbital (IX) was more effective against PTZ-induced seizure and less against electroshock seizure than mephobarbital and was not hypnotic. The replacement of the 1-methyl group on mephobarbital by morpholinomethyl (X) or piperidinomethyl (XI) groups resulted in retention of anticonvulsant activity against MES and PTZ-induced seizures. These compounds showed weaker hypnotic activity than phenobarbital [189]. The 1-alkyl, 1-alkoxymethyl, 1,3-dialkyl and 1-alkyl-3-alkoxymethyl derivatives of phenobarbital and barbital were as potent as mephobarbital against MES and PTZ-induced seizures. Substitution at N-1 in mephobarbital by another methyl group did not produce any change in anticonvulsant activity and the compound 1,3-dimethylphenobarbital (XII) was as potent as mephobarbital against MES and PTZ-induced seizures, and almost as hypnotic as mepho-barbital. Substitution at 1- and 3-positions by bulkier groups like ethyl (XIII) or benzyl (XIV) led to a substantial reduction in anticonvulsant and hypnotic activities [190].

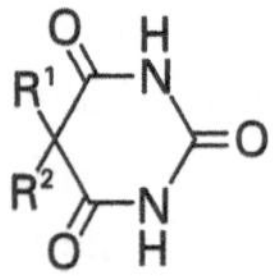

XV	$R^1 = R^2 = Ph$	
XVI	$R^1 = CH(Me)Pr$, $R^2 = Et$	
XVII	$R^1 = CH_2CH(Me)Et$, $R^2 = Et$	
XVIII	$R^1 = C(Me)=CHC_2H_5$, $R^2 = Et$	
XIX	$R^1 = C_4H_9$, $R^2 = Et$	
XX	$R^1 = CH_3C=CH[CH(Me)_2]$, $R^2 = Et$	
XXI	$R^1 = CH_2-CH=CMe_2$, $R^2 = Et$	
XXII	$R^1 = CH(Me)CH=C(CH_3)_2$, $R^2 = Et$	
XXIII	$R^1 = CH(Me)CH_2CH(CH_3)_2$, $R^2 = Et$	

XXIV $R^1 = CH_2CH_2$—⬡ , $R^2 = Et$

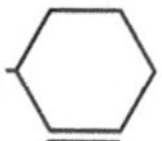

XXV $R^1 = CH_2CH$=⬡ , $R^2 = Et$

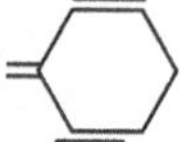

XXVI $R^1 = CH_2CH$=⬠ , $R^2 = Et$

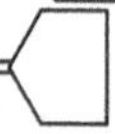

XXVII $R^1 = CH_2CH_2Ph$, $R^2 = Et$
XXVIII $R^1 = CH_2Ph$, $R^2 = Et$
XXIX $R^1 = CH_2CH(Me)Ph$, $R^2 = Et$

A large number of 5,5-disubstituted barbiturates have been investigated for their CNS effects including anticonvulsant effects [191–196]. Among these, 5,5-diphenylbarbituric acid was compared with phenobarbital and found less potent against MES and PTZ-induced seizures in mice [191]. The other compounds which have shown significant anticonvulsant activity are pentobarbital (XV), amytal (XVI) and vinbarbital (XVII). The interesting observation is that some of these compounds, particularly butethal (XIX), XX, XXI and XXII showed convulsant activity. The optical isomers of many of the 5,5-dialkyl barbituric acids have also been studied [168, 196, 197]. Sometimes one enantiomer showed convulsive action and the other anticonvulsant effect, e.g. the S(−) isomer of XXIII is anticonvulsant while the R(+) isomer and the racemic compound are potent convulsants. In order to study the role of the conformation of the 5-alkyl chain in the 5,5-dialkyl barbituric acids, the molecular conformations were studied using classical [198], molecular orbital [199] potential energy calculations [199, 200], ^{1}H and ^{13}C NMR spectrometry [201, 202] and X-ray crystallography [203–205]. Though the studies provide the details of conformations in solution, crystal and gas phases they do not directly identify the conformations responsible for convulsant and anticonvulsant actions. Studies using computer-graphic based pattern-recognition techniques have been reported on two series of 5-ethyl-5-substituted barbiturates [206] to find a correlation between molecular conformation and convulsant and anticonvulsant activities. These studies on barbiturates of type XVI–XXIII related to pentobarbital (trial set) revealed a region of space in which at least one low energy conformation of the hydrocarbon sidechain of each of the anticonvulsant barbiturates resides. Another region is occupied by a low energy conformation of each of the convulsant barbiturates. The biologically active conformations of anticonvulsants are near $\tau_1 = 180°$ and $\tau_2 = 180°$ (Fig. 2) while those of convulsants are $\tau_1 = 60°$ and $\tau_2 = 140°$ (Fig. 2).

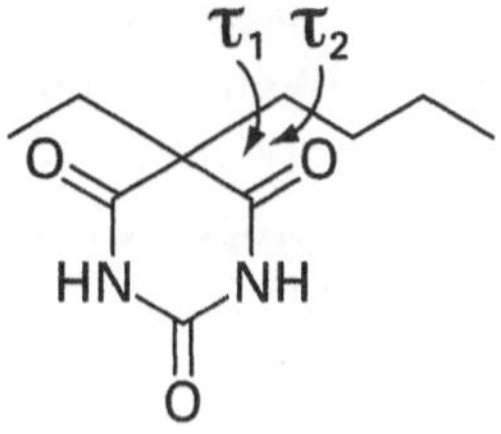

Fig. 2
Torsion angles τ_1 & τ_2 defined in clockwise rotations around the appropriate bond in barbiturates (**XIX**)

The aforesaid information regarding the spatial conformation of the pharmacophores also explains [206] the pharmacological activity in two other series of barbiturates in which minor structural changes convert the anticonvulsant XXIV [207] to the convulsants XXV and XXVI [208] and the anticonvulsant phenobarbital (I) and XXVII to the convulsants XXVIII and XXIX [207, 209, 210].

Several studies have been carried out to find the mechanism underlying the diverse effects of barbiturates. The main actions of barbiturates which may be important for the anticonvulsant effect are; (i) to enhance the GABA-mediated inhibitory response and (ii) to reduce the glutamate-mediated excitation. The former effect is due to their specific interaction with GABA$_A$ receptor Cl$^-$ channel complex [211]. Some studies suggest that the actions of barbiturates on GABA are important for the depressant action and not for the anticonvulsant action [210]. The observation that pentobarbital can directly activate GABA$_A$ receptor subunits in xenopus oocytes conclusively shows that barbiturate-induced Cl$^-$ current specifically involves the GABA receptor-channel complex [212]. The anaesthetic barbiturates have been shown to be (in comparison with GABA augmentation) more potent as direct agonists of Cl⁻ current than phenobarbital. Based on these studies it has been proposed that the anticonvulsant effects of barbiturates are related to GABA augmentation while the CNS depressant action is due to their GABA augmentation and their direct agonist activity [213]. In view of these results the role of direct or modulatory effects on GABA receptor function in the clinical action of antiepileptic drugs is uncertain.

In addition to pre- and post-synaptic inhibition, barbiturates reduce the depolarization-evoked neurotransmitter release in a wide variety of systems probably due to blockade of voltage-dependent Ca^{++} channels in nerve terminals [214–218]. It has been shown that barbiturates can inhibit the depolarization-stimulated Ca^{++} influx into synaptosomes [219–221], and also the Ca^{++}-dependent release of radiolabelled neurotransmitters from synaptosomes [222, 224] and reduce the maximal rate of rise and duration of Ca^{++}-dependent action potential [224–226].

Recently Gross and McDonald [227] have reported that the barbiturates selectively affect a new class of N-type Ca^{++} channel possessing different kinetic properties and voltage dependency and may be predominantly reponsible for Ca^{++} influx and neurotransmitter release. However, in view of the fact that phenobarbital inhibits Ca^{++} current at concentrations higher than the therapeutic antiepileptic level in brain, the importance of Ca^{++} channels for antiepileptic effects of barbiturates is also uncertain [211]. Wilson has shown that barbiturates at low doses enhance a voltage-dependent K^+ current in aplysia neurons [225]. In view of this observation and the similar effect of structurally related antihypertensive on K^+ current in hippocampal neurons [226], it has been proposed that K^+ channel activation could be a probable novel mechanism of antiepileptic drug action [228, 229].

Barbiturates also inhibit the responses mediated by excitatory amino acid (EAA) receptors preferably of non-NMDA type [230, 231]. Barbiturates potentiate the anticonvulsant effects of EAA antagonists while diazepam does not [232]. In view of these results and the observation that phenobarbital has weaker effects on GABA-receptor-mediated responses and voltage-sensitive Ca^{++} channels than the anaesthetic pentobarbital but is equipotent in inhibiting EAA responses [233] suggest that the anticonvulsant activity of barbiturates unlike their depressant action may be partly due to their ability to block excitatory transmission.

A number of studies have been made to correlate different topological (molecular connectivity, Wiener index, vertex indices of molecular graphs, electrotopological-state index) and physicochemical parameters like log P, gas chromatographic retention index, and HPLC retention time of barbiturates among themselves [234–240] and with pharmacokinetic parameters [241–245] or with biological activity parameter like barbiturate-cyclodextrin inclusion complex stability [246] or with anticonvulsant activity [237, 247, 248]. The topological indexes have mostly correlated well with lipophilic parameters. Hydrophobic parameters have shown good correlation with pharmacokinetic parameters and other biological activity parameters including anticonvulsant activity.

4.2   Deoxybarbiturates

The deoxybarbiturate 5-ethyldihydro-5-phenyl-4,6[1H,5H]-pyrimidinedione (primidone, XXX) may be viewed as the congener of phenobarbital (I) in which the carbonyl group of the urea moiety is replaced by a methylene group.

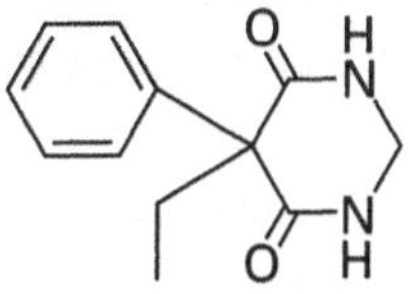

It is a widely used antiepileptic drug and metabolizes to the active metabolites phenobarbital and phenylethylmalonamide (PEMA, XXXI) [249, 250]. Primidone itself is almost as active as phenobarbital against MES but much less potent against PTZ-induced seizures. In contrast, PEMA has a similar spectrum of anticonvulsant activity to that of phenobarbital as it is active against both MES and PTZ-induced seizures, but its potency is one-sixteenth to one-thirteenth that of phenobarbital [251, 252]. However, the actual role of primidone and its active metabolites in the clinical antiepileptic activity of primidone has not been determined [249]. Primidone is given in divided doses of 750–1500 mg/day per adult. It is useful against generalized tonic-clonic and both simple and complex partial seizures. It is ineffective against absence seizures but is sometimes useful against myoclonic seizures in children. The common complaints associated with its use are sedation, vertigo, dizziness, nausea, autaxia, vomiting etc. Sometimes a patient experiences an acute feeling of intoxication immediately after its administration, i.e. before there is any significant metabolism.

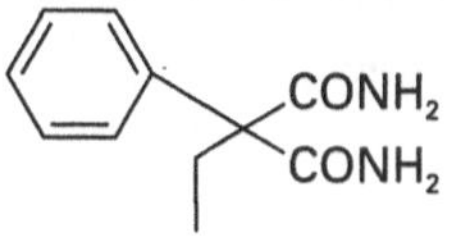

It has no serious side-effects and many of these are common to phenobarbital. The relationship of adverse effects to dosage is complex because they result from primidone and its two active metabolites. The side-effects are occasionally severe during initial therapy since tolerance develops only during long-term therapy.

4.3   Hydantoins

5-Ethyl-5-phenylhydantoin (phenytoin, XXXII), the oldest and most important member of this class, was the result of a search by Merritt and Putnam [72] for a non-sedating analogue of phenobarbital capable of suppressing electroshock-induced seizures in animals. At a normal therapeutic serum concentration of 10–20 µg/ml (40–80 µM), it protects against seizures without causing sedation [122, 253]. It abolishes the tonic phase (ED_{50} = 9.5 mg/kg i.p. in mice) and increases the clonic phase of the electroshock seizure. Unlike phenobarbital, phenytoin is ineffective against seizures induced by chemoconvulsants such as PTZ, bicuculline, picrotoxin, penicillin and strychnine [122, 254]. Its protective action against myoclonic responses in photosensitive baboons [255] and generalized seizures in alumina cream-lesioned cats is weak and variable against amygdaloid-kindled seizures in rats [173, 256]. Phenytoin exerts a wide variety of pharmacological actions on neurons compatible with its anticonvulsant activity. Its TD_{50} in rotarod ataxia test is 60 mg/kg in mice and its protective index (TD_{50}/ED_{50}) is 6.9. Phenytoin is a weak acid with pKa of about 8.3. Its pharmacokinetic characteristics are influenced by its limited solubility in water and by dose-dependent excretion. Its main metabolite, the p-hydroxyphenyl derivative (XXXIII), is inactive. The diverse neuronal actions of phenytoin have been reviewed in recent years [254, 257–259]. It has been demonstrated that it can interact with the voltage-dependent Na^+ channel in a highly specific voltage- and frequency-dependent manner. This is the only action which can explain its ability to suppress seizures without causing CNS depression at therapeutical concentrations (<10 µM). Phenytoin acts mainly by blockade of Na^+ channel. However, its effect on voltage-dependent Ca^{++} channel and K^+ current have also been implicated. It reduces the magnitude and duration of Ca^{++}-dependent action potential in cultured neurons at 20 µM [260]. It rapidly affects the inactivating type of Ca^{++} channel in neurons [260], and its inhibitory effect is intensified by membrane depolarization [261].

	XXXII	$R^1 = R^2 = Ph, R^3 = R^4 = H$
	XXXIII	$R^1 = 4\text{-OH–}C_6H_4, R^2 = Ph, R^4 = H$
	XXXIV	$R^1 = Ph, R^2 = Et, R^3 = H, R^4 = Me$
	XXXV	$R^1 = Ph, R^2 = Et, R^3 = H, R^4 = Et$
	XXXVI	$R^1 = R^2 = Thienyl, R^3 = R^4 = H$
	XXXVII	$R^1 = R^2 = Pyridyl, R^3 = R^4 = H$
	XXXVIII	$R^1 = R^2 = Ph, R^3 = H, R^4 = CH_2OMe$
	XXXIX	$R^1 = R^2 = Ph, R^3 = H, R^4 = CH_2OPh$
	XL	$R^1 = R^2 = Ph, R^3 = H, R^4 = CH_2OC_4H_9$
	XLI	$R^1 = R^2 = Ph, R^3 = H, R^4 = CH_2OCOMe$
	XLII	$R^1 = R^2 = Ph, R^3 = R^4 = CH_2OMe$
	XLIII	$R^1 = Ph, R^2 = Et, R^3 = H, R^4 = CH_2OCOMe$
	XLIV	$R^1 = Ph, R^2 = Et, R^3 = H, R^4 = CH_2OMe$

At concentrations >10 μM it delays the activation of outward K^+ current during action potentials in nerves leading to an increased refractory period [259]. Phenytoin has been reported to depress excitatory transmission by both pre- and post-synaptic mechanisms and to augment synaptic inhibition. These effects have been related to its effect on Ca^{++} and Na^+ channels. There have been controversial reports about the ability of phenytoin to enhance GABA-mediated synaptic inhibition or responses to exogenously applied GABA [260, 262]. In view of the fact that these effects on GABA responses have been reported to occur at concentrations substantially higher than therapeutic concentrations, it appears that the effects of phenytoin on GABA system do not significantly contribute to its anticonvulsant activity. Phenytoin is still the drug of choice in the treatment of generalized tonic-clonic grand mal epilepsy and is as effective as carbamazepine or valproate [263]. In multicentric trials phenytoin and carbamazepine have been found to be drugs of choice for the treatment of partial seizures [264]. It is not efficacious in the treatment of absence or myoclonic seizures. The toxic effects of phenytoin depend upon the route of administration, duration of treatment and dosage. Cardiac toxicity has been observed more frequently in older patients or those suffering from cardiac diseases, but rarely in young healthy patients [263]. At high doses it can produce marked cerebellar atrophy [264]. The other dose-related side-effects are nystagmus incoordination, ataxia, gingival hyperplasia, osteomalacia, megaloblastic anaemia and hirsutism.

The other hydantoins marketed but used infrequently are 3-methyl-5-ethyl-5-phenylhydantoin (mephenytoin, XXXIV) and 3-ethyl-5-phenylhydantoin (ethotoin, XXXV). Mephenytoin or mesantoin is active against tonic seizures in the maximal electroshock test. It has a somewhat different spectrum of anticonvulsant activity in the animal seizure model than phenytoin [265]. Unlike phenytoin it is active against PTZ-induced seizure and is sedative. At high doses it inhibits clonic seizures induced by bicuculline and picrotoxin. Mephenytoin is metabolized to give the N-dealkylated product-5-ethyl-5-phenylhydantoin (nirvanol). Although the latter is an effective anticonvulsant more potent than mephenytoin, it gets hydroxylated like phenytoin to give 5-(4-hydroxyphenyl)-5-ethylhydantatoin. Mephenytoin shows dose-related side-effects like nystagmus, diplopia and ataxia similar to phenytoin but apparently does not cause hirsutism and gingival hyperplasia. It shows high incidence of skin rashes, fatal aplastianaemia and other idiosyncratic toxicities [266–268]. Its topical daily dose is 200–600 mg in adults and 100–400 mg in children, but it is rarely advised in patients who fail to respond to other safer drugs.

Ethotoin (XXXV) was introduced in 1957 and is effective in complex partial and generalized tonic-clonic seizures. It has an almost similar profile of anticonvulsant action as that of mephenytoin [265]. It is generally well-tolerated and does not cause gingival hyperplasia or hirsutism similar to mephenytoin; however, it is used mostly as an adjunct to other drugs because of its relatively low potency compared with that of phenytoin. Its usual daily dose for adults is 2–3 g. It also gets N-dealkylated and p-hydroxylated *in vivo* similar to mephenytoin [253].

Among other 5,5-substituted hydantoins, the 5,5-dithienyl (XXXVI) and 5,5-dipyridyl (XXXVII) analogues showed anticonvulsant activities comparable to that of diphenylhydantoin [269, 270]. Among the 3-alkyl, alkoxy, acyloxy, alkylaryloxy, alkylaryl and piperazinoalkyl derivatives of 5,5-diphenylhydantoin studied for their anticonvulsant activity [184, 272], the 3-methoxymethyl derivative of (XXXVIII) was as active as the parent compound against MES test in mice and had weak anti-PTZ activity. The derivatives active against both MES and PTZ tests were 3-benzyloxymethyl (XXXIX) and 3-butoxymethyl (XL), while 3-acetoxymethyl (XLI) was active against MES but inactive against PTZ.

In another study, 3-acetoxymethyl and 1,3-diacetoxymethyl derivatives of 5-ethyl-5-phenylhydantoin and 1,3-dialkoxymethyl and alkylalkoxymethyl derivatives of 5,5-diphenylhydantoin and 5-ethyl-5-phenylhydantoin were evaluated for anticonvulsant activity in mice. Among these, 1,3-dimethoxymethyl)-5-diphenylhydantoin (XLII) and 3-acetoxymethyl-5-ethyl-5-phenylhydantoin (XLIII) were effective against MES and 3-methoxymethyl-5-ethyl-5-phenylhydantoin (XLIV) was active against both MES and PTZ-induced seizures in mice. However, none of them was more active in MES test than the parent compounds [273]. Substitution at the 3-position in diphenylhydantoin by groups like OC_2H_5, OH, NH_2, NHC_2H_5 and $NHNH_2$ did not result in loss of anticonvulsant activity [274].

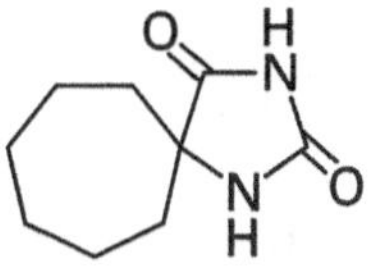

XLV 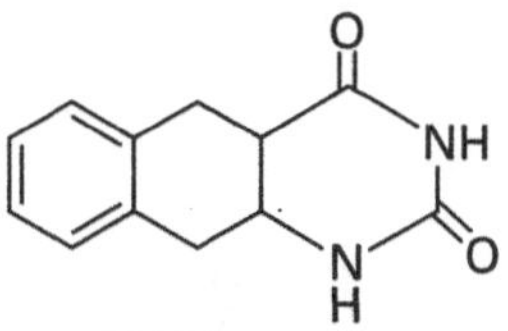   XLVI

Among the cycloalkanespiro-5-hydantoins, the cycloheptanospiro-5-hydantoins were active against PTZ-induced seizures. The cyclopentanospiro-5-hydantoins showed little anticonvulsant activity except at near toxic doses when they caused sedation. The cyclooctanospiro-5-hydantoins showed both anticonvulsant activity and sedation [275]. Among other spirohydantoins investigated, 5,5-heptamethylenehydantoin (XLV) and spirohydantoin derived from 2-tetralon (spirodon, XLVI) were active against MES and PTZ-induced seizures; the latter was more promising than the former being effective against grand mal epilepsy but it was toxic [276].

In a series of spirohydantoins (XLVII) derived from tricyclic ketones, compounds having X = $-CH_2-CH_2$, $-CH = CH-$, $(CH_2)_3-$ did not show anticonvulsant activity, rather the compound XLVII (X = $-(CH_2)_3$) was a potent convulsant [277]. Among the thio and dithiohydantoins resulting from the replacement of oxygen atom by sulphur in diphenylhydantoin, 5,5-dimethyldithiohydantoin (XLVIII) and 5,5-heptamethylene-2,4-dithiohydantoin (XLIX) were active against electroshock seizure in mice but 2-thiohydantoin was sedative and hypnotic. The replacement of oxygen by sulphur in diphenylhydantoin also resulted in the reduction of anticonvulsant activity [276, 23]. Albutoin (L) was active against all seizures but was most effective against grand mal epilepsy [278]. Among the 3-phenyl and 3-tolyl-5-arylidine-2-thiohydantoins, LI showed some activity against PTZ-induced seizures in mice [279].

In a recent study Kwon et al. synthesized and evaluated 5-substituted 2-iminohydantoins and their 1-carbobenzoxy derivatives for anticonvulsant activity in mice. The more lipophilic 1-carbobenzoxyiminohydantoins were more potent than the unsubstituted counterparts. Among chiral iminohydantoins, the activity resided mainly in compounds with S-absolute stereochemistry. The most active anticonvulsant compound of this series was

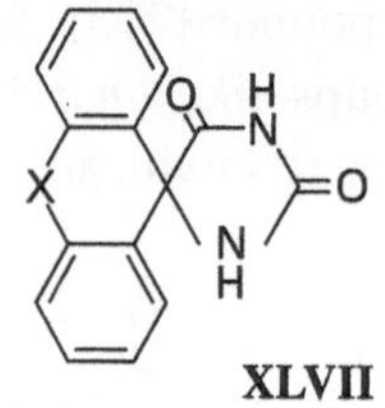

XLVII

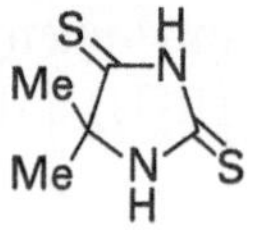

XLVIII

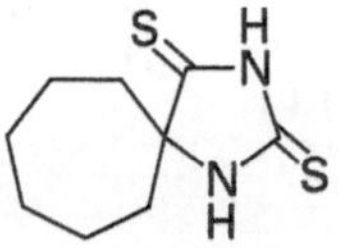

XLIX

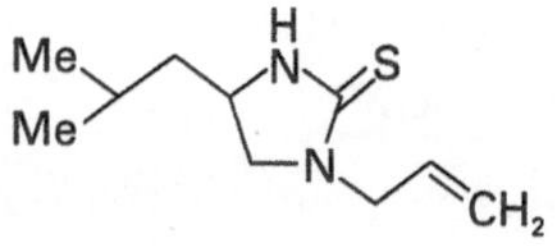

L

found to be (S)-(+)-1-carbobenzoxy-5-isobutyl-2-iminohydantoin (LII). It was not as active as phenytoin against electrically-induced convulsions, but was active against PTZ-induced seizures, suggesting that it may have a broader clinical potential. The closest analogue of phenytoin, i.e. 5,5-diphenyl-2-iminohydantoin (LIII) was inactive. The compounds obtained'

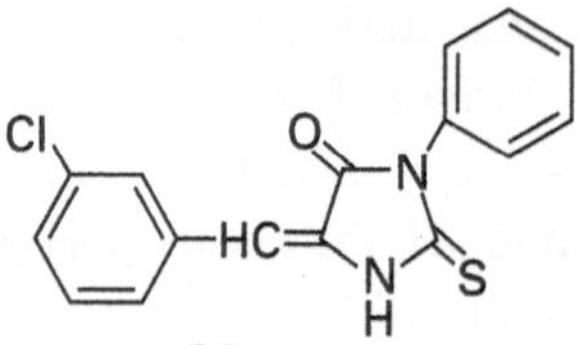

LI

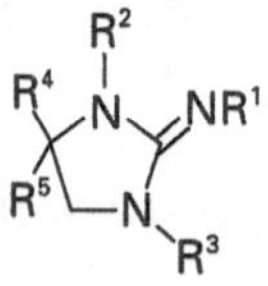

LII $R^1 = R^2 = R^4 = H$, $R^2 = COOCH_2Ph$, $R^5 = C_4H_9$ (iso)
LIII $R^1 = R^2 = R^3 = H$, $R^4 = R^5 = Ph$

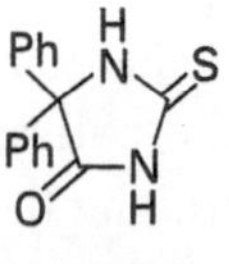

LIV

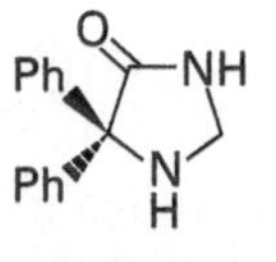

LV

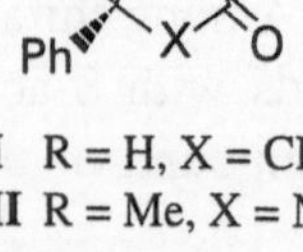

LVI R = H, X = CH_2
LVII R = Me, X = NH

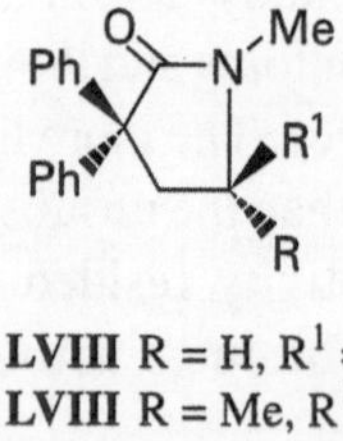

(R) **LVIII** R = H, R^1 = Me
(S) **LVIII** R = Me, R^1 = H

by methylation of N-3 or the imino nitrogen also did not show any significant activity. 2-Thiophenytoin (LIV) showed weak activity against PTZ-induced seizures and was inactive against electroshock seizures [280].

In order to study the effect of H-bonding on the antiepileptic activity of phenytoin in the MES test in mice, a series of compounds (LIV–LVII) was studied. Reduction in the ability to form H-bond by the replacement of a carbonyl or an NH group by a methylene (CH_2) group led to compounds which were less active than the parent diphenylhydantoin, as shown by the ED_{50} values of doxenitoin (LV, $ED_{50} = 129$ μmol/kg) and 3,3-diphenylsuccinimide (LVI, $ED_{50} = 107$ μmol/kg). The N-methylation also resulted in compounds which also had less ability to form H-bond than phenytoin. Thus, the compound 3-methyl-5,5-diphenylhydantoin (LVII, $ED_{50} = 149$ μmol/kg) had lower activity than phenytoin (XXXII, $ED_{50} = 228$ mg/kg). The pharmacological data, analyzed in terms of SAR, of the above compounds and of the racemic RS, R (LVIII) and S (LVIII) compounds indicated the importance of the H-bonding ability of these compounds and a certain degree of motional freedom of their phenyl groups for their antiepileptic activity [281].

4.4   Ureas

Phenylacetylurea (phenacemide, Phenurone, LIX), the oldest and the important member of this class was introduced by Gibbs et al. in 1949 [282]. It may be considered as ring-opened analogue of phenytoin. It is active against MES and PTZ-induced seizures, but its clinical use is limited due to adverse toxic reactions, including behavioural effects, gastrointestinal symptoms, rash, hepatitis, aplastic anaemia and nephritis etc. However, in a recent study it was found to be well-tolerated and effective in patients with refractory complex partial seizures [283]. Phenylethylacetylurea (LX, pheneturide) also has a similar profile of anticonvulsant activity and toxicity as phenacemide. Its use is limited to temporal lobe epilepsy refractory to other agents [284]. The α-chlorophenylacetylurea (LXI) obtained by the replacement of the C_2H_5 group in LX by Cl, also showed good anticonvulsant activity [276], but its replacement by a phenyl group, as in aromatic substitution or N-methylation in phenacemides, decreased the anticonvulsant activity. Diphenylacetylurea (LXII), which is an acyclic analogue of diphenylhydantoin, showed complete loss of anticonvulsant activity.

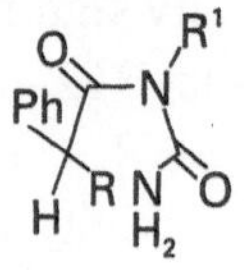

LIX   R = R^1 = H
LX   R = Et, R^1 = H
LXI   R = Cl, R^1 = H
LXII R = Ph, R^1 = H

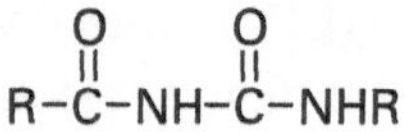

LXIII

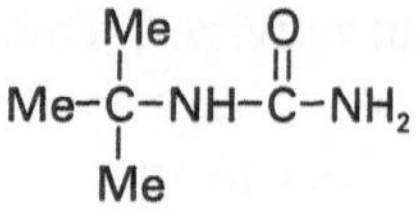

LXIV

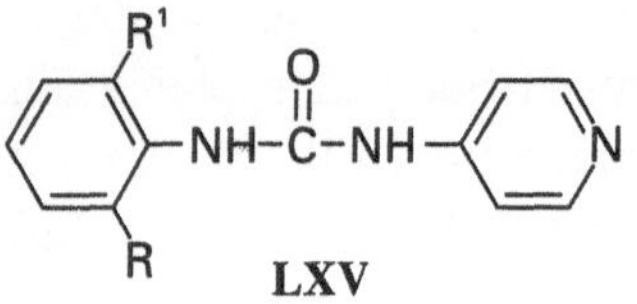

LXV

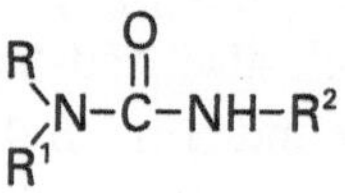

LXVII

Among a series of acylureas of type LXIII, where R = CH(CH$_3$)$_2$, CH(CH$_3$)C$_6$H$_5$, CH(CH$_3$)CH$_2$C$_6$H$_5$, iso-C$_5$H$_{11}$ or CH(C$_3$H$_7$)C$_6$H$_5$, and R^1 = CH$_3$, C$_2$H$_5$, C$_3$H$_7$, CH(CH$_3$)$_2$, C$_4$H$_9$, CH$_2$CH(CH$_3$)$_2$, C$_6$H$_5$ or CH$_2$C$_6$H$_5$, compounds having R = CH(CH$_3$)C$_6$H$_5$, CH(CH$_3$)CH$_2$C$_6$H$_5$ and R^1 = n-alkyl were the most effective against MES and PTZ-induced seizures [285]. The tert. butylurea (LXIV) has shown pronounced activity against PTZ-induced seizures in mice and rats [286]. In a recent study on N-phenyl-N'-pyridinylureas, optimal anticonvulsant activity was shown by the N-(2,6-disubstituted phenyl)-N'-(4-pyridinyl)urea (LXV) series. Among these compounds LXV (R^1 = CH$_3$, R = Cl) showed the best overall profile of anticonvulsant activity. It was effective in MES test in mice but did not protect them from PTZ-induced clonic seizures. The overall pharmacological profile suggested that LXVI would be of therapeutic use in the treatment of generalized tonic-clonic and partial seizures and it was selected for phase 1 clinical trials [287].

A pattern recognition SAR study using topological geometric and physicochemical descriptors has been carried out on 27 acyclic ureides of type LXVII, (R^1 = H, CH$_3$, C$_2$H$_5$, C$_4$H$_9$, CH$_2$C$_6$H$_5$, C$_6$H$_5$; R^2 = H, C$_3$H$_7$, (C$_6$H$_5$)$_2$CH; R = C$_4$H$_9$, C$_6$H$_5$, CH$_2$C$_6$H$_5$, tert. C$_5$H$_{11}$, (C$_6$H$_5$)$_2$CH, tert. C$_4$H$_9$, n-C$_4$H$_9$, n-C$_3$H$_7$, (CH$_3$)$_2$CHCH$_2$CH(CH$_3$)$_2$, CH$_2$C(CH$_3$)$_2$C$_6$H$_5$, fluorenyl, CH$_2$CH(C$_6$H$_5$)$_2$). Twelve topological descriptors were used as variables in a discriminant function analysis to categorize the ureide analogue with respect to their bioactivity [288]. The analysis suggested that one end of the ureide analogue must bear a bulky substituent. The high correlation of second order topological index and importance of the physi-cochemical log P values to the discriminant function indicate that this bulky substituent should be both branched and lipophilic. The other end of the ureide analogue must be sterically unencumbered. Thus, the antiepileptic bioactive fragment consists of an amide moiety, with both hydrogens sterically unrestricted, bonded via the carbonyl carbon through the remain-ing ureide nitrogen atom to a large, preferably aromatic, lipophilic group. This bioactive fragment is similar to that described for imidazolidindione (phenytoin) and iminostilbene (carbamazepine) anticonvulsants [289, 290].

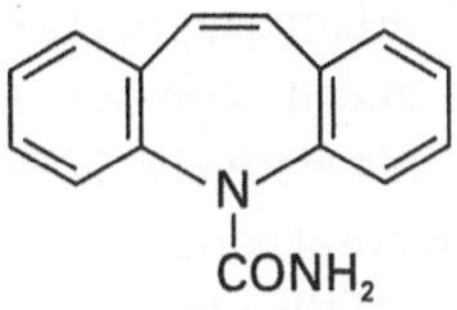

CONH₂

LXVIII

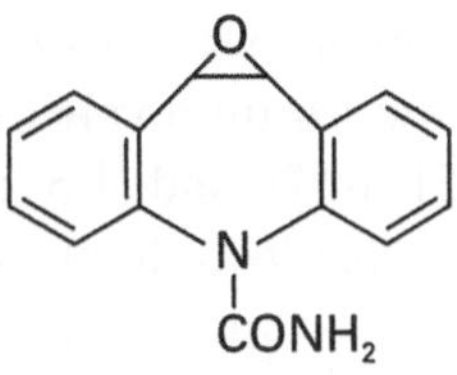

CONH₂

LXIX

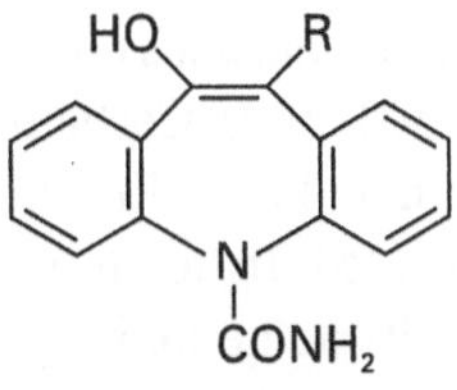

CONH₂

LXX   R = OH
LXXII R = H

CONH₂

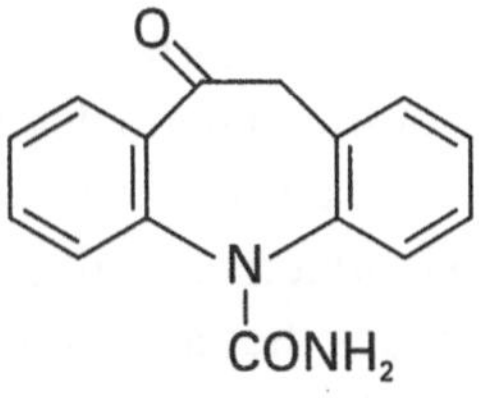

LXXI

5-Carbamyliminostilbene (LXVIII, carbamazepine) may also be consid-ered as a urea derivative where one of the urea nitrogens is part of a tricyclic system. Its synthesis was based on SAR studies carried out to maximize the anticonvulsant activity of a series of iminodibenzyl derivatives in 1950s [291].

It was approved for use as an anticonvulsant in 1974. However, it had been used for the treatment of trigeminal neuralgia since 1960s. It has a similar spectrum of anticonvulsant activity as phenytoin in many ways, both being effective against MES in mice. However, its ED50 in the mouse MES test is 8.8 mg/kg i.p. [292] and the protective index (TD50/ED50) is 8.1 which is a little higher than that of phenytoin. Carbamazepine reduces the severity and duration of amygdaloid-kindled seizure in rats at a dose of 30 mg/kg i.p. [122]. Like phenytoin, carbamazepine is highly effective in protecting against the spread of activity from the experimental focus and is less effective against initiation of epileptic discharges from the focus [293, 294]. Carbamazepine is more effective than phenytoin in blocking PTZ-induced seizures [295].

The pharmacokinetics of carbamazepine is complex and is influenced by its limited solubility in water and its increased ability to be converted by hepatic oxidative enzymes to an active 10,11-epoxide derivative (LXIX) which is further metabolized to inactive compounds [296]. The epoxide LXIX has a similar spectrum of activity to that of carbamazepine [297, 298]. The therapeutic serum levels of carbamazepine and its epoxide are 4–12 μg/ml (17–51 μM) and 1.5 μg/ml (6 μM), respectively [299]. Carbamazepine is absorbed slowly and erratically after oral administration. The CSF levels for carbamazapine may range 17–31% of the plasma concentration. The CSF to plasma ratio for carbamazapine epoxide (LXIX) are higher and range 45–55% [300].

Carbamazepine is well-tolerated by most patients and is as effective as phenytoin and phenobarbital in preventing partial and generalized tonic-clonic seizures. Both carbamazepine and phenytoin cause less impairment in the quality of life of patients than barbiturates [301, 302]. Carbamazepine produces less behavioural toxicity than phenytoin and also does not cause phenytoin-like hirsutism and gingival hyperplasia [5]. Its teratogenicity is similar to that of other antiepileptic drugs [303]. Its acute toxic symptoms are hyperirritability, convulsions and respiratory depression, which can lead to stupor or coma. The adverse effects include vomiting, eosinophilia, haematological toxicity and hypersensitivity reactions. Administration of carbamazepine along with phenytoin alters the pharmacokinetics of the latter [304], while combination therapy with phenobarbital does not have any advantage over either drug alone [305].

Carbamazepine and phenytoin have identical actions on Na^+ channel [306]. At clinically relevant concentrations (>4 μM), carbamazepine limits the sustained high frequency repetitive firing of cultured mammalian central neurons. This effect has been attributed to its action on Na^+ channels and is shared by its active metabolite LXIX but not by the inactive metabolite LXX [307]. The Na^+ channel block is voltage- and frequency-dependent. Like phenytoin, carbamazepine shifts the h_a curve for Na^+ currents to more negative membrane potentials and slows the recovery from inactivation

[308]. It also blocks the batrachotoxin site Na^+ channels like phenytoin [309, 310]. These observations support the view that carbamazepine acts on voltage-dependent Na^+ channels at therapeutic concentrations. However, how far this effect is specifically related to its anticonvulsant activity is not certain, because many other drugs which are more potent blockers of Na^+ channel than carbamazepine fail to specifically affect the epileptiform discharge at concentrations at which carbamazepine is strongly active [311]. Similarly, many drugs like butyrophenones, phenothiazines etc. which are more potent antagonists of (^{3}H)batrachotoxin binding than carbamazepine do not show anticonvulsant activity [312]. Carbamazepine also shows high affinity for both adenosine A_1 and A_2 receptors and acts as an antagonist [313, 314]. The anticonvulsant activity of a series of carbamazepine did not show correlation with adreno-receptor binding affinity [315] suggesting that adreno-receptor binding affinity is not necessary for anticonvulsant activity. Carbamazepine also interacts with the peripheral type of benzodiazepine receptors. Although one specific ligand (R05-4864) for these receptors blocks the anticonvulsant effect of carbamazepine in amygdaloid-kindled seizure in rats [316], the importance of this interaction for the anticonvulsant effect of carbamazepine is not yet established. Thus, there is no one single mechanism which unequivocally accounts for the anticonvulsant activity of carbamazepine. However, keeping in view its phenytoin-like effects, its action on voltage-dependent Na^+ channels may perhaps be the most plausible mechanism.

10,11-Dihydro-10-oxo-carbamazepine (LXXI, oxcarbazepine) is an analogue of carbamazepine in which a keto group has been introduced at the 10-position of the azepine ring. Although both carbamazepine and oxcarbazepine are ultimately metabolized to the inactive trans-diol LXIX, the keto group at 10-position prevents the formation of the epoxide intermediate (LXVIII). It is metabolized in humans to 10,11-dihydrocarbazepine (LXXII) [317]. The antiepileptic potency of oxcarbazepine as well as of its metabolite LXXII is similar to those of carbamazepine and phenytoin [318]. Oxcarbazepine has some advantages over carbamazepine. It is a weaker inducer of hepatic microsomal enzymes [319] and does not form an epoxide (LXIX) so the side-effects believed to be caused by this metabolite like nausea, headache, dizziness and drowsiness are eliminated [320]. The incidence of adverse side-effects including diplopia, ataxia, nystagmus, epigastric discomfort has been found to be lower in the case of oxacarbazepine than of carbamazepine [321]. The frequency of reactions too was less. According to a recent retrospective survey of 947 patients treated with oxacarbazepine only 18% discontinued the treatment because of adverse effects [322]. In clinical studies by Grant and Faulds [323], it was found safe and only one patient developed leukopenia. In some cases of elderly patients receiving high doses hyponatraemia has been observed [322, 324]. The non-oxidative metabolism of oxcarbazepine makes it less liable than carbamazepine to interact with other drugs [325]. A recent study has shown that oxcarbazepine may reduce the efficacy of oral contraceptives [326]. The existing clinical data on oxcarbazepine in adult patients with partial and generalized tonic-clonic seizures, the lower incidence of allergic reactions caused by it compared to carbamazepine and the low risk of interaction with other epileptic drugs support the adjunctive use of oxcarbazepine in the treatment of resistant patients. Its usual total daily dose is 600 to 1200 mg divided into 2–3 doses.

4.5   Oxazolidine 2,4-diones

Oxazolidine-2,4-diones (LXXIII–LXXIX) may be considered as structural analogues of hydantoins in which the NH at 1-position has been replaced by an oxygen. Substitution at 5-position is associated with anticonvulsant activity as in hydantoins. 3,5,5-Trimethyloxazolidine-2,4-dione (trimethadione, LXXIII) was the first compound of this class to be marketed as an antiepileptic drug for the treatment of absence or petit mal seizures. Its analogue 3,5-dimethyl-5-ethyloxazolidine-2,4-dione (paramethadione, LXXIV) has similar, but somewhat lesser activity and lesser toxicity than LXXIII. The alkyl substituents on the carbon in 5-position appear to be important for the selectivity of oxazolidine-2,4-diones both as antagonists of PTZ in animals and as clinically effective agents against absence seizure [23].

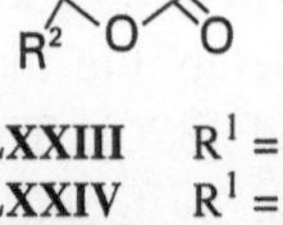

LXXIII	$R^1 = R^2 = R^3 = Me$
LXXIV	$R^1 = R^3 = Me$, $R^2 = Et$
LXXV	$R^1 = R^2 = Me$, $R^3 = Et$
LXXVI	$R^1 = H$, $R^2 = Me$, $R^3 = alkyl$
LXXVII	$R^1 = R^2 = Ph$, $R^3 = H$
LXXVIII	$R^1 = R^2 = Me$, $R^3 = H$

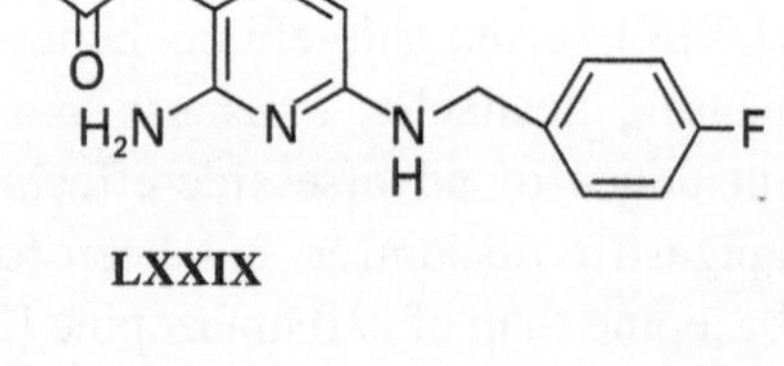

LXXIX

Substitution in the 5-position by lower alkyl groups leads to compounds active against petit mal seizure while substitution by aryl groups leads to agents effective against grand mal seizure. The other clinically useful oxazolidine-2,4-diones are 3-ethyl-5,5-dimethyloxazolidine-2,4-dione (dimidione, LXXV) and 3-alkyl-5-methyloxazolidine-2,4-dione (malidione, LXXVI) effective against petit mal and 5,5-diphenyloxazolidine-2,4-dione (LXXVII) against grand mal seizures [23, 276].

Alkylation of the imido-N at 3-position is mandatory for activity against petit mal seizure. This substitution either increases the lipophilicity or prevents the dissociation of the imido H, leading to effective transport of dimidione and malidione to the CNS. However, it has been observed that these compounds get N-dealkylated during metabolism. Thus it appears that N-alkyl substituents are not essential at the site of action and that N-dealkylated metabolites are important for activity. Trimethadione gets rapidly demethylated by hepatic microsomal enzyme to its active metabolite dimethadione (DMO, LXXVIII) [327]. Like trimethadione, dimethadione is also more effective against PTZ-induced seizures than against MES in mice and rats, and none of them binds to plasma proteins. According to studies by Frey and Kretschmer on the effect of chronic administration of trimethadione on the PTZ seizure threshold in mice, the anticonvulsant activity of trimethadione is mainly due to dimethadione [328]. Their use has become uncommon due to high incidence of sedation and visual disturbances (hemeralopia) and other toxic reactions [329]. The anti-absence seizure activity of DMO is considered to be due to blockage of the T-type Ca^{++} current in thalmic neurons (40–52% reduction at 4–8 mM concentration). DMO failed to alter the kinetic properties of this current or its h_∞ curve [330]. Recently, a novel pyridine oxazolidinone (D19274, LXXIX) has been reported to be an effective anticonvulsant agent which is active in the MES test (ED_{50} = 28 mg/kg i.p. in mice) [331]. It has relatively low motor toxicity (Rotarod TD_{50} = 150 mg/kg) and suppresses spontaneous spike and wave discharges in rats even at a dose of 10 mg/kg. It is expected to be effective against absence seizure.

4.6   Imides

The succinimides evolved from a systematic search for more effective and less toxic anticonvulsant agents against absence seizure than oxazolidinediones. The α,α-diphenylsuccinimide (LXXX), a close analogue of diphenylhydantoin, was active against MES. The effects of N-alkylation of LXXX and phenytoin were similar and the N-alkylated derivatives were found to be less effective than the parent compounds. N-Methyl-α-phenylsuccinimide (phensuximide, LXXXI) was the first succinimide introduced for the therapy of absence seizure when compared clinically with oxazolidinediones, it was found to be less potent than trimethadione. It is active against both MES in mice (ED$_{50}$ = 183 mg/kg p.o.) and PTZ seizure in rats (ED$_{50}$ = 125 mg/kg p.o.) [332]. The poor anticonvulsant activity of phensuximide may be due to its rapid metabolism and poor accumulation of its demethylated metabolite, desmethylphensuximide (LXXXII) [333]. LXXXII is deactivated by dihydropyriminidase to 2-phenylsuccinamic acid. The half-lives of phensuximide and its metabolite LXXXII in plasma are similar (approx. 8 hr). Its 2-methylated analogue, N,α-dimethyl-α-phenylsuccinimide (methsuximide, LXXXIII) is more active than phensuximide in the MES test in mice (ED$_{50}$ = 84 mg/kg p.o.) and in PTZ test [332]. It is more active than phensuximide in the treatment of petit mal and psychomotor seizures but is more toxic. Methsuximide has a broader spectrum of clinical antiepileptic activity than ethosuximide [333]. It is also metabolized by demethylation to N-desmethylmethsuxi-' mide (LXXXIV), but unlike LXXXII the succinimide ring of LXXXIV does not get opened by dihydropyrimidinase due to the protection provided by the additional methyl group. So it accumulates in plasma and hence the plasma half-life of LXXXIV is 40 hr. It was found to be effective in a wide variety of seizures in a majority of 34 paediatric patients [334].

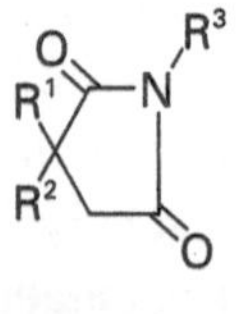

LXXX $R^1 = R^2 = Ph, R^3 = H$
LXXXI $R^1 = Ph, R^2 = H, R^3 = Me$
LXXXII $R^1 = Ph, R^2 = R^3 = H$
LXXXIII $R^1 = Ph, R^2 = R^3 = Me$
LXXXIV $R^1 = Ph, R^2 = Me, R^3 = H$
LXXXV $R^1 = Et, R^2 = Me, R^3 = H$

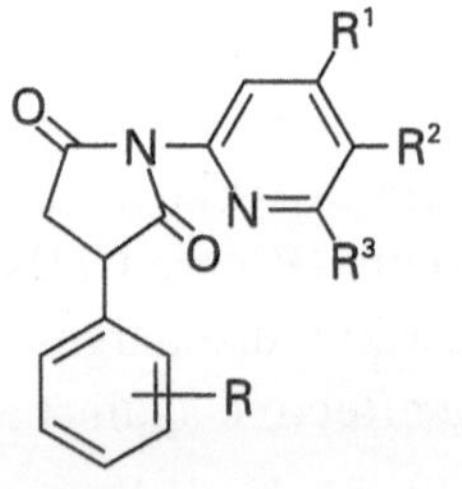

LXXXVI $R = R^1 = R^3 = H, R^2 = Cl$
LXXXVII $R = R^2 = H, R^1 = R^3 = Me$

α-Ethyl-α-methylsuccinimide (ethosuximide, LXXXV) is the drug of choice in the treatment of absence or petit mal seizures. It specifically blocks PTZ and bicuculline-induced clonic seizures in mice (ED$_{50}$ = 130 mg/kg i.p.) but does not show activity against tonic seizure in the MES test except at an anaesthetic dose [111]. It is effective in a variety of other models of generalized absence seizures [335–338]. Ethosuximide is more effective against absence seizure and less toxic than trimethadione.

The clinical efficacy of ethosuximide has been established in patients with absence seizure [339, 340]. The most common dose-related side-effects are nausea, vomiting, anorexia, CNS-effects like drowsiness, lethargy, euphoria, dizziness, headache. It has a unique profile of activity and a novel mechanism of action. Unlike phenytoin and carbamazepine it fails to limit sustained high frequency repetitive firing of neurons at clinically effective concentrations and hence it presumably does not block the voltage-gated Na^+ channels [341]. It also does not potentiate the post-synaptic actions of GABA responses [342, 343] similar to other drugs effective in the treatment of absence seizure. It may, however, interact with the picrotoxin site on $GABA_A$ receptor channel complex [345]. Unlike other prototype antiepileptic drugs, ethosuximide is a selective antagonist of T type voltage-dependent Ca^{++} channels in thalamic neurons [345–347].

4-Alkylphenyl-N-methyl succinimides were more active against MES than other types of seizure. The substitution of the alkyl group by the iso-alkyl group tends to increase the activity against PTZ-induced seizures [348]. The compounds α-methylalkoxyphenylsuccinimides were more active than alkoxybenzylsuccinimides against PTZ-induced seizures, while the latter were more active against MES [349].

Different aryl succinimides particularly those substituted by a 5-chloro-2-pyridyl (LXXXVI) or 4,6-dimethyl-2-pyridyl (LXXXVII) group at imide N have been investigated for their anticonvulsant activity [350, 351]. The conformations of the active and inactive molecules differ in the relative positions of the pyridyl ring and succinimide moiety. The anticonvulsant activity and toxicity of 20 arylsuccinimides has been quantitatively correlated with the hydrophobicity, and the steric and electronic parameters of the substituents in the benzene ring and on the N-atom. The activity was optimum when the benzene ring substituent X had a hydrophobic fragmental constant (fx) value of 1.0–1.7, while the toxicity increased with (fx) [352].

Among other succinimides, spiro(dibenzo(a,d)cycloheptadiene-5,2-succinimide (LXXXVIII) showed activity against MES and PTZ-induced seizures in mice at 1/20th LD_{50} dose [277]. The enlargement of the 5-membered imide ring to a six-membered glutarimide derivative did not lead to the abolition of anticonvulsant activity. α-Methyl-α-phenylglutarimide

(LXXXIX) showed activity against PTZ-induced seizures in mice, but its ethyl analogue (XC, glutethimide) is more useful as a sedative-hypnotic whereas α-(4-aminophenyl)-α-ethylglutarimide (XCI, aminoglutethimide) is effective as an anticonvulsant in grand mal and to some extent in petit mal seizures, but has no sedative action. Aminoglutethimide has shown activity comparable with that of diphenylhydantoin against grand mal seizure but has a relatively higher incidence of side-effects than phenylhydantoin. The glutethimide metabolite, 4-hydroxy-2-ethyl-2-phenylglutarimide (XCII), showed anticonvulsant activity against MES in mice along with potent sedative hypnotic-activity. Its 4-amino analogue (XCIII) also showed increased anticonvulsant activity relative to sedative and hypnotic activities similar to XCI w.r.t. XC [353].

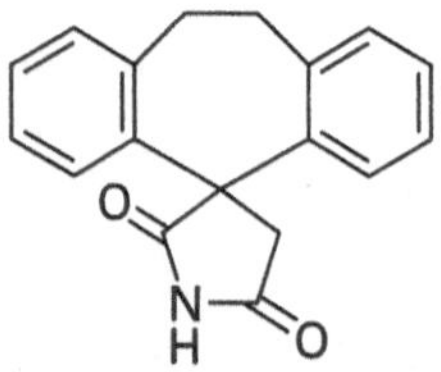

LXXXVIII

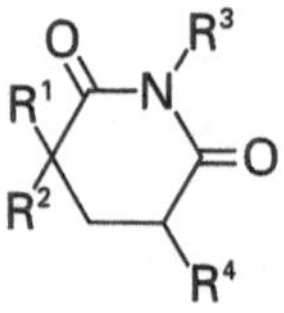

LXXXIX	R^1 = Me, R^2 = Ph, R^3 = H, R^4 = OH
XC	R^1 = Et, R^2 = Ph, R^3 = R^4 = H
XCI	R^1 = Et, R^2 = C_6H_4-4-NH_2, R^3 = R4 = H
XCII	R^1 = Et, R^2 = Ph, R^3 = H, R^4 = OH
XCIII	R^1 = Et, R^2 = C_6H_4-4-NH_2, R^3 = H, R^4 = OH
XCIV	R^1 = Et, R^2 = Me, R^3 = CH_2Ph, R^4 = H
XCV	R^1 = Et, R^2 = Me, R^3 = O-xylyl, R^4 = H
XCVI	R^1 = R^2 = R^3 = H, R^4 = CH_2Ar
XCVII	R^1 = R^2 = R^3 = H, R^4 = $CH_2 \cdot C_6H_4$-4-Cl

Several acetyl -D(R) and L(S)-N-(4-substituted phenyl)-succinimides and glutarimides have been evaluated for their anticonvulsant activity in mice [354]. Among the succinimides the D(R)-unsubstituted and chloro derivatives were active in MES and scMet tests in mice while L(S) isomers showed CNS-stimulant effects. The L(S) and D(R) methoxy derivatives showed neither anticonvulsant nor CNS-stimulant effects. Among the glutarimides the D(R) isomers were more active in MES tests in mice than the corresponding L(S) isomers. In the scMet test stereoselectivity was observed for the nitrophenylglutarimides. SAR studies showed the importance of hydrophobic, electronic and steric factors [354]. In an extension of this work more 4-substituted-N-acetyl-L(S) and D(R)-α-amino-N-phenylglutarimides having 4-substituents like $COCH_3$, I, CN, C_2H_5 and C_4H_9 were studied for anticonvulsant activity (MES and scMet ED_{50}s), neurotoxicity (TD_{50}) and protective indices ($PI = TD_{50}/ED_{50}$) and minimal seizure threshold (ivMet) in comparison to the other clinically useful anticonvulsants. A parallel relationship was found between neurotoxicity (TD_{50}) and anticonvulsant potency (ED_{50}) in the case of R and S isomers. In most cases the R isomers had a more rapid onset of action and possessed greater anticonvulsant potency and neurotoxicity than the S isomers [355]. In a series of N-allyl, benzyl and N-o-xylyl glutarimides, N-benzylbemergide (XCIV) and N-o-xylylbemergide (XCV) showed some anticonvulsant activity at 20 mg/kg i.p. in mice [356]. A series of twenty-two, 2-benzylglutarimides (XCVI, Ar = C_6H_4-X where X = H, 4-OCH_3, 2-Br, 4-Br, 4-I, 4-CF_3, 2,4-$(Cl)_2$, 3,4-$(Cl)_2$, 4-$Si(CH_3)_3$ etc.) and its N-methyl analogues (XCVI, $R_3 = CH_3$) was designed using Topliss scheme for selection of the benzyl substituent for optimum anticonvulsant activity against MES and scMet-induced sei-zures in mice. Among these compounds 2-(4-chlorobenzyl)glutarimide (XCVII) was the most effective both in MES and scMet tests and also had low neurotoxicity. In drug differentiation tests, it was also effective against seizures induced by bicuculline, picrotoxin and strychnine. In a comparison with other clinically useful anticonvulsants it exhibited an overall profile most closely resembling that of valproate [357].

4.7   Acids

Dipropylacetic acid (XCVIII, valproic acid) may be considered as the most important member of this class. Its activity was discovered serendipitously during its use as a vehicle for the screening of anticonvulsant compounds. Although initially it was found as active as trimethadione and ethosuximide in the PTZ-induced seizure threshold test, and slightly active in the MES test [358], later it was shown to have anticonvulsant activity in a wide variety of animal seizure models with minimum sedation and other side-ef-fects. It is active against tonic-clonic seizures induced by a variety of chemoconvulsants (PTZ, bicuculline, picrotoxin, strychnine, isonicotonic acid, 3-mercaptopropionic acid, penicillin, aminophylline), reflex seizures induced by sensory stimuli and kindling models [359–362] but is weakly protective against seizures induced by excitatory amino acids [359, 363]. It inhibits the spread of seizures from a cortical lesion produced by the implantation of cobalt or alumina cream from the site of kindling. Its efficacy has been tested against the homocysteine and thiolactone-induced secondary generalized tonic-clonic seizures in rats, where its ED_{50} was 211.9 mg/kg, i.p. [364]. Based on the comparison of these results in terms of serum concentration with other anticonvulsants in this model it has been predicted that a serum concentration of 270 μg/ml of VPA would be required for the control of generalized convulsive seizure in human patients; however, its safety at this concentration has not been studied [364]. Valproate shows an anticonvulsant effect in mice only at high doses of 150–400 mg/kg, i.p. but this is not due to its inability to cross the blood-brain barrier less effectively than other anticonvulsant drugs, because its concentration in CSF is almost the same as that of phenytoin (approx. 10%) [365]. In mice it causes motor toxicity at a dose close to its ED_{50} (272 mg/kg i.p.) in the MES test so that the protective index (TD_{50} for motor toxicity/ED_{50}) is only 1.6 compared to 6.9 for phenytoin [122]. However, it is well tolerated in man and its toxic side-effects are few in clinical practice. The two major metabolites of the drug formed are 2-propyl-2-pentenoic acid (XCIX) and 2-propyl-4-pentenoic acid (C) by β and ω oxidation, respectively [366], which are as potent as valproic acid. However, only the 2-ene trans isomer of the former has been found in measurable quantities in brain. The half-life of valproate is 15 hr [359]. It has a broad spectrum of anticonvulsant activity and has been found to be as effective as ethosuximide in a double-blind, response-conditional crossover study of absence seizures in 45 patients [367]. In recent years its clinical efficacy against partial seizures [368] and other generalized types of seizure [369] has been demonstrated. The most common side-effects of valproic acid are transient gastrointestinal symptoms like anorexia, nausea, vomiting and CNS effects like sedation, ataxia, tremor, while rare side-effects are rash, alopecia and hepatitis [370]. Teratogenicity of VPA and its metabolites XCIX and C in humans and experimental animals has been studied in recent years [371–376].

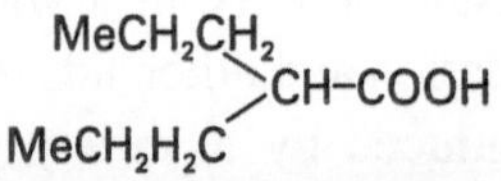

$$MeCH_2CH_2 \diagdown CH\text{-}COOH$$
$$MeCH_2H_2C \diagup$$

XCVIII

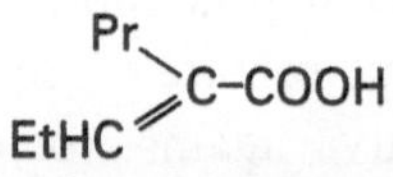

$$Pr \diagdown C\text{-}COOH$$
$$EtHC \diagup$$

XCIX

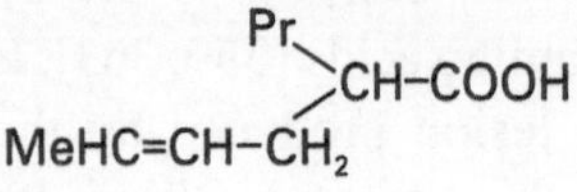

$$Pr \diagdown CH\text{-}COOH$$
$$MeHC\text{=}CH\text{-}CH_2 \diagup$$

C

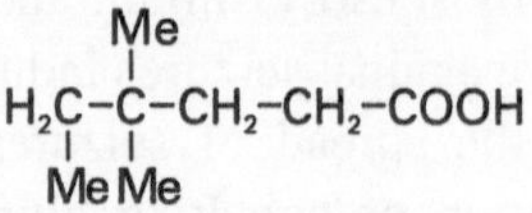

$$H_2C\text{-}\underset{\underset{Me}{|}}{\overset{\overset{Me}{|}}{C}}\text{-}CH_2\text{-}CH_2\text{-}COOH$$

CI

These studies have opened up the possibility for development of novel antiepileptic agents of this class with low teratogenicity. Two hypotheses have been proposed for the mechanism of action of valproate. According to the first, its administration increases the GABA level in whole brain and nerve terminals and this increase is related to the drug's anticonvulsant activity [370, 377–379]. According to the second theory, valporates acts on voltage-dependent Na^+ channels because, like phenytoin and carbamazepine, it markedly inhibits the repetitive firing of cultured neurons at therapeutical concentrations (2–10 μg/ml) [376]. However, valproate does not show any effect as these concentrations on batrachotoxin-stimulated 22 Na^+ flux [380] or on batrachotoxin-binding [381]. In view of these observations, it seems that the clinical activity of valproate is due to a combination of two mechanisms. The phenytoin-like effect on Na^+ channels may be responsible for its action against electroshock seizure and partial seizure, whereas its interaction with the GABA-ergic system may explain its broader spectrum of activity than phenytoin and carbamazepine. However, today's data is insufficient to establish conclusively either of these mechanisms.

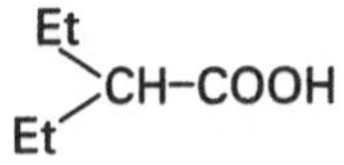

$$\begin{array}{cc} \underset{Et}{\overset{Et}{>}}CH\text{–}COOH & \underset{Me}{\overset{Me}{\underset{|}{\overset{|}{Me\text{–}C\text{–}CH_2\text{–}COOH}}}} \\ \textbf{CII} & \textbf{CIII} \end{array}$$

$$\begin{array}{cc} \underset{Me}{\overset{Me}{>}}HC\text{–}CH_2\text{–}COOH & \underset{Me}{\overset{Me}{>}}CH\text{–}COOH \\ \textbf{CIV} & \textbf{CV} \end{array}$$

$$\underset{Pr}{\overset{Pr}{>}}CH\text{–}COOR$$

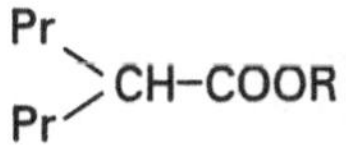

CVI

$$\underset{R^2}{\overset{R^1}{>}}CH\text{–}COOH$$

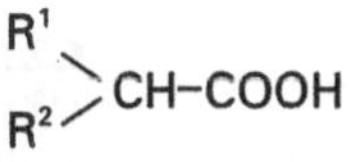

CVII $R^1 = R^2 = C_4H_9$
CVIII $R^1 = Pr, R^2 = CH_2COMe$

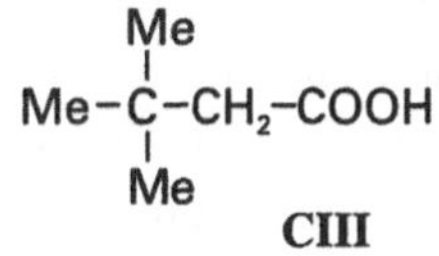

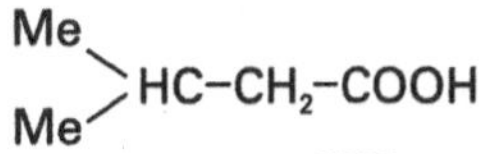

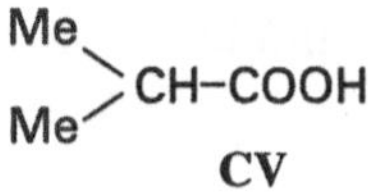

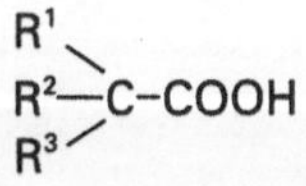

$$\underset{R^3}{\overset{R^1}{\underset{}{\overset{}{R^2\text{–}C\text{–}COOH}}}}$$

CIX $R^1 = R^2 = Me, R^3 = Et$
CX $R^1 = R^2 = R^3 = Me$

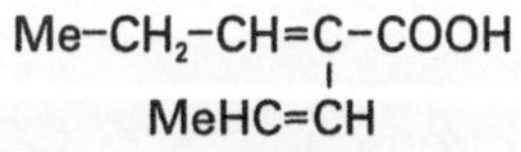

$$Me\text{–}CH_2\text{–}CH=C\text{–}COOH$$
$$MeHC=CH$$

CXI

Among several analogues of valproic acid studied earlier [382], the compound 3,3,4-trimethylpentanoic acid (CI) was as active as VPA. Diethylacetic acid (CII), 2,2-dimethylbutyric acid (CIII) and 2,2-dimethylpropionic acid (CIV) showed 80% of the activity of VPA while the isobutyric acid (CV) was only 20% as active. Other analogues like dibutylacetic acid, isovaleric acid, vinylacetic acid, isocrotonic and triglic acid and those in which CH_2 adjacent to CO_2H group has been oxidized to CO like $C_2H_5COCO_2H$, $C_3H_7COCO_2H$ and $C_4H_9COCO_2H$ were inactive as anticonvulsants. In a series of dialkylalkanoic acids, (<14 C atom) and some of their alcohol and amide analogues, anticonvulsant activity was found to increase with increase in chain length. The introduction of a double bond decreased the activity while the introduction of a sec. or tert. OH group or replacement of the CO_2H group by an OH group had no effect [382]. The conversion of acid into esters or amides sometimes increased the activity. These esters or amides have been found to act as prodrugs of VPA. Among the five esters, propyl (CVI, R = C_3H_7), butyl (CVI, R = C_4H_9), isobutyl (CVI, R = iso-C_4H_9) and hexyl (CVI, R = C_6H_{13}) valproate, only the propyl ester showed anticonvulsant activity and was less neurotoxic than VPA [383]. Several other analogues of valproic acid have been studied for their anticonvulsant activity in recent years [359, 379, 384, 385]. Most of these compounds showed a correlation between structure and anticonvulsant potency; the larger molecules were in general more active. These compounds reduced cerebral aspartate levels and most of them elevated cerebral GABA levels [379]. The valpromide will be discussed in the next section along with other amides.

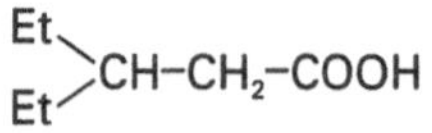

Et
  \
   CH–CH$_2$–COOH
  /
Et

CXII

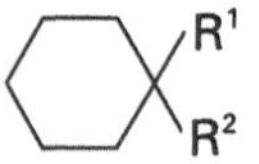

CXIII R^1 = Me, R^2 = COOH
CXIV R^1 = H, R^2 = CH$_2$COOH

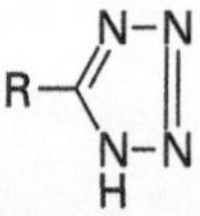

CXV   R = C_7H_{15}
CXVI R = (CH$_3$)$_2$CHCH$_2$CH$_2$–

R
  \
   N–C–CH$_2$–CH$_2$COOH
  /   ‖
R   O

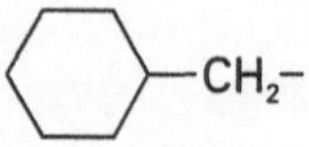

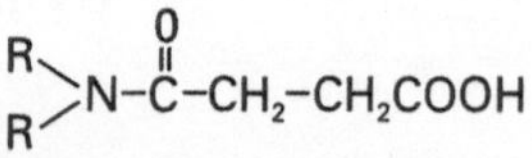

CXVIII   R = Et
CXIX   R = C$_4$H$_9$

CXVII R = –CH$_2$–

In QSAR studies on valproic acid analogues (XCIX, CI, CV, CVII–CXIX) and other analogues in which the CO_2H group was replaced by the isosteric tetrazole, Abbott and Acheampong demonstrated that anticonvulsant potency as measured in the PTZ test in mice, within a class of compounds like carboxylic acids can be correlated with lipophilicity and pKa. However, the anticonvulsant potency of compounds of other classes with diverse polarities could be correlated with dipole moment and lipophilicity [386]. The most active compounds among these were 5-heptyltetrazole (CXV, $ED_{50} = 0.31$ mmol/kg i.p.), and 2-butylhexanoic acid (CVII, $ED_{50} = 0.57$ mmol/kg i.p.) as compared to $ED_{50} = 0.70$ mmol/kg i.p. for VPA [486].

A series of 1-phenylcycloalkanecarboxylic acids based on the anticonvulsant 2-[2-(diethylamino)ethoxy]ethyl-1-phenyl-1-cyclopentylcarboxylate (CXX, carbetapentane) has been tested against MES in mice; of these compounds, CXXI ($ED_{50} = 16$ µmol/kg i.p.), CXXII ($ED_{50} = 86$ µmol/kg i.p.) and CXXIII ($ED_{50} = 173$ µmol/kg, i.p.) were found to be effective anticonvulsants, CXXI was more potent than the parent compound CXX ($ED_{50} = 48$ µmol/kg i.p.) and was twice as potent as diphenylhydantoin [387].

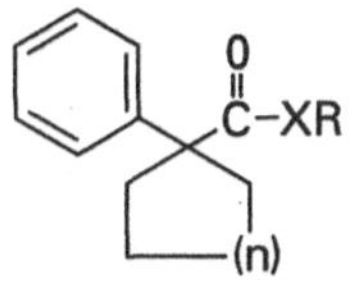

CXX	$R = (CH_2)_2O(CH_2)_2N(Et)_2$, X = O, n = 1
CXXI	$R = (CH_2)_2O(CH_2)_2N(Et)_2$, X = CH_2O, n = 1
CXXII	$R = (CH_2)_2O(CH_2)_2N(Et)_2$, X = CH_2O, n = 2
CXXIII	$R = (CH_2)_2O(CH_2)N(Et)_2$, X = COO, n = 2

Recent advances in the physiology and pharmacology of excitatory amino acid (EEA) transmitter systems have shown that EEA receptors are implicated in epilepsy and are the targets for anticonvulsant drugs [388]. Of the three types of EEA receptors viz. quisqualate, kainate and NMDA, the third plays an important role in many types of seizures and is involved in some forms of epilepsy [156, 389]. Selective NMDA receptor antagonists and compounds that otherwise depress the responses mediated by NMDA receptors have been found to have anticonvulsant activity in many seizure models and good correlation has been observed between the affinity of NMDA receptor antagonists and their anticonvulsant potency [390]. Most of the NMDA receptor antagonists which have shown anticonvulsant activity are carboxylic acids containing primary or secondary amino group at the α-carbon, noteworthy compounds being APH (CXXIV, AP5), APV (CXXV, AP7), CXXVI (CGS 37849), CXXVII (CGP 39551), CXXVIII (CPP), CXXIX (CPP-ene), CXXX (CGS 19755), CXXXI (NPC 19626), CXXXII and CXXXIII.

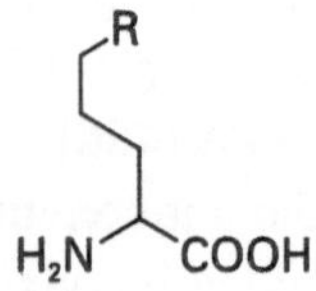

CXXIV   R = PO₃H₂
CXXV   R = CH₂PO₃H₂

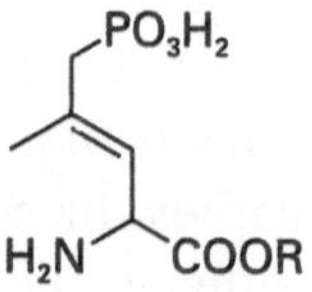

CXXVI   R = H
CXXVII R = Et

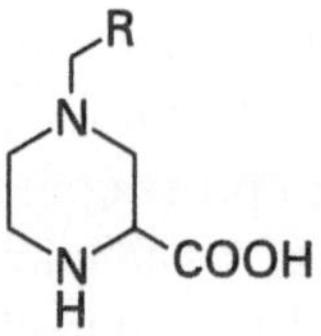

CXXVIII R = (CH₂)₂PO₃H₂
CXXIX   R = CH
                  ‖
                  CH–PO₃H₂

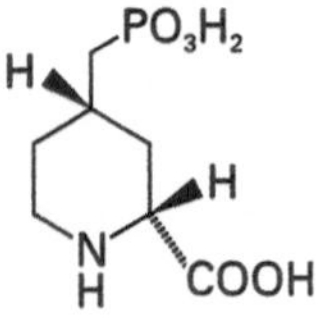

CXXX

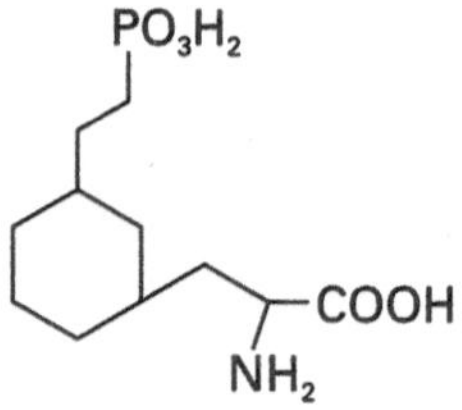

CXXXI

APV and APH were initially found to block reflex seizures in DBA/2 mice [391] and later in baboons [392] and epileptic fowl [390]. They were active against seizures induced by NMDA and picrotoxin [393] and in MES tests in mice [394]. These compounds are inactive orally, but show potent activity when given i.c.v. or tested *in vitro* preparations [392, 395], though they are less active than phenytoin and phenobarbital when administered systemically, because of their limited blood-brain barrier permeability. This permeability was overcome in the 3-unsaturated analogues of APV viz. CGP 37849, its ester CGP 39551 [396, 397] and the D-enantiomer of 1-unsaturated derivative of CPP (CXXIX) [398, 399]. These compounds showed potent oral anticonvulsant activity in rats, mice and baboons. CGP-37849 and D-CPP-ene showed high affinity for the NMDA recognition site and a long duration of action *in vivo*, whereas CGP-39551 showed lower affinity for receptor but was more active orally, perhaps due to its better absorption

as an ester and deesterification *in vivo* to CGS-37849. Two conformationally restricted analogues of APV and APH viz. CPP and CGS-19755
respectively, and a distinct cyclic analogue of APH, viz. NPC-12626 have
been described [400]. These compounds have been found to be more potent
than APV or APH both as NMDA antagonists and in MES test in mice. The
ED_{50} values of CPP, CGS-19755 and NPC-19755 were 2.6 and 20 mg/kg,
i.p., respectively compared with 156 mg/kg, i.p. for APH [401–403]. (±)
CPP depressed the behaviour seizure (amygdala binding) in male Wistar
rats at 10 mg/kg, i.p. dose [404]. In a study on the analogues of 4-(phosphe-
noalkyl) and alkenyl-2-piperidine carboxylic acids of type CXXXIII (R_1–
R_5 = H, CH_3, n = 0, 2) for their binding to NMDA receptor and *in vivo*
activity in NMDA seizure model in mice, the phosphenopropenyl analogues
CXXXII and CGS-19755 showed anticonvulsant activity at 12 mg/kg, i.p.
[405]. Using computer-aided modelling the bioactive conformation of APH
and preliminary model of the antagonist preferring state of NMDA receptor
have been described. Despite the high anticonvulsant activity of these
NMDA receptor antagonists, they have the drawback of causing behavioural or neurological side-effects, particularly those related to their effect
on EAA transmission including effects on motor performance and memory
function [406, 407].

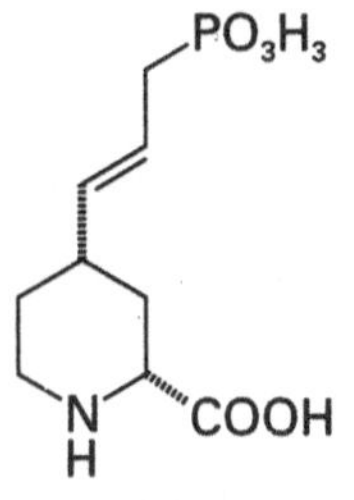

CXXXII

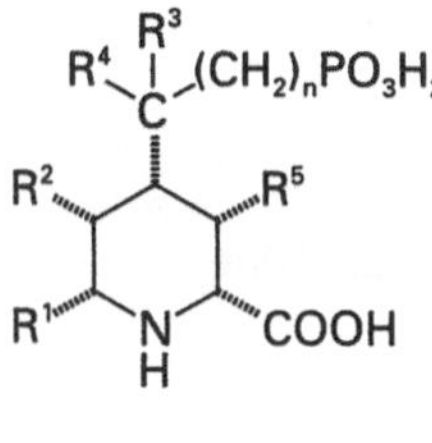

CXXXIII

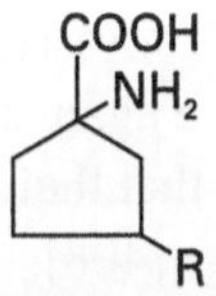

CXXXIV R = H
CXXXV   R = Me

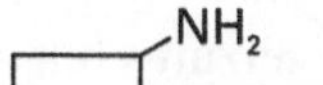

CXXXVI

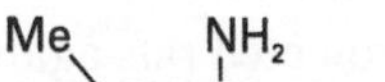

CXXXVII

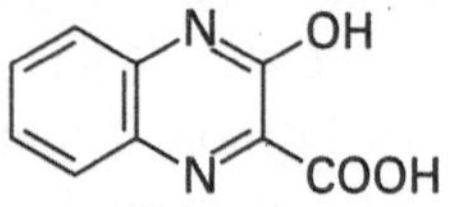

CXXXVIII

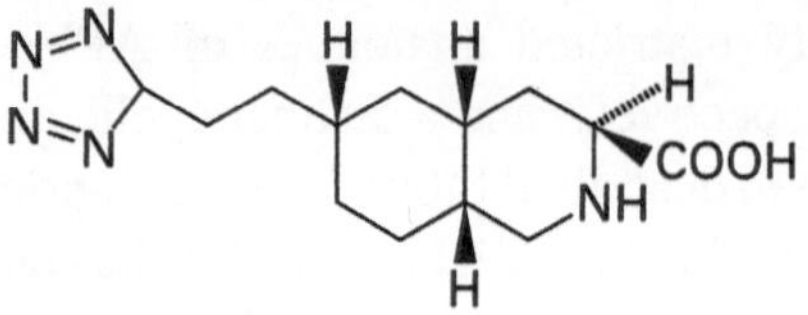

CXXXIX

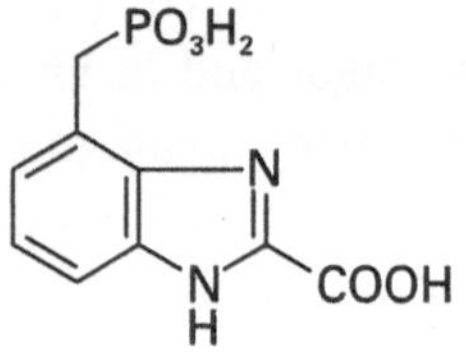

CXL

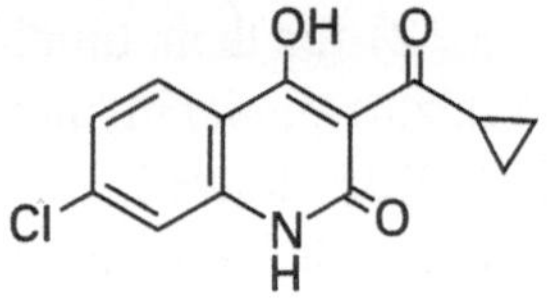

CXLI

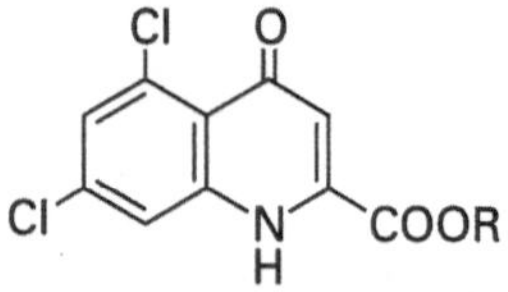

CXLII   R = H
CXLIII   R = CH(Me)CH$_2$NMe$_2$

Apart from these compounds other analogues like cyclopentano amino acids have been investigated for anticonvulsant activity in MES test in mice. Of these, 1-aminocyclopentane carboxylic acid (CXXXIV), 1-amino-3-methylcyclopentane carboxylic acid (CXXXV), 3-aminotetrahydrothiophene carboxylic acid (CXXXVI) and α-aminoisobutyric acid (CXXXVII) protected rats against electroshock seizures but did not protect mice against PTZ-induced seizures. SAR studies on these compounds suggest that their lipophilicity or hydrophobic interactions are important for activity [408]. Among the other acids studied as EAA receptor antagonists, the 3-hydroxy-2-quinoxaline carboxylic acid (HQC, CXXXVIII) [409], (–)-decahydroisoquinoline carboxylic acid (CXXXIX) [410], 4-phosphonomethylbenzamidazole-2-carboxylic acid (CXL) [411], 3-acyl-4-hydroxyquinolin-2(1H)-one (CXLI) [412], 5,7-dichlorokynurenic acid (CXLII) and 1-methyl-(2-di-methylamino)ethyl ester of CXLII (CXLIII) [413, 414] have shown promising anticonvulsant activity. HQC suppressed the NMDA response (Ki = 0.27 nM) and provided protection against picrotoxininduced convulsions and death [409]. CXXXIX is a competitive AMPA receptor antagonist and showed selective affinity for the receptors of the excitatory amino acids, AMPA (2-amino-3-(5-methyl-3-hydroxyisooxazol-4-yl)propionic acid) (IC_{50} = 4.81 µM), NMDA (IC_{50} = 26.4 µM) and kainic (IC_{50} = 247 µM) isolated from cortical slice preparations using [^{3}H] AMPA, [^{3}H] CGS-19755 and [3H] kainic acid radioligands, respectively. It also antagonized the AMPA (IC_{50} = 6 µM), NMDA (IC_{50} = 31.7 µM) and kainic acid (IC_{50} = 61 µM)-induced depolarizations in the cortical slice assay. It was tested for anticonvulsant activity in maximal electroshock and in AMPA-induced rigidity tests in mice in which its ED_{50} values were 9.0 and 3.6 mg/kg i.p., respectively. These doses were 1/2 to 1/5 of those required to produce the neurological impairment in mice in a horizontal screen assay suggesting that the compound is a promising candidate for development. Among the two (–) and (+) enantiomers, only CXXXIX (3S, 4aR, 6R, 8aR) showed affinity for AMPA (IC_{50} = 1.35 µM) and NMDA (IC_{50} = 12.1 µM) while the (+) isomer did not show significant inhibition of [3H] AMPA or [^{3}H] NMDA-binding at doses up to 100 µM [410]. CXL at 56 mg/kg, s.c. provided 20–50% protection to mice against tonic hind limb extensor seizures [411]. In 4-hydroxyquinolin-2(1H)-one (CXLI) the anionic functionality corresponding to the acid group is a vinylogous acid. The compound CXLI showed strong affinity for NMDA receptor and protected DBA/2 mice from audiogenic seizures (ED_{50} = 4.1 mg/kg i.p.) [412]. The 5,7-dichlorokynurenic acid (CXLII) and its ester (CXLIII) have shown good anticonvulsant activity in the DBA/2 mouse audiogenic seizure model; the latter showed no behaviour stimulation at the anticonvulsant dose (ED_{50} = 62 mg/kg, i.p.) [414].

In view of the importance of GABA in the CNS for anticonvulsant activity, compounds incorporating the GABA substructure have been investigated for their anticonvulsant action. Some of the promising compounds now under development as drugs are SL-75102 (CXLIV), its prodrug progabide (CXLV), vigabatrin (CXLVI), SKF-84976A (CXLVII), CLXVIII, CL-966 (CXLIX) tiagabine (–) R CLXVIII (CL) and gabapentin (CLI).

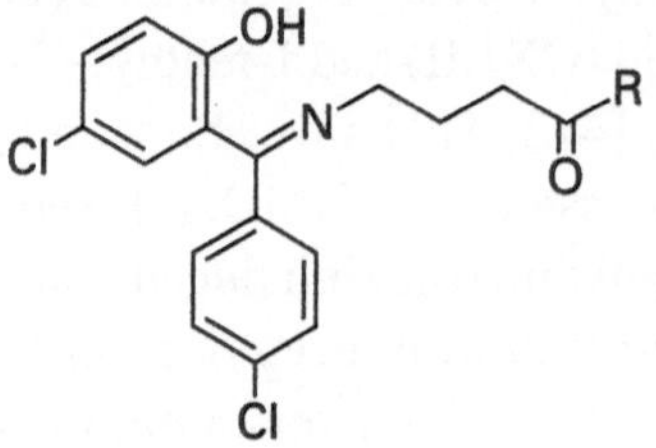

CXLIV R = OH
CXLV R = NH$_2$

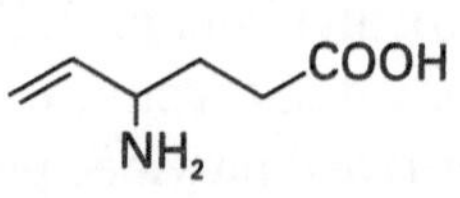

CXLVI

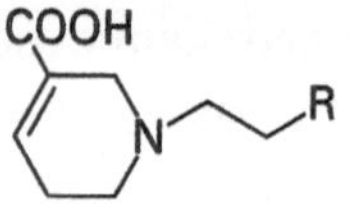

CXLVII R =

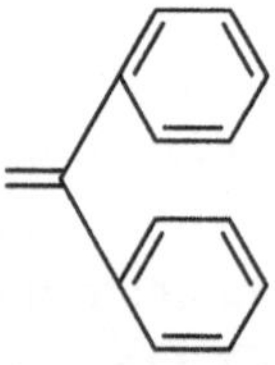

CXLVIII R =

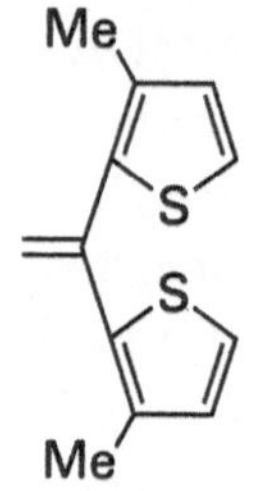

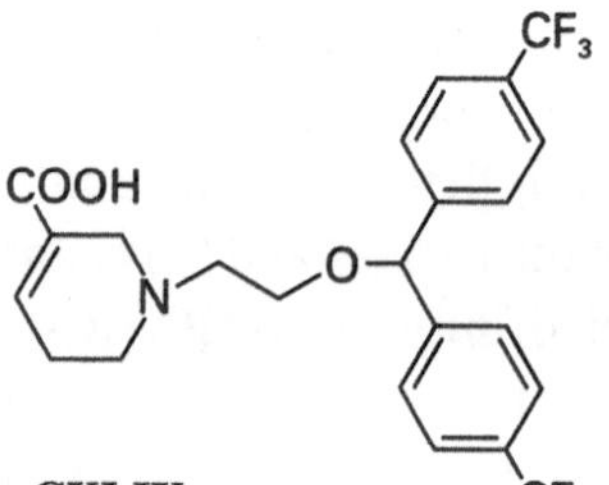

CXLIX

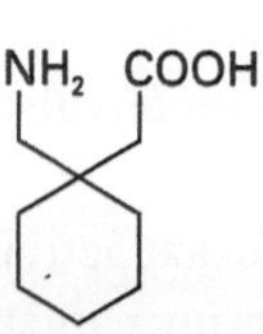

CLI

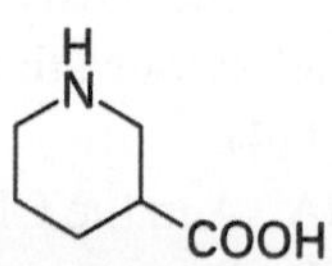

CLII

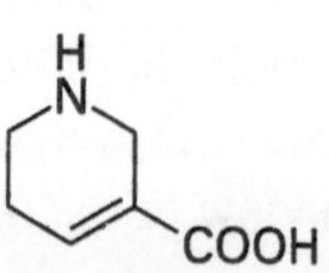

CLIII

Progabide is a lipid-soluble derivative of gabamide which is able to cross the blood-brain barrier and undergoes metabolic transformation by deamidation to SL75102. Both these compounds are agonists of the brain GABA-receptor. The IC$_{50}$ values for CXLIV and CXLV in displacement assay using [3H] GABA are 35 and 1.5 μM, respectively [415]. Progabide and SL75102 are highly specific for the GABA receptor system and do not significantly influence GABA synthesis, metabolism and reuptake. It has been suggested that SL75102 acts as a full agonist at both $GABA_A$ and $GABA_B$ receptors [416].

γ-Vinyl GABA (Vigabatrin, CXLVI) elevates GABA levels by irreversible inhibition of GABA transminase [417]. It can cross the blood-brain barrier as shown by its detection in the cerebrospinal fluid (CSF) after a single oral dose (approx. 3–12 μM) [418–420]. The drug is effective as an anticonvulsant in a variety of seizures including the kindling model [421], chemically-induced seizures [422] and perforant pathway stimulation model [423]. The effect of vigabatrin in the MES model is controversial [422]. Of its two optical isomers, only the S(+) isomer has anticonvulsant activity [424]. Clinical studies have demonstrated that it has antiepileptic activity and is well tolerated even up to 7 years of treatment [423, 425–27]. The usual daily dose was 2–4 g. It has proved effective in partial epilepsy in mentally retarded patients [428] and in children with partial epilepsy and infantile spasms [429]. Vigabatrin as add-on therapy improved cognitive processing, attention and memory after a 4-week treatment [430]. Furthermore, it did not show any adverse effects on a broad range of cognitive and quality-of-life measures during 12-week follow-up studies in a placebo-controlled double-blind add-on study [431]. Vigabatrin monotherapy appears to show a more favourable cognitive profile than carbamazepine monotherapy [432]. However, its use presented a toxicological dilemma. Toxicity studies in rodents and dogs revealed microvacuolation in white matter tracts at doses over 30–50 mg/kg/day [433], while in monkey at a dose of 50–100 mg/kg/day [433] and in humans treated with vigabatrin no microvacuolation was observed [434].

SKF 89976-A (CXLVII) was synthesized as a GABA re-uptake blocker. On oral administration, racemic CXLVII inhibited various parameters of kindled seizure activity; the D-enantiomer was more potent than the L isomer when given intraperitoneally [435, 436]. The anticonvulsant activity profile of the racemate was good [437]. However, the problem of blood-brain barrier penetration by GABA uptake blockers like guvacine, nipecotic acid etc. was solved by Cl-966 (CXLIX) which had a higher potency ($IC_{50} = 0.30$ μM) as a GABA re-uptake blocker than nipecotic acid (CLII, 5.2 μM) and guvacine (CLIII, 6.8 μM); it was also behaviourally active when given orally, suggesting that it can cross the blood-brain barrier. In mice, it was effective against PTZ-induced clonic seizures ($ED_{50} = 0.5$–1.0

mg/kg p.o.) and prevented MES at a higher dose (2.6 mg/kg p.o.) [438]. It caused ataxia in mice at a dose of 64 mg/kg i.m., and in monkeys and dogs even at 3 and 5 mg/kg i.m., respectively. In two human volunteers it caused neurological side-effects at 50 mg p.o. dose. [439].

1-(Aminomethyl)cyclohexane acetic acid (Gabapentin, CLI) is a conformationally rigid analogue of GABA. It was originally designed as a centrally acting GABA agonist capable of crossing the blood-brain barrier because of higher lipophilicity than GABA [440, 441]. However, in spite of a structural similarity to GABA, it does not interact with any of the GABA receptors, and the precise mechanism of its action is not clear [442]. A possible mechanism may be an increase in GABA synthesis induced by it [443]. Gabapentin has been shown to interact with binding sites on neuronal membranes in areas with excitatory synapses [444]. It has a broad spectrum of anticonvulsant activity similar to that of valproate. It is effective in preventing tonic seizures in mice induced by various chemoconvulsants like bicuculline, picrotoxin, isonicotinic acid semicarbazide, strychnine and PTZ (ED_{50} = 5–57 mg/kg p.o.). It is active in the MES test in rats (ED_{50} = 9.4 mg/kg p.o.) but is not in mice. It blocks reflex seizures in DBA/2 mice and in genetically epilepsy-prone rats, and produces a minimal prolongation of the latency to seizure on set and death following i.p. injection of NMDA [442, 445]. It has shown clinical efficacy in patients with primarily generalized tonic-clonic seizures or absence seizures [446, 447], partial seizures [448, 449] and refractory partial seizures [450]. It controlled seizures in 10 out of 20 patients treated for up to 6 months but it was found less effective than carbamazapine 1200 mg/day or the combination of both drugs in this trial [451]. It has been found safe in a study on 800 patients with refractory partial seizures [450]. No difference was observed in a study comparing the neuropsychological performance of patients taking gabapentin or carbamazepine in monotherapy for 4 to 8 months [452]. However, in long-term open-label studies, somnolence (36%), dizziness (27%) and ataxia (26%) have been reported [446].

4.8   Amides

Certain dialkylmalondiamides have shown anticonvulsant activity along with sedative and hypnotic activities [453], while the disubstituted cyanoacetamides used in their synthesis showed anticonvulsant but no sedative-hypnotic activity. Among these cyanoacetamides and their N-alkylated and N-cyclic derivatives, the 2-ethyl-2-propyl (CLIV) and 2,2-diethylcyanoacetamides (CLV) showed significant anticonvulsant activity against MES and PTZ-induced seizures in mice [453, 454]. Valpromide or dipropyl-acetamide (VPD, CLVI), a primary amide of valproic acid (XCVIII), has been found to be 2–5 times as potent as VPA [385]. It is widely used as an antiepileptic drug in several countries. It gets rapidly metabolized to VPA in humans when given orally or i.v. [25, 455].

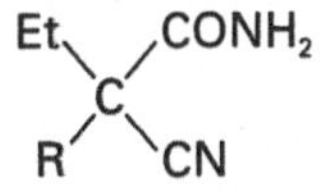

CLIV R = Pr
CLV   R = Et

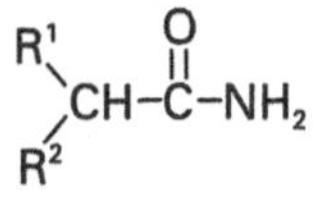

CLVI $R^1 = R^2 = Pr$
CLVII $R^1 = C_4H_9, R^2 = Et$
CLVIII $R^1 = Me, R^2 = C_5H_{11}$

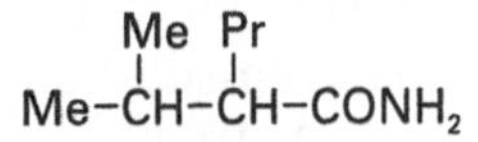

CLIX

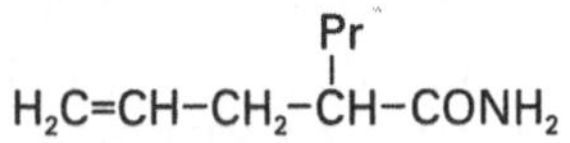

CLX

In view of its potent anticonvulsant activity, valpromide and its different derivatives viz. ethylbutylacetamide (EBD, CLVII), methylpenty-lacetamide (MPD, CLVIII), propylisopropylacetamide (PID, CLIX) and propylallylacetamide (PAD, CLX) were synthesized and evaluated for their anticonvulsant and pharmacokinetic properties in comparison to VPD and valnoctamide (VCD, CLXI) [456]. Among these compounds MPD was the least branched, showed the maximum clearance and shortest half-life and was least active. All other amides had similar pharmacokinetic parameters. Unlike the other amides, PID and UCD were not metabolized to their respective acids and were the most active compounds. The study showed that amide-acid biotransformation requires an unsubstituted β-position in the aliphatic side chain. All amides were more active than their respective acids. Among a series of (E) and (Z)-N-alkyl-α,β-dimethylcinnamides, the E-isomers exhibited CNS-depressant activity and marked anticonvulsant activity in PTZ tests in mice, whereas the Z-isomers caused marked CNS stimulation with tremors and convulsions [457]. Subsequently, the effect of substitution in the phenyl ring among selected compounds of E series viz. (N-cyclopropyl, N-allyl and N-propargyl) and of Z series (N-cyclopropyl and N-allyl) was studied [458]. In the E series anticonvulsant activity was

increased by electron-withdrawing substituents like halogens and was reduced or abolished by electron donating ones (methyl, methoxy and 3,4,5-
trimethoxy). A halogen substituent at *p*-position in *Z* series was found to
increase anticonvulsant activity and reduce CNS-stimulant activity. The
effect was marked in the case of N-cyclopropyl-α,β-dimethylcinnamide
where the 4-chloro- (CLXII) and 4-bromo-(CLXIII) derivatives showed
marked anticonvulsant activity. However, this increase in anticonvulsant
activity substitution was accompanied by a parallel increase in toxicity. In
a study to verify if introduction in the phenyl ring of a *m*-CF3 group which
has the same electronic effect as a halogen, can lead to equally active
anticonvulsant compounds, (*E*) and (*Z*) *m*-(trifluoromethyl)-α,β-dimethyl-
cinnamides and some of their N-alkyl derivatives and some (*E*)-*m*-(trifluoromethyl) α-methyl- and non-methyl-substituted cinnamides were synthesized and examined for their anticonvulsant activity in mice [459]. In the
α,β-dimethyl series, *m*-CF3 yielded compounds which were more active
than the unsubstituted ones but still less active than the halogen-substituted
compounds CLXII or CLXIII. In the α-methyl and non-methyl substituted
series, compounds with a *m*-CF3 group were less toxic and, in some cases,
more active, than the corresponding amides discussed before. (*E*)-N-Cyclo-
propyl-*m*-(trifluoromethyl)cinnamide (CLXIV) was the most active and
least toxic compound of this series.

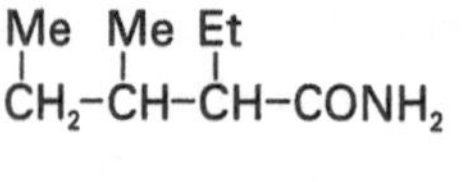

Me Me Et
| | |
CH2–CH–CH–CONH2

CLXI

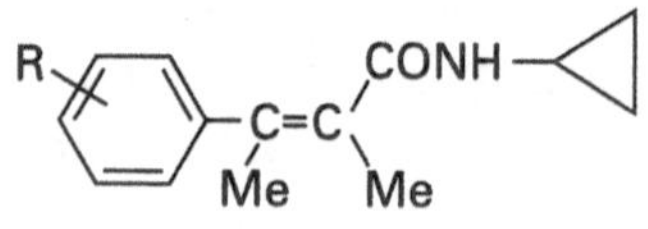

CLXII   R = 4-Cl
CLXIII   R = 4-Br

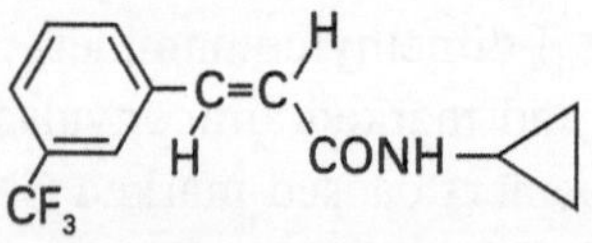

CLXIV

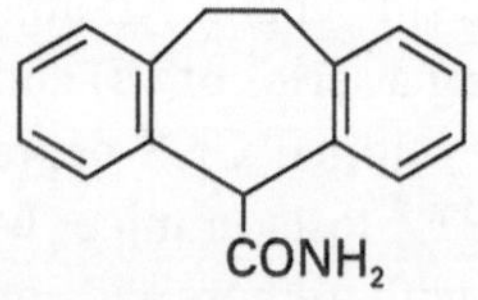

CLXV

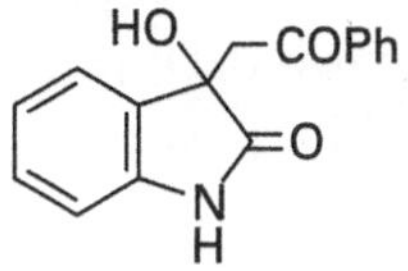

CLXVI

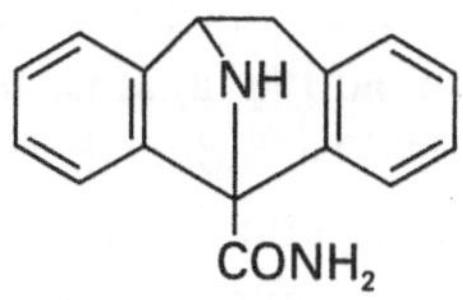

CLXVII

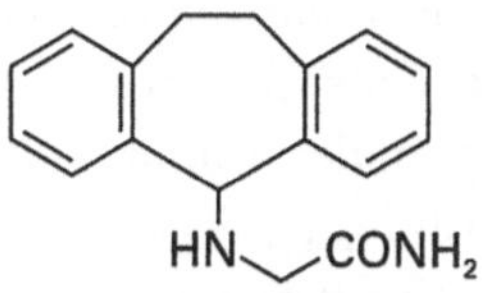

CLXVIII

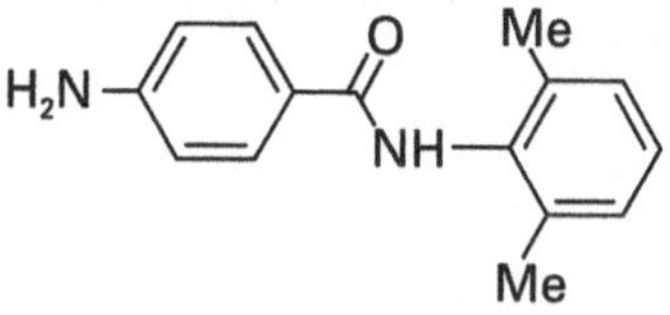

CLXIX

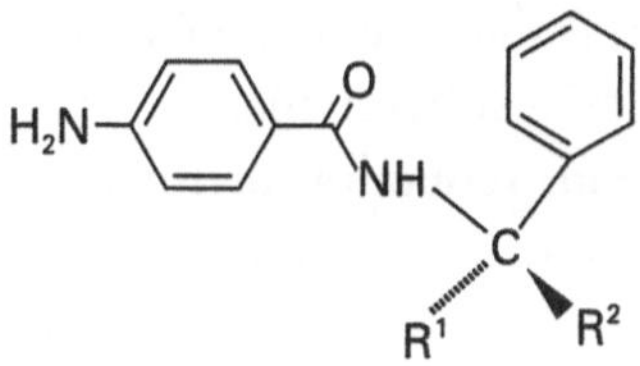

CLXX R^1 = Me, R^2 = H
CLXXI R^1 = H, R^2 = Me

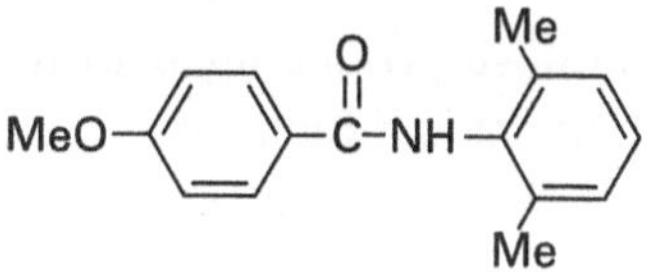

CLXXII

Dibenzo(a,d)cycloheptadiene-5-carboxamide (cyheptamide, CLXV) may be considered an analogue of carbamazepine, in which the N of the tricyclic ring has been replaced by CH. It showed good anticonvulsant activity in PTZ and MES tests in mice. Though it has some stereochemical features in common with carbamazepine and phenytoin, it is much less potent on an i.p. dose, but the difference in potency was much less when blood or brain concentrations were compared [289, 460]. The structural and electronic features of cyheptamide, carbamazepine, diphenylhydantoin and '3-hydroxy-3-phenacyloxindole (CLXVI) have been analyzed and correlated with anticonvulsant activity [290].

ADCI (CLXVII) is another tricyclic amide structurally similar to carbamazepine. It showed potent anticonvulsant activity, almost equal to that of carbamazepine, in the MES test in mice (ED_{50} = 8.9 mg/kg i.p.) and motor toxicity at 1/3 to 1/4 of the dose used for the protection against MES (TD_{50} for motor toxicity = 0.38 mg/kg). It has a protective index of 5.5

which is similar to that for carbamazepine [228]. Unlike carbamazepine, ADCI is also active against PTZ-induced clonic seizures ($ED_{50} = 37$ mg/kg) and NMDA-induced seizures ($ED_{50} = 15$ mg/kg) [461]. Recently, among some tricyclic glycinamides, CLXVIII was found effective as an inhibitor of 3-mercaptopropionic acid-induced convulsions in mice and also inhibited 1-(1-(2-thienyl)cyclohexyl)piperidine-binding to rat brain synaptic membranes with an $IC_{50} = 38$ μM [462].

Extensive structure-activity relationship studies have been carried out on the anticonvulsant activity of aminobenzamides of arylalkylamines and arylamines by Clark et al. [463–469]. Of these compounds, 4-amino-N-(2,6-dimethylphenyl)benzamide (LY201116 or ameltolide, CLXIX), and 4-amino-N-(1-phenylethyl)benzamide are as or more active than phenobarbital, diphenylhydantoin and valproic acid. LY20116 is the most potent in the MES test in mice ($ED_{50} = 2.6$ mg/kg i.p.). Its protective index value of 5.8 is slightly less than that of phenytoin (6.9). It is inactive in the PTZ test. There is good separation between its dose producing anticonvulsant effects, and the dose producing neurological impairment, reduction of tolerance development and induced sleeping time. This would suggest that it may be effective against partial seizures and generalized tonic-clonic seizures [470, 471]. N-(2,6-Dimethylphenyl)-4-(diethylamino)acetylamino)benzamide has been described as a prodrug of ameltolide with longer duration of action [472]. It is inactivated *in vivo* by metabolic acetylation and addition of a hydroxy group to one of its methyl substituents leading to formation of its major metabolite N-(4-(2-hydroxymethyl)-6-(methylphenyl)aminocarbonyl)phenylacetamide. Both these metabolites are less active than ameltolide [473]. The racemic LY1885445, corresponding to the optical antipodes of CLXVIII and CLXIX, is active in the MES test ($ED_{50} = 103$ mg/kg i.p.) and in the scMet test ($ED_{50} = 41.7$ mg/kg, i.p.) in mice [463, 467]. Out of the enantiomers S (LY188545, CLXX) and R (LY188546, CLXXI) the S isomer is more potent than the R isomer against MES [465, 467]. But the overall results suggest that the latter has a better anticonvulsant profile than the former [468]. Subsequently a series of mono-, di- and trimethylated derivatives of 4-methoxy and 4-chlorobenzanilides were synthesized and evaluated for anticonvulsant activity by Clark et al. 4-Methoxy-2,6-dimethylbenzanilide (CLXXII) was the most active compound in MES test in mice ($ED_{50} = 18.58$ mg/kg i.p.) and its toxicity was $TD_{50} = 133.72$ mg/kg, i.p. The oral ED_{50} and TD_{50} values in mice were 27.50 and 342.58 mg/kg, respectively [474]. Molecular modelling and crystallographic studies on the above five MES-active N-phenylbenzamides have been carried

out to identify the common conformational features responsible for anticonvulsant activity [475]. The four major features are: (i) an N-phenyl ring
which is nearly perpendicular to the central amide region, resulting in the
formation of strong intermolecular hydrogen bonds between them, (ii) an
o-methyl substituent oriented toward the NH group of the central amide
plane, (iii) a hydrogen bond acceptor in the central region on the side of the
central plane opposite to the o-methyl group, and (iv) an approximately
coplanar arrangement of the aminophenyl ring to the central amide plane.
Whether the substituent methyl group plays any role other than orienting
the phenyl ring with respect to the amide region is uncertain; however, given
the preferential orientation of a single o-methyl group, it has been suggested
that it acts as a hydrophobic pocket at the binding site.

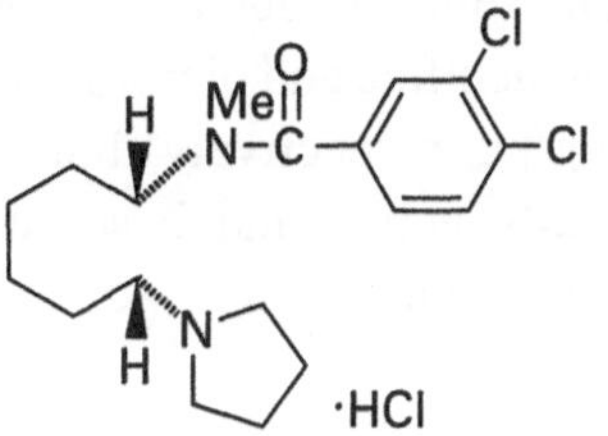

CLXXIII

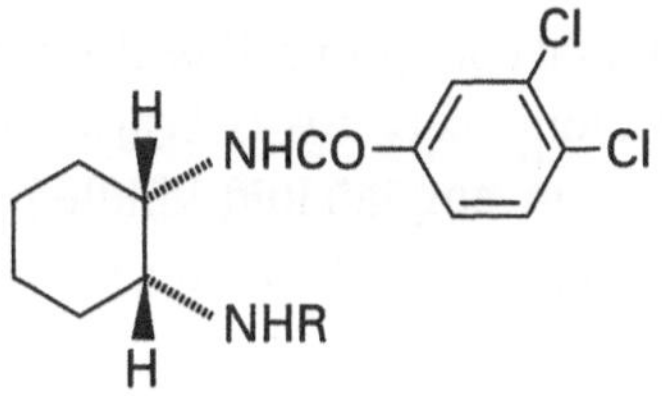

CLXXIV   R = H
CLXXV   R = Me

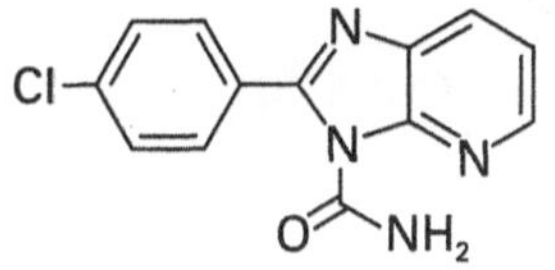

$C_4H_9-CH_2-NH-CH_2-CONH_2$

CLXXVII

CLXXVI

The compound CLXXIII (U-54494A) belongs to a series of benzamide
κ-opioid agonists with anticonvulsant activity, but unlike other members
of the series it is devoid of analgesic and sedative properties and shows
activity in MES tests in mice ($ED_{50} = 36$ mg/kg, i.p.) [476]. It is an
excitatory amino acid antagonist and blocks seizures induced by kainate
($ED_{50} = 28$ mg/kg), NMDA (79 mg/kg) and quisqualate (28 mg/kg) s.c., in
mice. U-54494A is a racemic mixture and both its enantiomers are almost

equiactive [477]; however, its overall anticonvulsant activity profile is better than that of either of the enantiomers, both on oral and i.c.v. administration. In addition, it has a long duration of action when given orally. The activity persists even after its concentration in brain has declined, which is attributed to two of its major metabolites CLXXIV (U-83892E) and CLXXV (U-83894A). Both show anticonvulsant activity in the MES test and also block the voltage-dependent Na^+ channel in NIE-115 neuroblastoma cells in a voltage- and use-dependent manner by interacting with the inactivated channels as well as with the channels in the resting state [478]. The imidazopyridine amide CLXXVI, (AHR-12245) has been found effective against PTZ-induced clonic seizures in mice ($ED_{50} = 29$ mg/kg, i.p.) and did not show motor toxicity up to a dose of 2000 mg/kg [479]. Based on these results its protective index (>69) has been calculated to be several fold higher than that of ethosuximide (3.4) determined under the same experimental conditions. It is also active against bicuculline and picrotoxin-induced clonic seizures ($ED_{50} = 174$ and 211 mg/kg, respectively) but is not active in amygdaloid-kindled rats. It is orally active and a serum concentration of 17.4 µM provides 50% protection against PTZ-induced seizures [480].

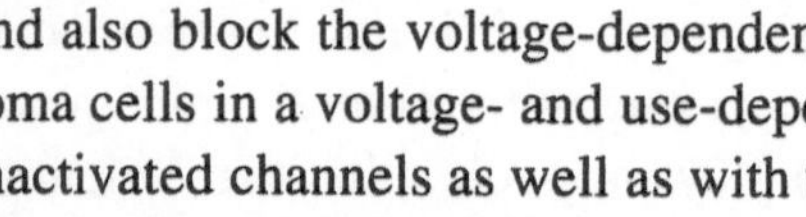

CLXXVIII R = Ph
CLXXIX R = furonyl
CLXXX   R = pyrrolyl
CLXXXI R = NH(OMe)
CLXXXII R = N(Me)OMe

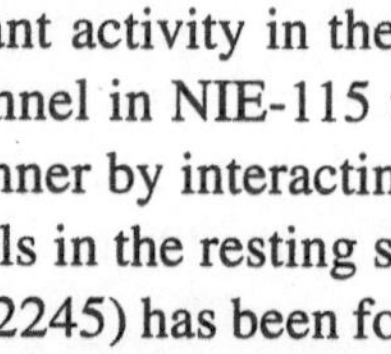

CLXXXIII

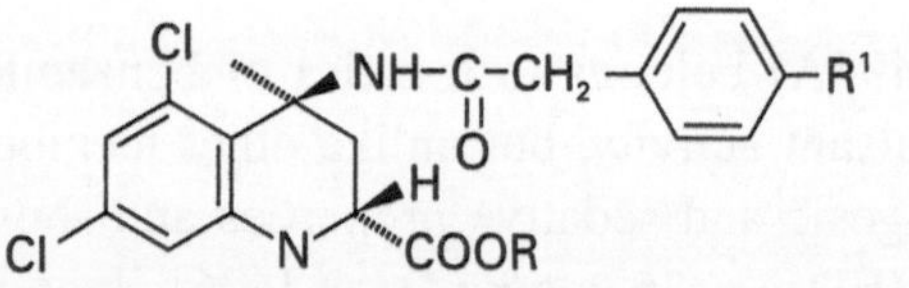

CLXXXIV R = H, R^1 = CH$_2$NH$_2$·HCl
CLXXXV R = Me, R^1 = CH$_2$NH$_2$·HCl
CLXXXVI R = H, R^1 = CH$_2$CH(NH$_2$·HCl)COOH

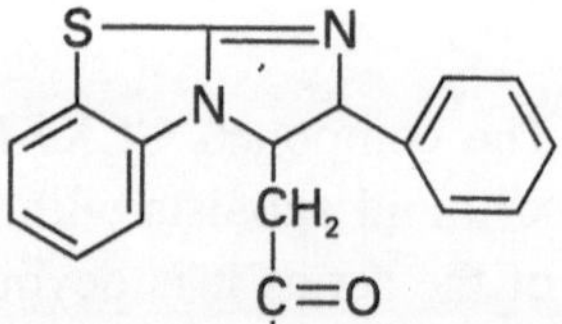

CLXXXVII

Several substituted acetamides have been synthesized and screened for their anticonvulsant activity [481–487]. The 2-N-pentylaminoacetamide (Milacemide, CLXXVII) is a potent anticonvulsant. At a low dose ($ED_{50} = 5.7$ mg/kg p.o.) it is active against bicuculline-induced seizures and at a high dose ($ED_{50} = 741$ mg/kg) in the PTZ test. Its activity is believed to be due to its metabolic conversion, first to glycinamide, primarily by MAO [488–490], and then to glycine, resulting in elevation of glycine level in brain [491]. However, the importance of this activity for anticonvulsant action is not clear. Its neurological toxicity is low, it does not cause ataxia in rats and does not prolong pentobarbital-induced sleeping time in mice up to a dose of 1000 mg/kg p.o. The drug has been evaluated clinically, but since it shows only marginal advantages over the existing anticonvulsants, it is no longer being followed up [492, 493]. The anticonvulsant activity of a series of functionalized α-aromatic and α-heteroaromatic amino acids has been evaluated in the MES test and horizontal screen (tox) test in mice. The replacement of the α-phenyl substituent in CLXXVIII by an electron-rich heteroaromatic moiety led to a substantial improvement in the anticonvulsant potency of the compounds. The most active compounds (R,S)-α-acetamido-N-benzyl-2-furan (CLXXIX), 2-pyrrole (CLXXX), 2-methoxyamino (CLXXXI), 2-methoxymethyl-amino (CLXXXII) acetamides showed ED_{50} values of 10.3, 16.1, 6.2, 6.2 mg/kg i.p., respectively in MES tests in mice and compared well with phenytoin ($ED_{50} = 9.5$ mg/kg). The anticonvulsant activity was confined to the R isomers. The low ED_{50} (3.3 mg/kg) of R-CLXXIX contributed to its high protective index (TD_{50}/ED_{50}) which was similar to that of phenytoin [482–484]. The (S)-α-ethyl-2-oxopyrrolidine acetamide (UcbL059, CLXXXIII) is a novel anticonvulsant agent incorporating the common features of various antiepileptic drugs. It is active both by oral or i.v. route in mice and rats with a unique profile of action. The compound inhibits audiogenic seizures, electrically-induced convulsions, and seizures induced by PTZ, bicuculline, picrotoxin and NMDA and has an ED_{50} of 5.0–30.0 mg/kg. It retarded the development of PTZ-induced kindling in mice. It showed low neurotoxicity in the Irwin observation test, rotarod test and open field exploration, even at a dose 50–100 times higher than the anticonvulsant dose. It is a safe, broad-spectrum anticonvulsant [485]. In a series of N-(substituted quinolin-4-yl)arylacetamides, compounds CLXXXIV (L-690590), CLXXXV (L-691470) and CLXXXVI (L-696833) were found to have ED_{50} values of 39, 31.5 and 29 mg/kg i.p., respectively in the DBA/2 mouse audiogenic seizure model. The correlation between the *in vitro* and *in vivo* activities suggests that the systemic anticonvulsant action of these glycine-site NMDA antagonists depends both on penetration of brain as well as access to receptors within the brain [486]. The substituted imidazo(2,1-b)benzothiazole-3-acetamides (CLXXXVII) where X=H, halo, CH_3, C_2H_5, Pr, MeO, EtO, MeS, $MeSO_2$, cyano, aminocarbonyl; R^1 = H, C_{1-4} alkyl; R^2 = H, linear, branched or cyclic C_{1-5} alkyl, possibly bearing by one or more F atoms, by MeO, Me_2N, Ph group, 2-propenyl, 2-propynyl; R^1R^2N = pyrrolidino, piperidino, hexahydroazepin-1-yl, 4-(phenylmethyl)piperidino, 4-methylpiperazino, 4-(phenylmethyl)piperazino, morpholino, thiomorpholino, exhibited type 1 and type 2 benzodiazepine receptor antagonistic activity and are claimed to be anticonvulsant and anxiolytics [487].

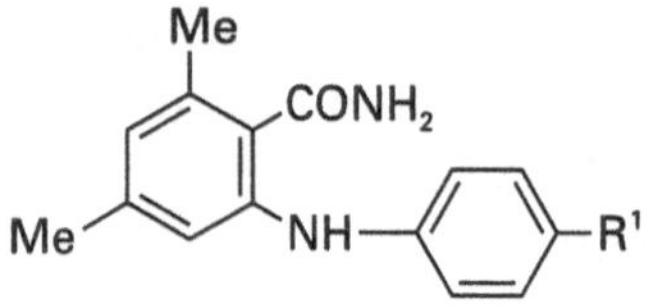

CLXXXVIII

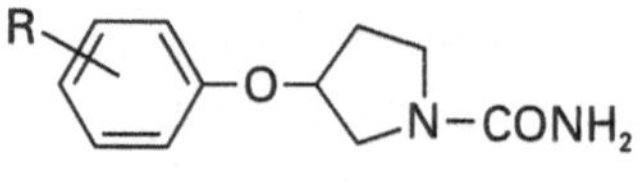

CLXXXIX

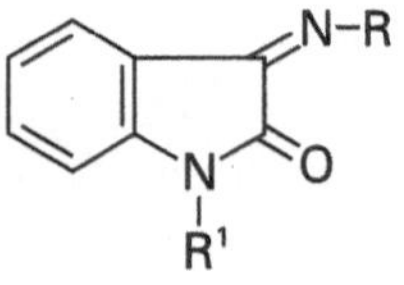

CXC

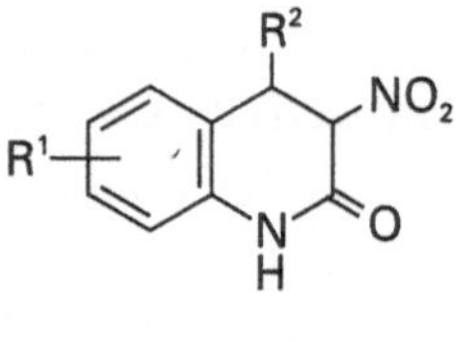

CXCI

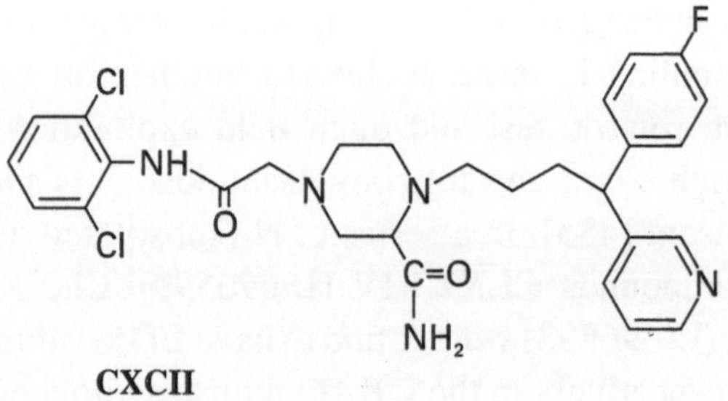

CXCII

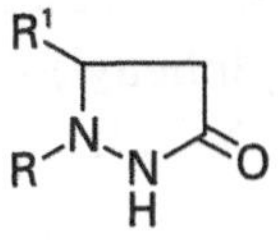

CXCIII

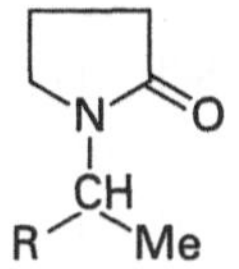

CXCIV   R =

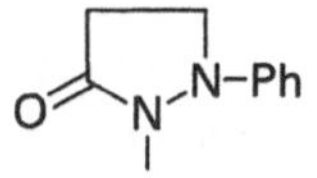

CXCV   R =

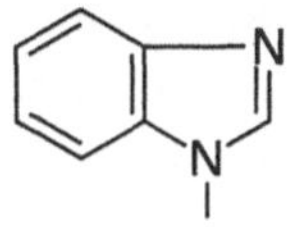

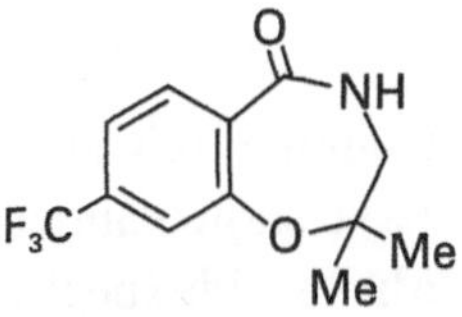

CXCVI

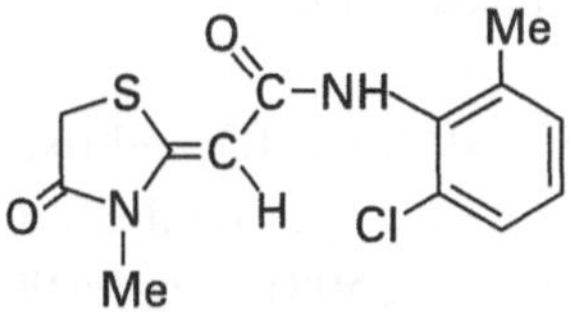

CXCVII

A number of other open and cyclic amides viz. 2-arylamino-4,6-dimethyl-nicotinamides (CLXXXVIII) [494] and other substituted nicotinamides [495], 3-aryloxy-1-azetidinecarboxylamides (CLXXXIX) [496], 3-aryl/alkylamino-1-methylindol-2-ones (CXC) [497] and substituted 3-nitro-3,4-dihydro-2(1H)quinolines (CXCI) [498] and other related compounds [499], soluflazine (CXCII) [500], 5-substituted 1-butyl-3pyrazolidinones (CXCIII) [501, 502], substituted 2-pyrrolidinones (CXCIV–CXCV) [503] and tetrahydropyridooxazepines (CXCVI) [504] have been tested for their anticonvulsant activity. CXCI (R^1 = 7-Cl, R^2 = H, L-698,544) has shown broad-spectrum excitatory amino acid antagonist activity (K_bNMDA = 6.7 μM, K_bAMPA = 9.2 μM). It is also active in the DBA/2 mouse anticonvulsant model and is claimed to be the most potent combined glycine/NMDA-AMPA antagonist *in vivo* [498]. The other interesting new class of anticonvulsants is soluflazine because it can increase the extracellular adenosine level in the CNS [500]. All the eleven 5-substituted-3-pyrazolidinones synthesized on the basis of QSAR studies, with a hydrophobic fragmental constant (ΣFr value of 3.91–6.76, showed potent anticonvulsant activity. Among these, CXCIII (R = 4-C_4H_9, R^1 = C_6H_4-4-Cl) was the most potent [501]. The other compounds CXCIV and CXCV showed activity in the bicuculline test [503] and CXCVI was active against metrazole-induced convulsions in mice [504]. The (Z)-N-(2-chloro-6-methylphenyl)-(3-methyl-4-oxothiazolidin-2-yl idene)acetamide (Ralitoline, CXCVII) has also shown potent anticonvulsant activity in the MES test in mice (ED_{50} = 2 mg/kg p.o.) but is not active in PTZ-induced seizure tests [505]. It is active against reflex epilepsy in Mongolian gerbils and in DBA/2 mice, and audiogenic seizures in photosensitive baboons. It also protects rats against hippocampal kindled seizures at high doses [361]. Its profile is similar to that of phenytoin but it is more potent in slowing the rate of increase of action potentials in cardiac muscle. Thus it may have a similar action on voltage-dependent Na^+ channels as phenytoin [506].

4.9   Sulphonamides

Acetazolamide (CXCVIII), ethoxzolamide (CC), disamide (CCI) and sulthiame (CCII) are old members of this class which have shown anticonvulsant activity [507, 508]. Among these, acetazolamide has a wide spectrum of activity in different seizure models. It is effective in MES tests and audiogenic seizures and at a high dose protects against PTZ and picrotoxin-induced seizures. It is effective against most types of seizures, including generalized tonic-clonic, complex partial and absence seizures. However, its clinical usefulness is limited by the rapid development of tolerance to it [509–510]. Its anticonvulsant action has been attributed to the inhibition of brain carbonic anhydrase which is localized mainly in the cytoplasm of glial cells [511]. At a clinically effective dose, acetazolamide causes >99% inhibition of brain carbonic anhydrase. Adverse effects are minimal when it is used in moderate doses for a limited period, but chronic administration may cause proliferation of glial cells. The other sulphonamides CC-CCII are also brain carbonic anhydrase inhibitors but, unlike disamide (anti-petit mal) which inhibits carbonic anhydrase located in the same area of the brain where acetazolamide acts, the location of the enzyme is different for ethoxzolamide (anti-grand mal) and for sulthiame which is effective in psychomotor epilepsy. In a recent study 2,4,6-tri-, 2,3,4,6-tetra- and 2,3,4,5,6-penta substituted 1-(2-sulphonamido-1,3,4-thiadiazol-5-yl)pyridinium perchlorates, which are acetazolamide analogues in which the 5-acetamido group is replaced by an arylpyridyl moiety, were tested for their bovine red cell carbonic anhydrase inhibitory activity. Among these compounds, the CXCIX (IC_{50} = 0.1 µM) was almost as effective as acetazolamide (IC_{50} = 0.08 µM); however, it has not been evaluated for anticonvulsant activity [512].

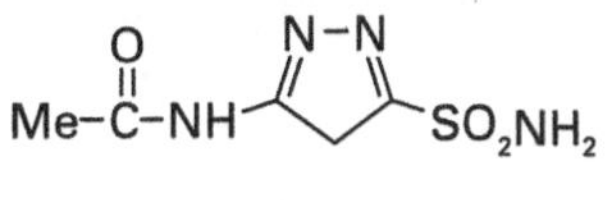

CXCVIII

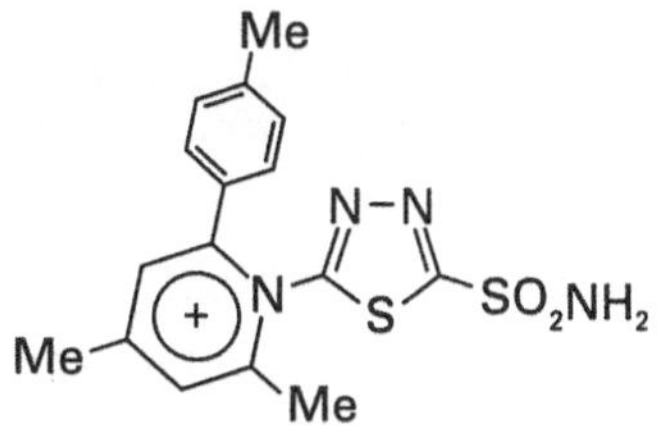

CXCIX

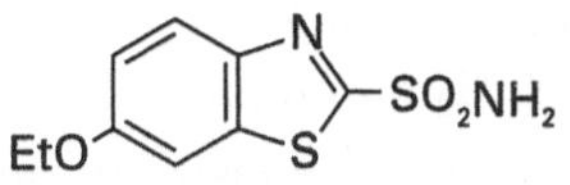

CC

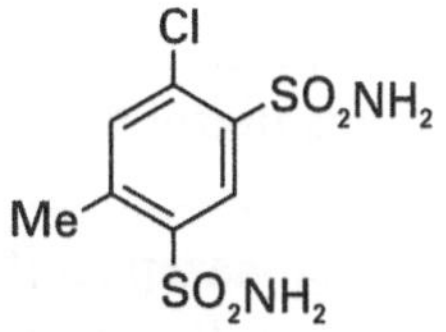

CCI

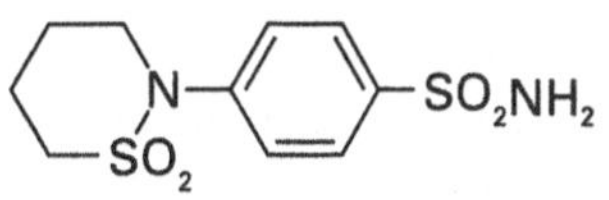

CCII

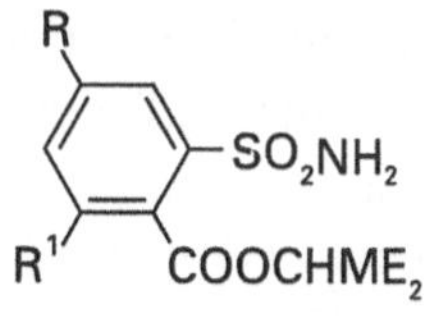

CCIII R = H, R^1 = Cl
CCIV R = Br, R^1 = H

A series of alkyl esters of 2-sulfamoyl and 4-amino-2-sulfamoyl benzoic acid exhibited anticonvulsant activity particularly against MES and strychnine-induced seizures [513]. The anticonvulsant activity was correlated with the rate of hydrolysis of ester which in turn was related to the effect of the substituent on the benzene ring. This was confirmed by the observed anticonvulsant activity in isopropyl 6-chloro-2-sulfamoyl benzoate (CCIII) and inactivity in isopropyl 4-bromo-2-sulfamoyl benzoate (CCIV): CCIII resists ester hydrolysis due to steric protection to the ester function by the bulky Cl group in the o-position while the same is absent in CCIV [513]. Other sulphonamides that have emerged as potent anticonvulsants and are in different stages of development are 1,2-benzisoxazole-3-methanesulphonamide (Zonisamide, CCV), 2,3,4,5-bis-O-(1-methylidine)-α-fructopyranose (Topiramate, CCVI) and 2-phthalimidoethanesulphon-N-isopropylamide (Taltrimide, CCVII). Zonisamide is effective in the MES test in mice (ED_{50} = 19.6 mg/kg p.o.) but is not active in the PTZ-induced seizure model of clonic seizures [505]. Its protective index value of in MES test (rotarod TD_{50}/ED_{50}) is 11.6 compared with the corresponding values of phenytoin (9.1) and of carbamazepine (10.6) [514]. It is also active against reflex and kindled seizures in Mongolian gerbils and rats, respectively [505, 515]. Similar to phenytoin and carbamazepine, it blocks certain chemically induced cortical seizure discharges [516, 517]. It stablizes Na^+-channels in their inactivated stage to phenytoin [518]. It blocks the sustained repetitive firing of cultured mouse neurons but has no effect on the responses to GABA or glutamate in these cells [519].

In receptor-binding studies it was found to inhibit the binding of [^{3}H]flunitrazepam (a benzodiazepine receptor agonist) and [^{3}H]muscimol ($GABA_A$ receptor agonist) to rat brain membrane and also gets displaced by the benzodiazepine clonazepam [520]. The physiological significance of these findings is not clear. Its effects on excitatory and inhibitory mechanisms in the cat spinal trigeminal nucleus are similar to those of valproate, suggesting that it has a GABAergic mechanism of action [521]. Recent studies on the effects of zonisamide on extracellular levels of monoamine and its metabolite on the striatum and hippocampus and on Ca^{++}-dependent dopamine release suggest that it facilitates dopaminergic and serotonergic neurotransmissions but does not affect Ca^{++}-dependent release at therapeutic plasma concentration [522]. In clinical studies zonisamide has been found effective in partial and refractory partial seizures and in myoclonus epilepsy [523–525]. Varying degrees of success have been observed in open trials [526–528], and it has also been found effective in a variety of seizures in children [529, 530]. However, the trials were terminated in the USA due to the high incidence of renal calculi observed in long-term trials.

Topiramate is a structurally distinct type of anticonvulsant compound with ED_{50} = 38 mg/kg i.p. in MES tests in mice and ED_{50} = 17.5 mg/kg p.o. in MES tests in rats, but it is inactive against PTZ-induced seizures [531]. It has a profile of anticonvulsant action similar to that of phenytoin but has longer duration of action. In clinical evaluation interaction of this compound with other anticonvulsants like phenytoin or valproate has not been observed [532]. It has been found effective in patients suffering from refractory partial seizures and showed no significant toxicity even on prolonged use for 1 year. The only side-effect observed is mild cognitive impairment [533].

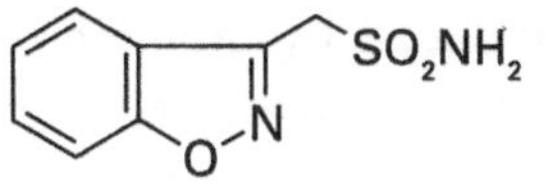

CCV

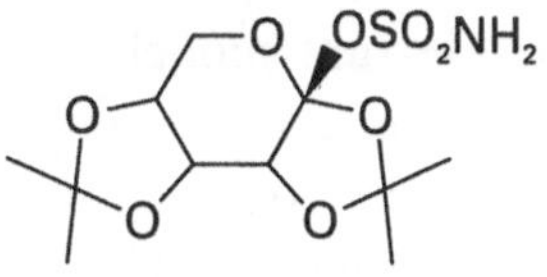

CCVI

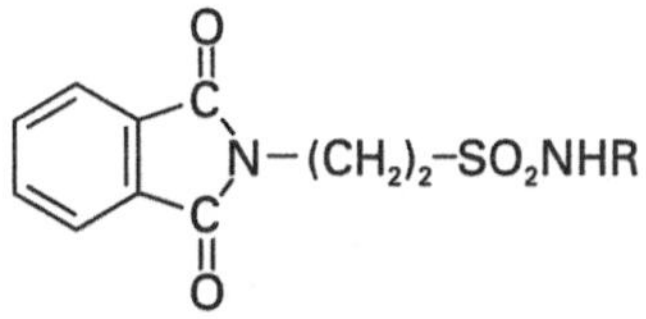

CCVII   R = Pr
CCVIII   R = H

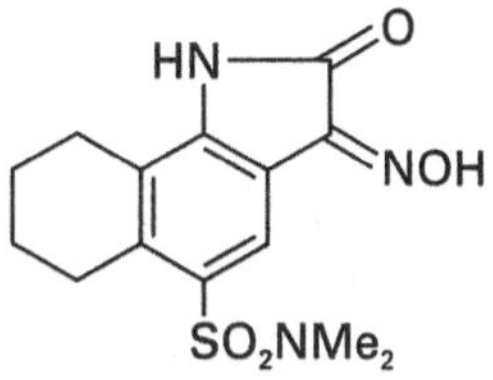

CCIX

Taltrimide has a broad spectrum of anticonvulsant activities. It is active in the MES test in mice and also inhibits PTZ-, bicuculline-, picrotoxin- and strychnine-induced seizures [534, 535]. Taltrimide and its dealkylated metabolite 2-phthalimidoethane-sulphonamide (MY-103, CCVIII) inhibit the binding of [^{3}H] taurine to brain membrane. Taltrimide has the same affinity as taurine [534–536]. It does not appear to bind to GABA$_A$ and benzodiazepine receptor [537]. Taltrimide and CCVIII enhance the K$^+$ depolarization-induced release of GABA from cerebral cortical slices and their anticonvulsant activity has been suggested to be due to this fact [534]. In clinical studies it was found to be as effective as valproate in primary generalized seizures [539] but was not active against myoclonus epilepsy and partial seizures [540]. Recently 5-(N,N-dialkylsufamoyl)-1H-6,7,8,9-tetrahydro-benz(g)-indol-2,3 -dione-3-oximes [540] have been synthesized and evaluated for anticonvulsant activity. Among these, the oxime CCIX has been found effective against AMPA-induced seizures in mice both orally (ED$_{50}$ = 30 mg/kg) and i.v. (ED$_{50}$ = 3 mg/kg).

4.10   Benzodiazepines

Benzodiazepines have been mainly used as sedative and antianxiety drugs. However, some of them have shown broad spectrum anticonvulsant action. The compounds are particularly effective against PTZ-induced seizures but are also effective against seizures induced by picrotoxin and fluoroethyl and in other seizure models including focal seizure induced by alumina or strychnine, in reflux epilepsies such as those occurring in photosensitive baboons or audiogenic mice, in kindled seizures and in absence-like seizures occurring in tottering mutant mice [335, 111]. Most of the benzodiazepines are inactive or active only in high doses in the MES test.

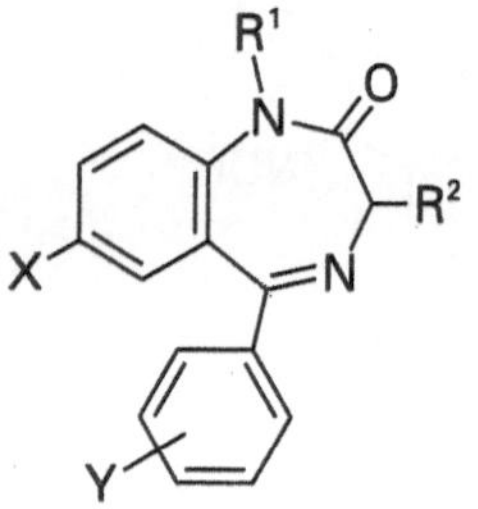

CCX   X = Cl, R^1 = Me, R^2 = H, Y = H
CCXI   X = NO_2, R^1 = R^2 = Y = H
CCXII   X = Cl, R^1 = H, R^2 = OH, Y = 2-Cl
CCXIII X = NO_2, R^1 = R^2 = H, Y = 2-Cl

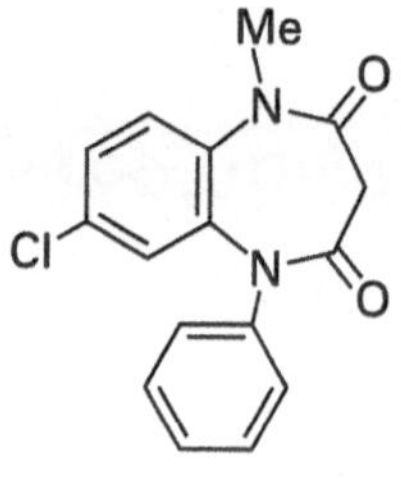

CCXIV

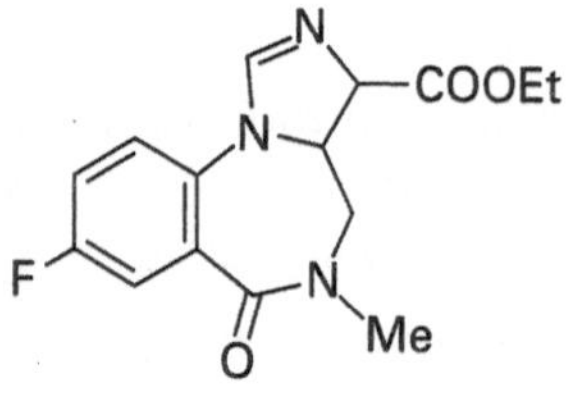

CCXV

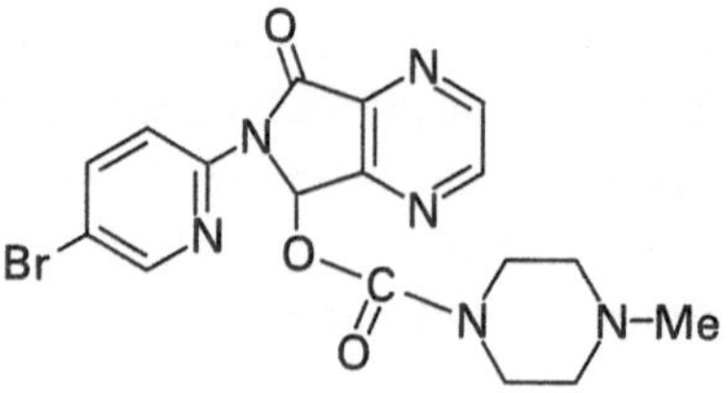

CCXVI

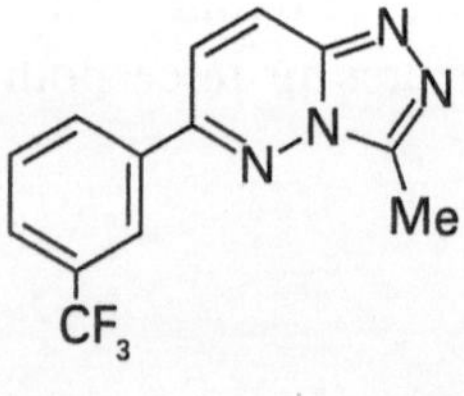

CCXVII

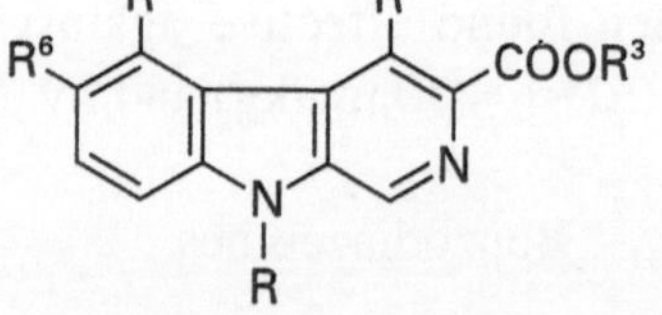

CCXVIII R^3 = Et, R^4 = R^5 = R^6 = R = H
CCXIX R^3 = Et, R^4 = CH_2OMe, R^5 = R = H,
         R^6 = OPr

Among several benzodiazepines investigated for their anticonvulsant activity, diazepam (Valium, CCX), nitrazepam (CCXI), lorazapam (CCXII), clonzapam (Klonopin, CCXIII), clobazam (CCXIV) and chlorozepate have shown interesting anticonvulsant activity. Diazepam is active against PTZ-induced seizures in mice ($ED_{50} = 0.3$ mg/kg), and at a higher dose ($ED_{50} = 19$ mg/kg) against MES in mice. The dose required to produce motor incoordination is higher than the doses required to protect against seizures in either of the above two anticonvulsant screens ($TD_{50} = 57$ mg/kg). However, the protective index is higher in the former test [122]. Diazepam is very widely used in the acute treatment of seizures especially status epilepticus. It is quite safe and very effective by the i.v. route. It is reported to stop initial seizures in 88% patients with various types of status epilepticus [541]. However, its limitation is the short duration of action (not >1 hour) [268]. Its N-desmethyldiazepam, major metabolite is less active than diazepam and has a greater plasma half-life (60 hours) than diazepam (1–2 days). It may sometimes cause cardiovascular and respiratory depression after i.v. administration, particularly if other anticonvulsants or CNS-depressants have been administered before. Diazepam is not useful for chronic therapy because intermittent dosing does not provide a stable blood level. Nitrazepam is also effective ($ED_{50} = 0.7$ mg/kg) in mouse [542] and has been evaluated for the treatment of infantile spasms. It is metabolized to the inactive 7-amino derivative and its half-life in plasma is about 1 day. Unlike diazepam, nitrazepam has been very commonly used in chronic therapy. Lorazepam is more effective ($ED_{50} = 0.2$ mg/kg) against PTZ-induced seizures in mice [542]. Though diazepam is used in acute management of seizures, lorazepam having an almost equal speed of onset of action but greater duration of action is gaining acceptance [543]. There is controversy about its effectiveness; some clinicians prefer it to diazepam because of its longer duration of action and lesser cardiorespiratory depressant effect while others consider it to be less effective. [268, 544]. Lorazepam is excreted mainly as its glucuronide and its half-life in plasma is about 14 hours. Clonzapam is one of the most effective anticonvulsant drugs approved in USA for long-term treatment of certain types of seizures. It is more effective in PTZ-induced seizures in mice ($ED_{50} = 0.06$ mg/kg) than diazepam but is far less active in MES test ($ED_{50} = 78$ mg/kg) with a low TD_{50} (3–4 mg/kg) [122]. It suppresses the spread of seizure activity produced by epileptogenic foci in the cortex, thalamus and limbic structures, but does not abolish the abnormal discharge of the focus. Both diazepam and clonazepam suppress stimulus-induced generalized convulsions in kindled rats but produce almost no reduction in stimulus induced after discharges [545]. It is also effective in the treatment of various forms of status epileticus [546].

Like nitrazepam, the major metabolite of clonazepam is its reduction product which is inactive. Clonazepam has a plasma half-life of 1 day similar to that of nitrazepam. The major side-effects of long-term therapy with clonazepam are drowsiness, lethargy as well as behavioural and personality changes [546].

Unlike the benzodiazepines mentioned earlier, clobazam is a 1,5-benzodiazepin. Its profile of anticonvulsant activity is like that of other benzodiazepines and it is effective against PTZ-, bicuculline-, picrotoxin- and strychnine-induced clonic seizures and MES-induced tonic seizures [547, 548]. Clobazam and its principal metabolite, N-desmethylclobazam, have been shown to protect against reflex seizures in DBA/2 mice and photosensitive baboons [549]. Clobazam has been found effective against amygdaloid kindled seizures in rats [550–552]. It is almost as potent as diazepam in the MES test, 1/5th as potent against PTZ-induced clonic seizures and 1/9th as potent in inducing motor toxicity as measured by the rotarod ataxia test. In clinical trials it was effective against partial and generalized seizures [553, 554]. However, the observation that it produces less sedation and motor toxicity than diazepam and nitrazepam in animals [555, 548] and also in humans [556] was not confirmed, in these studies. It has been suggested that the metabolite N-desmethylclobazam is clinically superior to clobazam [557]. Development of tolerance to the sedative and anticonvulsant action on chronic administration in animals and in humans limits its clinical usefulness in most patients [558, 559], but in a few patients clobazam was effective on long-term therapy [560].

All benzodiazepines show a similar profile of anticonvulsant action and are likely to act by a common mechanism that is stimulation of GABA-mediated synaptic inhibition. Benzodiazepines interact with the allosteric high affinity sites (benzodiazepine receptors) on the GABA$_A$-receptor complex. The effect of such action is to enlarge GABA-induced changes in membrane potential which are associated with increased frequency of opening of chloride channels [561, 562]. High correlation has been observed between the anticonvulsant potencies of benzodiazepine receptor agonists in animal seizure models and other pharmacological effects and their receptor-binding affinities [563–565]. The involvement of benzodiazepine receptors in the anticonvulsant activity of benzodiazepines is supported by studies with the benzodiazepine receptor antagonist, flumazenil (CCXV), which blocks

the anticonvulsant action of diazepam but does not reduce that of phenobarbital, valproate or progabide [566, 567]. The various benzodiazepine
receptors and their different physiological functions has been reviewed
[568]. The discovery that the GABA receptor consists of different α-sub-
units ($\alpha_1\beta_1\gamma_2$, $\alpha_2\beta_1\gamma_2$, $\alpha_3\beta_1\gamma_2$) which may possess distinct pharmacological
properties [569], has led to the suggestion that drugs targeted to the receptor
of composition $\alpha_1\beta_1\gamma_2$ are likely to be better anticonvulsants than the
benzodiazepines in clinical use at present.

In view of the importance of benzodiazepine (Bz) receptors, qualitative and
quantitative structure-activity relationship studies have been carried out to
identify the molecular determinants of such receptors [570–574]. In most
of these studies benzodiazepine receptor ligands of various chemical types
including zopiclene (CCXVI), Cl,218,872 (CCXVII), β-CCE (CCXVIII)
have been used. Borea et al. have proposed a stereochemical model which
accounts for both the binding ability of a drug and its biochemical and
pharmacological activities. It is based on the assumption of a diffuse and
substantially planar recognition site where the drug-receptor interactions
are mediated by carboxylic or imino groups via hydrogen bonding, and
differences in pharmacological profiles are accounted for by the different
localizations of various ligands at the unique binding site [570].

Another study showed that 1,4-benzodiazepines interact with positively
charged receptor sites through two hydrogen bonds one of which is accepted
by the carbonyl oxygen at position 2 and the other by the N4-atom of the
diazepine ring; a third interaction is that of the phenyl ring at C-5 with a
hydrophobic pocket on the receptor [571]. Villar has proposed a model for
receptor recognition, which involves two anchoring hydrogen bond-recep-
tor sites, and for activation involving interaction of the most lipophilic
aromatic region of a compound with the receptor. The model systematically
accounts for the three different types of behaviour, namely agonist, antagonist and inverse agonist, observed in these molecules [574]. Gilda et al. have
calculated the conformational and electronic properties of 1,4-ben-
zodiazepine analogues of types CCX–CCXIII using empirical energy and
semiempirical orbital methods for identifying molecular properties and
modes of receptor interaction. These studies have led to the conclusion that
three cationic receptor sites are required for high affinity analogues. The
specific cationic interactions involve electron-withdrawing groups at C_7,
the $C_2 = O$ group and the imine nitrogen N_4. The interactions of N_4 with a
model cationic receptor site are enhanced by halogen substituent at C_2, but
only when the phenyl ring is rotated by 30° to provide a more planar

conformer [575]. The Free Wilson analysis of 39 benzodiazepines for their receptor binding affinity showed the importance of the carbonyl group at position 2 and of the nitrogen atom at position 4 of the diazepine ring for optimum binding [576]. Based on the structural and stereochemical requirements of benzodiazepine receptor ligands of different chemical classes and using computer-aided molecular modelling, 3-D models have been proposed for the agonist pharmacophore [570, 577–581]. Using one of these models (Figure 3) which consists of sites H_1 and H_2 for hydrogen bond donating groups, and L_1–L_3 for hydrophobic and S_1 for repulsive steric interactions, a new selective β-carboline type agonist CCXIX was studied. It showed both anticonvulsant and anxiolytic activities and was devoid of myorelaxant/ataxia properties associated with benzodiazepines [581].

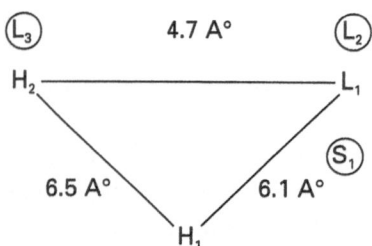

Fig. 3
Schematic representation of the agonist pharmacophore model for Bz-receptor.

Structure-activity relationships of 1,4-benzodiazepines as anticonvulsants have been extensively studied. In a study by Lucek et al. where attempts were made to correlate anti-Met activity with lipophilicity, electronic molecular indices such as total electronic charge on atomic centres, and highest occupied and lowest occupied molecular orbital energies, the most significant descriptor was found to be the electron density on an orbital of the aromatic carbon adjacent to the amide nitrogen [582]. In other studies the negative dependence of anti-Met activity on the total molecular dipole moment has been reported [583–589]. The results were consistent with studies on other miscellaneous anticonvulsants [584–586]. Other QSAR studies have indicated the importance of electronic parameters and overall lipophilicity for anticonvulsant activity [587–590]. Structure-activity correlation studies in a series of 1,3-dihydro-2H-1,4-benzodiazepin-2-ones for activity in PTZ test using a computer-automated structure evaluation programme based on artificial intelligence have led to the identification of the three structural units a, b, c which activate with 100% probability, and a unit d, deactivating with 87.5% probability [591].

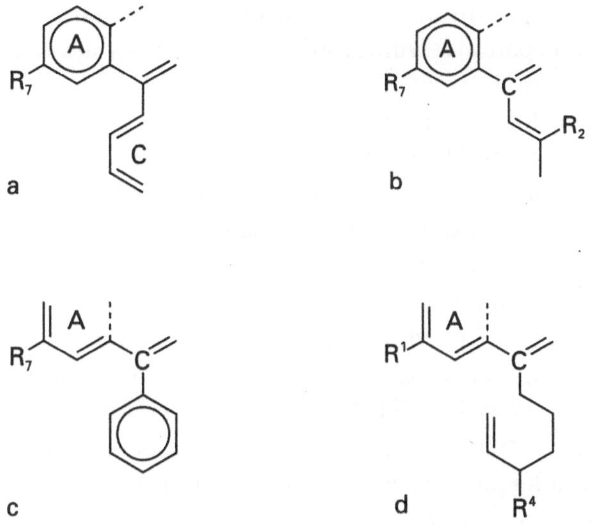

Fig. 4
Structure of most relevant descriptors of anti-Met activity.

4.11   Imidazoles

This new class of anticonvulsants was discovered in the early eighties. Its two most important members are N-{β-(4-(β-phenylethyl)phenyl)-β-hydroxyethylimidazole (Denzimol, CCXX) and (1-(2-naphthoylmethyl)imidazole (Nafimidone, CCXXI). Both these compounds are active in MES tests in mice with ED_{50} values of 5.3 and 15 mg/kg i.v., respectively but are ineffective against PTZ-induced clonic seizures. The protective indexes in the MES test (TD_{50} in rotarod ataxia test/ED_{50}) in mice are 5.2, for CCXX (1 hr after oral administration) and 6.3 for CCXXI (30 min. after oral administration) and which are lower than that for phenytoin (8.4) but greater than that for phenobarbital (2.6) and valproic acid (1.3) [592–595]. Denzimol is also effective against audio seizures in DBA/2 mice and this protective action is inhibited by pretreatment with purine (aminophylline) and benzodiazepine (RO15-1788) receptor antagonists [596]. Denzimol is clinically effective in complex partial seizures and no serious side-effects have been observed, except for nausea and vomiting [597, 598]. Nafimidone at a 25–50 mg/kg i.p. dose showed moderate protective activity against amygdaloid kindled seizures in rats with side-effects of sedation and ataxia

[599]. However, it showed promising results in a add-on clinical trial in an adult male with intractable partial seizures [600]. Robertson has shown that apart from phenylethylphenyl, naphthalenyl and aryl moieties in nafimidone and denzimol, analogues carrying other groups like fluorenyl, benzo(b)thienyl and benzofuraryl have provided several highly active (arylalkyl)imidazole anticonvulsants like denzimol and nafimidone. These compounds were active in MES test in mice but had little or no effect on PTZ- or bicuculline-induced seizures in mice [601]. Based on SAR studies in this series it has been proposed that in arylalkylimidazole anticonvulsants, the pharmacophore is the alkylimidazole and the aryl portion helps in increasing the lipophilicity for crossing the blood-brain barrier. The most active compound of this series is 1-(9H-fluoren-2-yl)-2-(1H-imidazol-1-yl)ethanone (CCXXII). It is twice as potent as nafimidone in MES tests in mice (ED$_{50}$ 25 and 50 mg/kg p.o., respectively, and the LD$_{50}$ values in rats are 4550 and 504 mg/kg p.o., respectively.

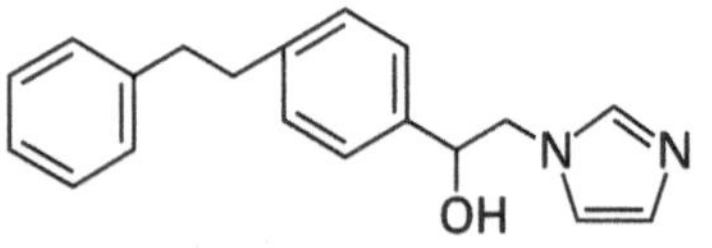

CCXX

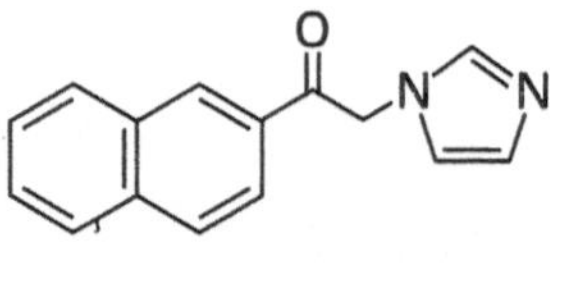

CCXXI

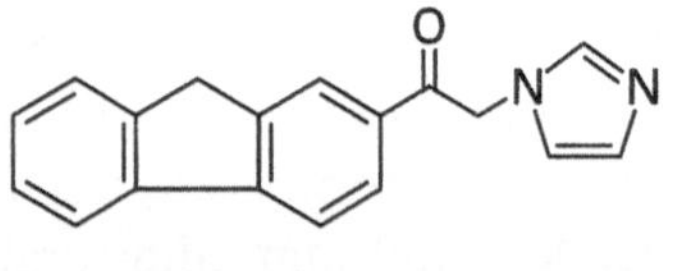

CCXXII

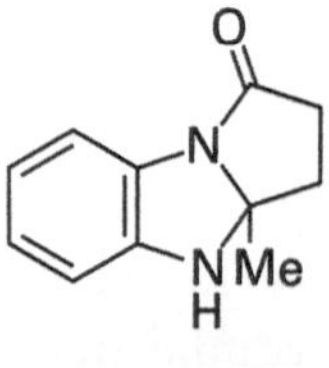

CCXXIII

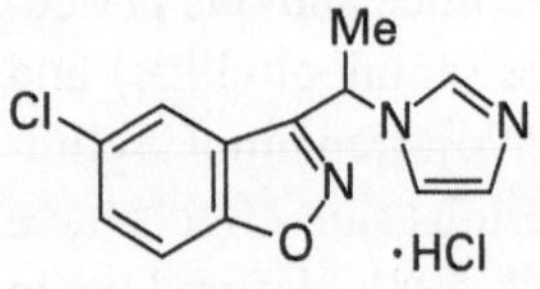

CCXXIV

In a series of 2,3,3a,4-tetrahydro-1H-pyrrolo(1,2a)benzimidazol-1-ones investigated for anticonvulsant activity in DBA/2 mice against sound-induced seizures and in rats against maximal electroshock seizures, compound CCXXIII has shown activity comparable to that of diphenylhydantoin in both tests [602]. Another compound CGS18416A (CCXXIV) which is similar to denzimol and nafimidone in terms of imidazole moiety and to zonisamide in terms of benzisoxazole structure, has shown promising anticonvulsant activity. It is effective in MES tests in mice (ED$_{50}$ = 17.3 mg/kg p.o.) but is inactive against PTZ-, picrotoxin- and bicuculline-induced seizures in mice [603].

4.12 Triazoles

Among the triazoles studied for their anticonvulsant activity [604–608], loreclezole (CCXXV) has shown anticonvulsant activity in rats of WAG/R strain against generalized absence epilepsy [606] and in patients with photosensitive epilepsy [607]. In recent studies on 5-aryl-3(alkylthio)-4H-1,2,4-triazoles [608, 609], the compound 5-(2-fluorophenyl)-4-methyl-3(methylthio)-4H-1,2,4-triazole (CCXXVII) has been found most potent against strychnine-induced convulsions in mice (ED$_{50}$ = 12.1 mg/kg i.p.) but less effective against MES (ED$_{50}$>200 mg/kg), PTZ (ED$_{50}$ = 61.3 mg/kg) or MPA (ED$_{50}$ = 100.0 mg/kg) induced seizures in mice, while 5-(3-fluorophenyl)-4-methyl-3-methylsulphonyl-4H-1,2,4-triazole (CCXXVI) was the most selective antagonist of strychnine-induced convulsions in mice (ED$_{50}$ = 8.8 mg/kg i.p.) and far less effective against MES, PTZ- or MPA-induced seizures in mice (ED$_{50}$>200).

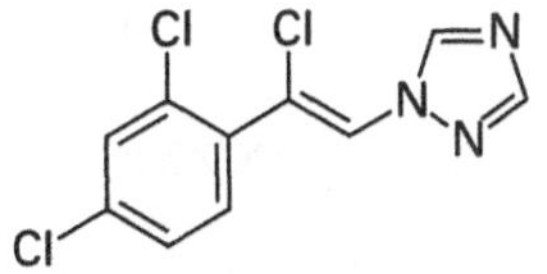

CCXXV

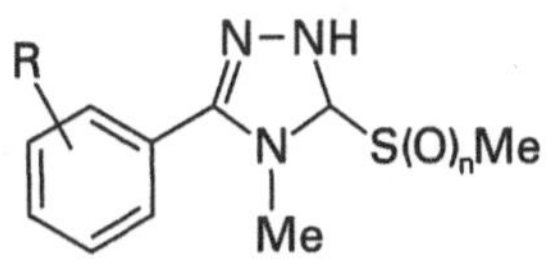

CCXXVI R = 3-F, n = 2
CCXXVII R = 2-F, n = o

4.13 Amines

Among a number of amines and imines investigated for their anticonvulsant activity the dibenzocycloalkenimines MK801 (CCXXVIII, dizocilpine), phencyclidine (CCXXIX), betamine (CCXXX), (+)-3-methoxy-N'-methylmorphinan (dextromethorphan) (CCXXXI) have shown potent anti-convulsant activity in several animal models. All these compounds are NMDA antagonists. MK801 antagonized bicuculline-induced tonic seizures in mice even at a dose of 0.023 mg/kg, p.o. and was active in the MES test (ED_{50} = 0.35 mg/kg i.v. or s.c.) and in PTZ-induced clonic seizures (ED_{50} = 11 mg/kg) [160, 389, 407]. It also protected against sound-induced seizures in DBA/2 mice [610] and pilocarpine-induced seizures in lithium pretreated rats [611]. It acts mainly via NMDA and is a potent non-competitive NMDA antagonist and may block the NMDA receptor channel complex in its open chain conformation [612, 613]. The molecular properties and the pharmacophore responsible for its recognition by NMDA receptors and PCP receptors have been identified [614–616]. MK-801 has been clinically evaluated in various types of seizures but the results have not been very promising [617]. Moreover, its clinical value is limited due to major side-effects like elevation of blood pressure, headache, dizziness and adverse behavioural effects [618, 619]. The anticonvulsant action of MK-801 has been recently reviewed [620]. A series of 1,3-dibenzo(a,d)cycloalkenimines has been studied for anticonvulsant activity in mice against NMDA-induced convulsions. The ED_{50} values for most of these compounds ranged between 0.22 and 7.76 mg/kg, but none was superior to MK-801 [621].

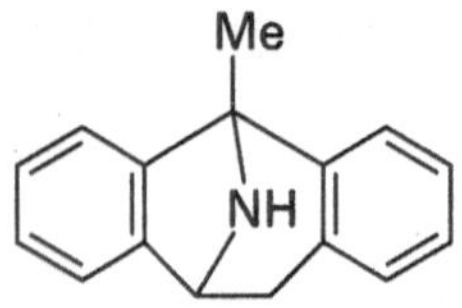

CCXXVIII 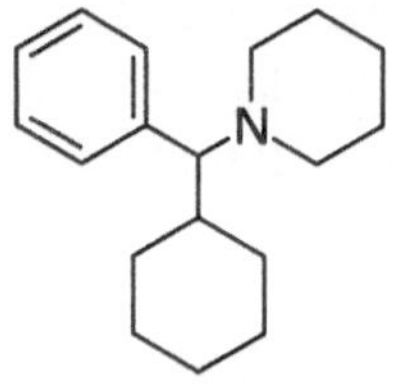   CCXXIX 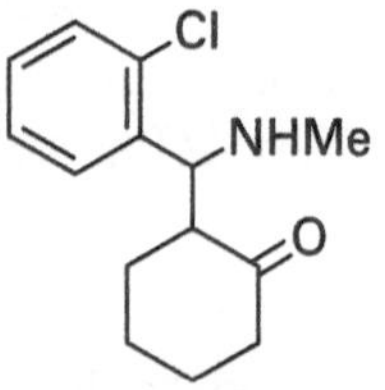   CCXXX

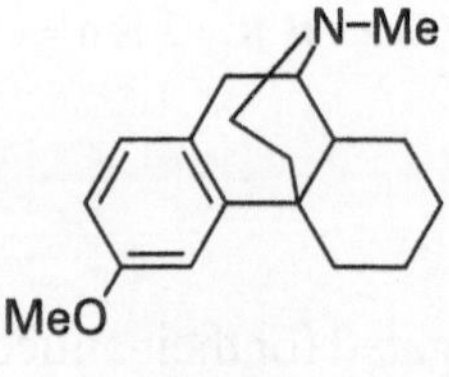

CCXXXI 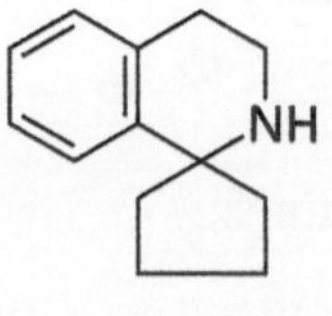   CCXXXII

Phencyclidine (PCP) and ketamine have also shown potent anticonvulsant activity in different animal seizure models [622]. PCP is highly active against MES in mice (ED$_{50}$ = 3 mg/kg i.p.) [623–625], audiogenic seizures in DBA/2 mice [610] and against seizures induced by various chemoconvulsants including NMDA [160, 407] and flurotyl [626]. Ketamine is active in the MES test in mice (ED$_{50}$ = 15 mg/kg i.p.) [624, 160]. It is also active against audiogenic seizures in DBA/2 mice [610] and seizures induced by chemoconvulsants like picrotoxin, mercaptopropionic acid and NMDA [624–627]. PCP and ketamine are also effective in amygdaloid kindled seizures in rats [628, 629] but are less effective in clonic seizures induced by PTZ [630]. Both ketamine and PCP act mainly via NMDA receptors [631]. The blockade of NMDA receptor channel by these compounds is voltage- and use-dependent [632, 633].

Among different analogues of PCP studied for anticonvulsant activity by Rogawaski, its conformationally restricted analogue 11-pentamethyle-netetrahydroisoquinoline (CCXXXII) has shown high activity in MES tests [625, 634]. The major side-effect of these compounds is motor toxicity. Dextromethorphan is active in MES tests [635] and also prevents amygdaloid-kindled seizures in rats and cats [636, 637]. It is metabolized to dextrophan which is several fold as potent both as a NMDA antagonist and as a anticonvulsant [610, 638, 639]. It was ineffective in double-blind clinical trials in patients with complex partial seizures, but at the test dose no adverse side-effects were noticed [640].

4.14   Miscellaneous

Apart from the classes of compounds discussed above, 2-phenyl-1,3-propanediol dicarbamate (CCXXXIII, Felbamate), 4,4-dimethyl-1-(3,4-(methylenedioxy)phenyl)-1-penten-3-ol (CCXXIV, Stiripentol), 3,5-diamino-6-(2,3-dichlorophenyl)-1,2,4-triazine (CCXXV, Lamotrigine), (E)-1(bis(4-fluorophenyl)methyl) phenyl-2-propenyl)piperazine (CCXXVI, Flunarizine), (Z)-N-(2-chloro-6-methylphenyl)-3-(4-oxothia-zolidine-2-ylidene) acetamide (CCXXXVII, Ralitoline) have shown promising anticonvulsant activity and are in different stages of drug development.

Felbamate is active in several animal seizure models, including MES tests (ED$_{50}$ = 50.1 mg/kg i.p.) and PTZ tests (ED$_{50}$ = 148 mg/kg i.p.) in mice [122]. It is active against picrotoxin and bicuculline seizures at high doses but is not active against strychnine seizures [641]. It has been found 10 times

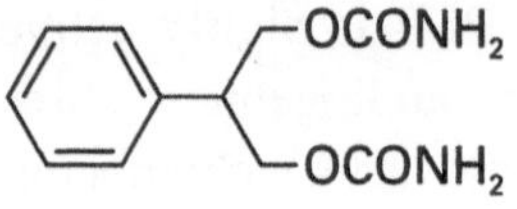

CCXXXIII

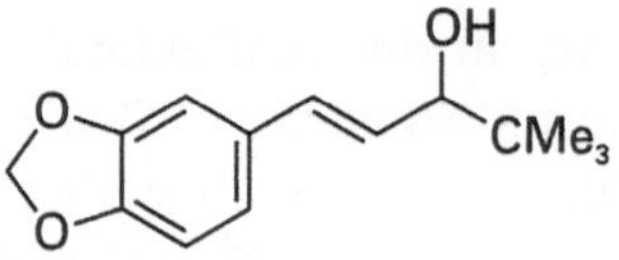

CCXXXIV

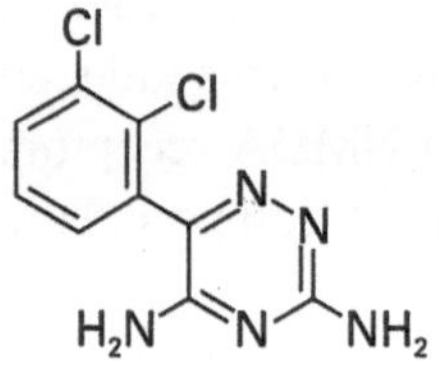

CCXXXV

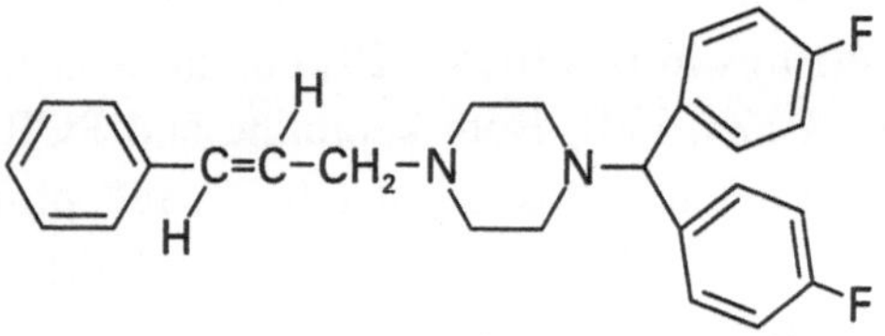

CCXXXVI

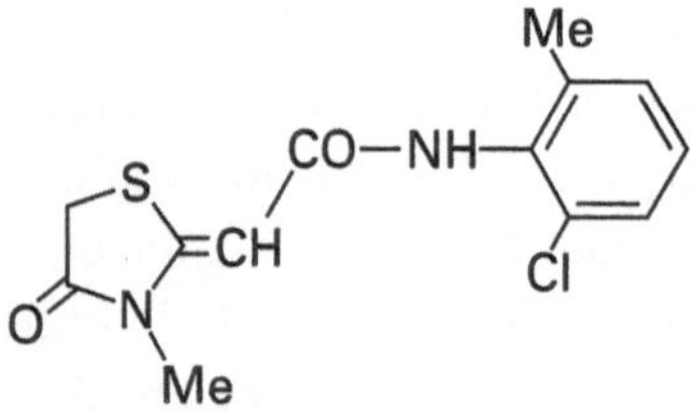

CCXXXVII

as potent against pilocarpine-induced seizures in lithium-treated rats than in untreated free animals [642]. It has low neurotoxicity and a wide spectrum of anticonvulsant activity as compared to conventional anticonvulsants [643]. It has shown reduction in seizure frequency in clinical trials [644–647]. Clinical studies indicate that it may be effective in idiopathic generalized epilepsies. The common side-effects are headache, nausea, vomiting and dizziness.

Stiripentol is also a broad-spectrum anticonvulsant active against electroshock seizures in rats (ED_{50} = 240 mg/kg i.p.) and PTZ-induced seizures in mice (ED_{50} = 200 mg/kg i.p.) [648, 649]. It possibly acts by inhibition of GABA uptake and blockade of GABA-T (691, 693]. It has shown encouraging results in clinical trials in atypical and refractory absence seizures [651, 652].

Lamotrigine, originally synthesized as an antifolate, has shown high potency in the MES tests in mice (ED_{50} = 1.9 mg/kg p.o.) and low motor toxicity. Its antiepileptic profile is similar to that of phenytoin and carbamazepine [653, 654]. In a recent study lamtotrigine and phenytoin did not affect the incidence or latency of minimal (i.e. predominantly clonic, non-generalized) seizures although pretreatment with phenytoin changed the seizure pattern without any influence on the clonic phase [655]. It possibly acts by stabilizing neuronal voltage-dependent sodium channels, thus reducing the presynaptic release of excitatory amino acids, principally glutamic [656–658]. It has shown encouraging results in several clinical trials and has been found most useful in tonic-clonic and atypical absence seizures [659]. Limited studies in children have shown its efficacy in children absence, atypical absence, tonic, atonic and myoclonic seizures [660–662]. It has shown low incidence of side-effects which include ataxia, diplopia, blurred vision, nausea and vomiting [663].

Flunarizine, a potent Ca^{++}-channel antagonist [664], is highly active in MES tests in mice (ED_{50} = 21 mg/kg p.o.) but is inactive against PTZ-induced clonic seizures, produced PTZ similar to phenytoin and carbamazepine [665]. It is active against audio seizures in DBA/2 mice [666, 667], kindled seizures in rats and dogs [668–670], tonic seizures induced by bicuculline [666] and provides partial protection against myoclonus in photosensitive baboons [667]. Other Ca^{++}-channel blockers like dihydropyridine also show anticonvulsant activity in different clinical models [667, 671], but their spectra of activity are different from that of flunarizine as they fail to block MES at doses that protect against PTZ-induced clonic seizures [673, 674], whereas flunarizine blocks MES but not PTZ-induced clonic seizures even when given i.c.v. Its profile of anticonvulsant activity is similar to that of phenytoin and thus the two drugs may have a common mechanism of action, that is interaction with voltage-dependent Na^+-channels [675]. It has been found effective in clinical trials in patients with drug-resistant complex partial seizures [676, 677]. The drug is safe and has only mild side-effects.

Ralitoline shows high activity against MES in mice (ED_{50} = 2 mg/kg p.o.) but is not active against PTZ-induced seizures. It also has a similar anticonvulsant profile as phenytoin and is effective against reflex seizures in DBA/2 mice and photosensitive baboons and against kindled seizures [505, 361]. It has been suggested that its action on voltage-dependent Na^+-channels is similar to that of phenytoin [506].

Besides these compounds, a number of other heterocyclics, viz. quinazolinones and quinazolines [678–687], alkyl substituted γ-butyrolactones

264   Anil K. Saxena and Mridula Saxena

[688, 689], cannabinol [690, 691], substituted cyclopentanones and cyclo-
hexanones [692], thiazolidines [693], substituted benzopyrans and ben-
zothiopyrans [694], thiadiazoles [695–697], oxazolidines [698], 3-aryl-4-
(3H)pyrimidinones [699–701], hydroxysteroids [702], pyridines [703,
704], piperidines [705–708], dihydrothienopyridines [708], aryl/alkylimi-
noindoles [709], arylsemicarbazones [710], isoxazolopyridines [711],
pyrazolopyridopyrimidines [712], thiadiazolidines [713], triazolopyridi-
nes [714], tetraoxatetracycloheneicosane [715], and benzomorphans
[716] have been investigated for anticonvulsant activity. Among these
compounds, 3-amino-3,4-dihydro-2(1H)-quinazolinone (CCXXXVIII antiMES ED_{50} = 30 mg/kg i.p. in mice) [686], 4-propyloxy (CCXXXIX);
4-pentyloxy (CCXL), and 4-heptyloxy-2-(4-methyl-1-piperazinyl)quina-
zolines (CCXLI) (antiMES ED_{50} = 10 mg/kg p.o. in mice) [687], α-di-
ethyl-γ-thiobutyrolactone (CCXLII; antiMES ED_{50} = 374 mg/kg i.p.,
antiPTZ ED_{50} = 104 mg/kg i.p., both in mice) [689], 2-methylcyclohex-
anone (CCXLIV; antiMES; ED_{50} = 216 mg/kg i.p., antiPTZ ED_{50} =
219 mg/kg i.p., both in mice) [692], (R),2,2-dimethyl-4-(2-hy-
droxypropylimino)-5-hydroxy-7-pentyl-4H -1-benzopyran (CCXLIV; antiMES ED_{50} = 13.8 mg/kg and antiPTZ ED_{50} = 14.0 mg/kg p.o., both in
mice) and 2,2-dimethyl-4-(2-hydroxypropylimino)-5-hydroxy-7-pentyl-
4H-1-benzothiopyran (CCXLV, antiMES ED_{50} = 20.6 mg/kg and antiPTZ
ED_{50} = 4.8 mg/kg p.o., both in mice) [694], 5-(2-biphenylyl)-2-(1-
methylhydrazino)1,3,4-thiadiazole (CCXLVI, antiMES ED_{50} = 18 mg/kg,
antiMMS (maximum metrazole seizures) ED_{50} = 27 mg/kg p.o., both in
mice) [695], 2-aminomethyl-5-(biphenylyl)-1,3,4-thiadiazole (CCXLVII,
antiMES ED_{50} = 10 mg (rat) and 22 mg (mice) /kg p.o., antiMMS
ED_{50} = 9 mg (rats) and 20 mg (mice) /kg p.o.) [696], 9,10-dioxo-7-
phenyl-1-aza-8-oxa-bicyclo(5,2,1)decane (CCXLVIII, antiMES ED_{50} =
66 mg/kg, anti ED_{50} = 45 mg/kg i.p., both in mice) [698], 3-(2-tri-
fluoromethylphenyl)-2-methylmercapto-4-(3H)-pyrimidinone (CCXLIX,
antiMES ED_{50} = 35.4 mg/kg, antiMet ED_{50} = 42.5 mg/kg, antistrychmine
ED_{50} = 52.9 mg/kg, i.p. all in mice) [701], 3-hydroxy-5-pregnan-20-one
(CCL, antiMES ED_{50} = 28.6 mg/kg in mice [702], α-methyl-α-
phenylpyridineethanamine (CCLI, antiMES ED_{50} = 10.4 mg/kg p.o. in
mice) [703], 1-(3'-amino-4'-pyridyl)-4-(m-trifluorophenyl)piperazine
(CCLII, antiMES ED_{50} = 25 mg/kg i.p. in mice) [704], 4-amino-1-(6-
chloro-2-pyridyl)piperidine (CCLIII, antiMES ED_{50} <30 mg/kg i.p. in
mice) [706], 4-substituted 1-(phenoxyalkyl)piperidines (CCLIV,
R1,R2 = H, halo, OCH_3, CF_3, n = 3,4; Y = CH_2, $(CH_2)_2$, OCH_2, CH_2O;

antiMES ED_{50} = 5–50 mg/kg i.p.) [707], methyl (+)-(4S)-4,7-dihydro-3-isobutyl-6-methyl-4-(3-nitrophenyl)thieno(2,3-b)pyridine-5-carboxylate (CCLV, anticonvulsant activity at 10–80 mg/kg) [708], 4-chlorophenyl-semicarbazones (CCLVI, antiMES ED_{50} = 74.84 mg/kg i.p., antiPTZ ED_{50} = 135.1 mg/kg i.p., TD_{50} = 252.2 mg/kg, all in mice and CCLVII, antiMES ED_{50} = 90.36 mg/kg i.p., antiPTZ ED_{50} = 177.3 mg/kg i.p., TD_{50} ⇒500 mg/kg i.p., all in mice) [710], 4,5,6,7-tetrahydroisoxa-zolo(4,5-c)pyridin-3-ol (THPO, CCLVIII), pyrazolo(1,5-a)pyrido(3,4-c)pyrimidin-6-(7H)-ones and related compounds (CCLIX, R = CO_2Na, $CO_2C_2H_5$, H; R' = H, $CH_2N(C_2H_5)_2$, CH_2CO_2Na, CCLX, antiPTZ activity at 100 mg/kg i.p. in mice) [712], 4-(4-methoxyphenyl)-3-(4-methoxyphenyl)amino-5-imino-1,2,4-thiazolidine (CCLXI) [713], 2,6-(difluorophenyl)methyl-4-aminomethyl-1H-1,2,3-triazolo(4,5-c)pyridine (CCLXII) [714] have shown promising anticonvulsant activity. Recently, Weaver et al. have applied computer-aided molecular modelling to model the receptor-regulated sodium channel protein and to deduce a model of the NMDA antagonist site. After an extensive series of experiments, a simple cyclic dipeptide (CDP15) consisting of D-phenylglycine and L-alanine was designed as a potential anticonvulsant capable of interacting with the putative receptor site influencing the channel function. CDP15 showed significant anticonvulsant activity in the MES test (ED50 <100 mg/kg i.p., and <50 mg/kg p.o.). It was inactive in the PTZ test, and in preliminary studies it showed binding to the Na^{++} channel [716, 717].

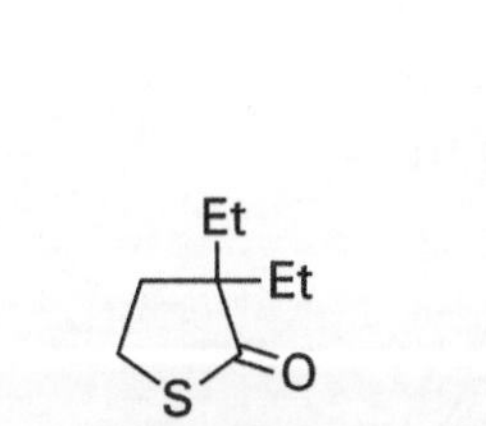

CCXXXVIII

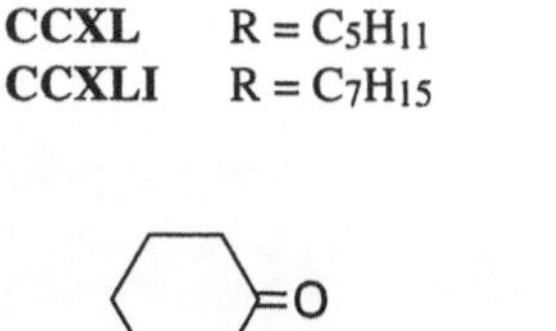

CCXXXIX R = Pr
CCXL R = C_5H_{11}
CCXLI R = C_7H_{15}

CCXLII

CCXLIII

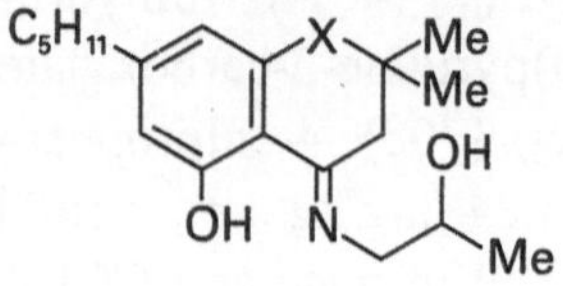

CCXLIV X = O
CCXLV   X = S

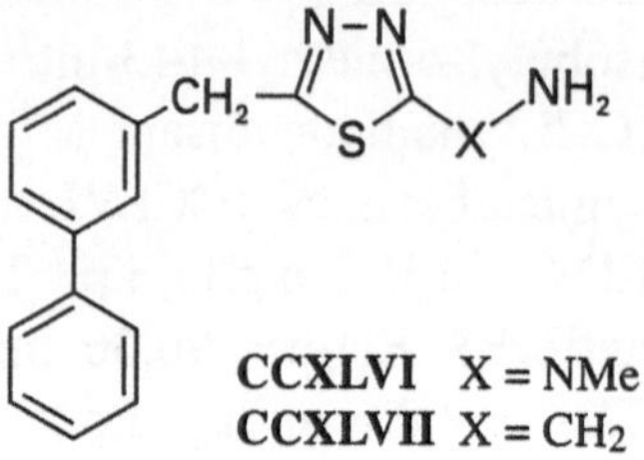

CCXLVI X = NMe
CCXLVII X = CH₂

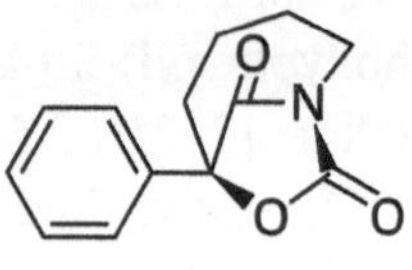

CCXLVIII

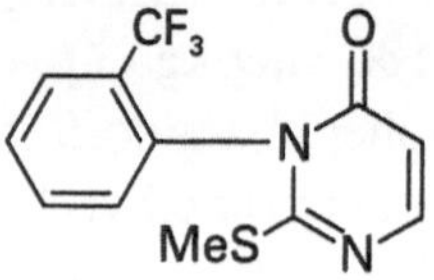

CCXLIX

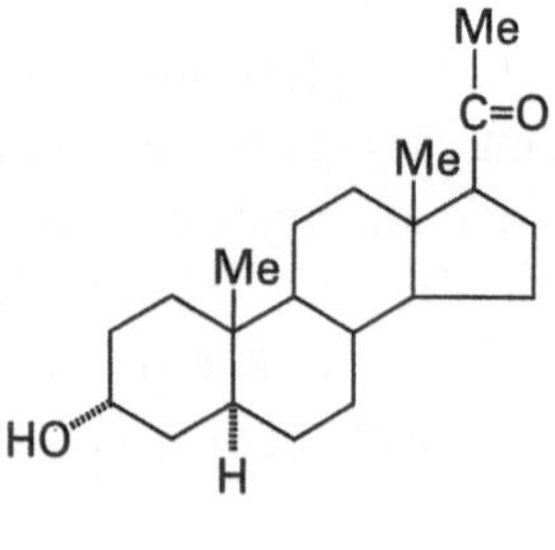

CCL

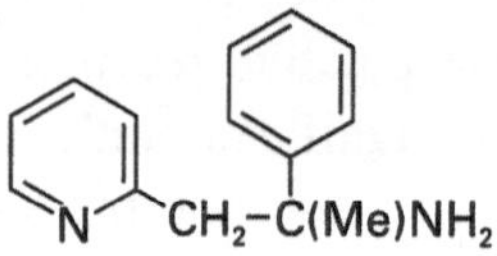

CCLI

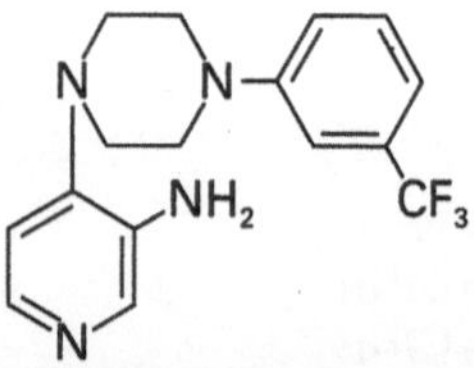

CCLII

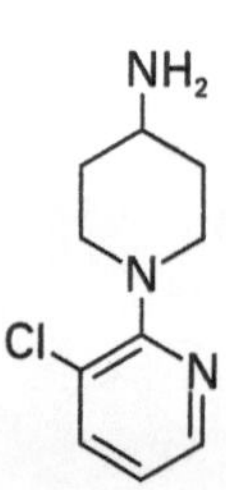

CCLIII

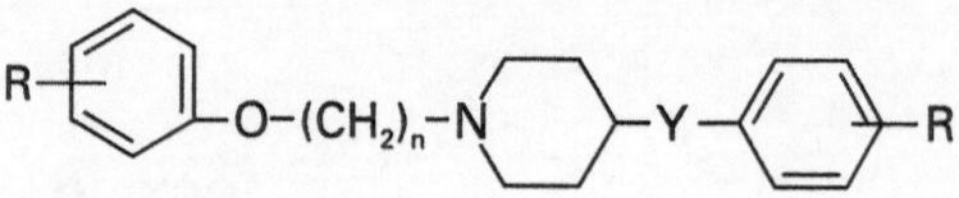

CCLIV

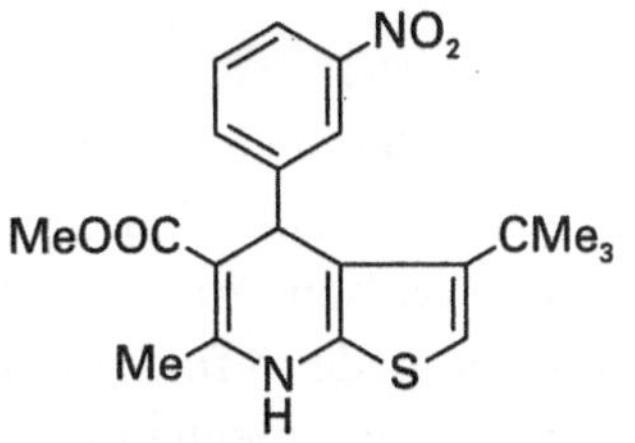

CCLV

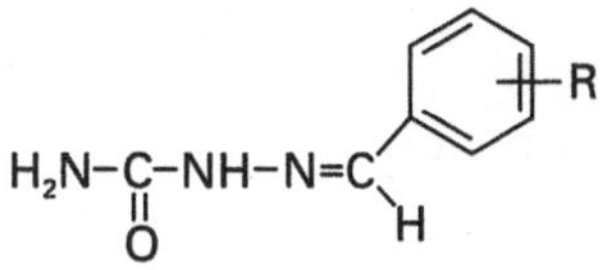

H₂N-C-NH-N=C

CCLVI   R = 4-Cl
CCLVII   R = 3-Cl

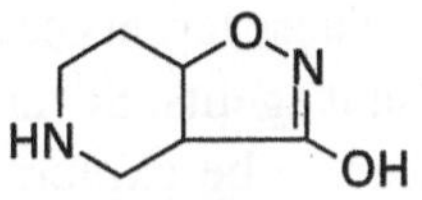

CCLVIII

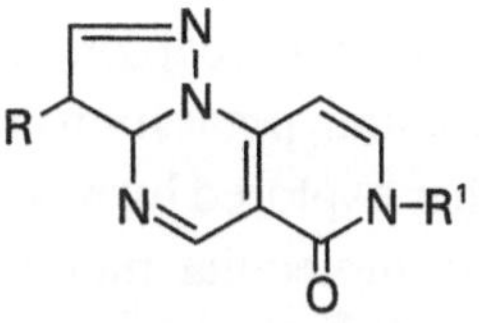

CCLIX

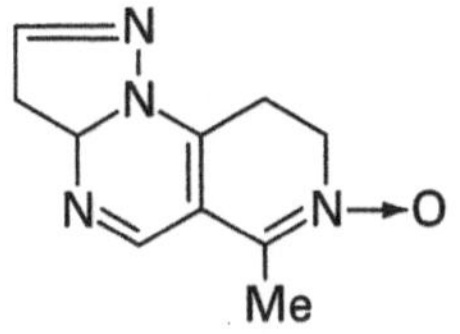

CCLX

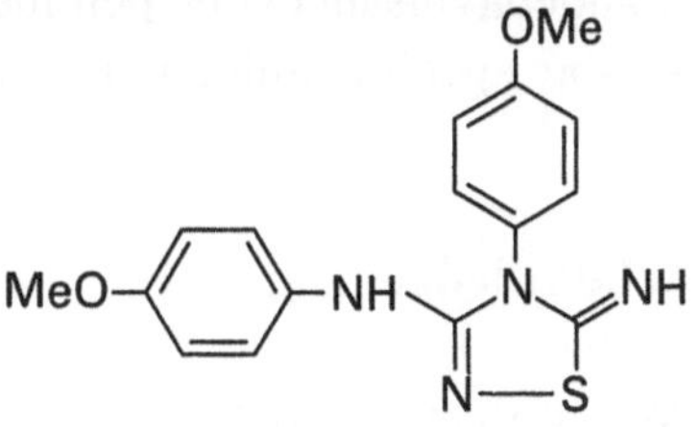

CCLXI

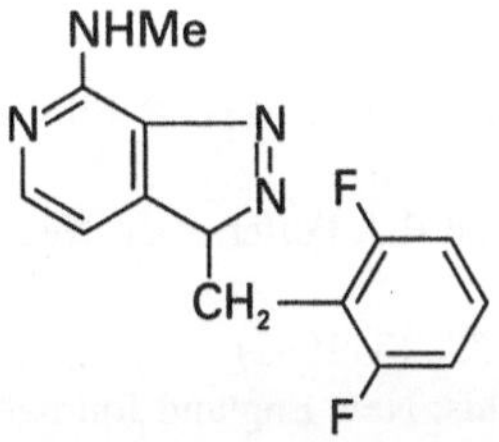

CCLXII

5   Conclusion

This review underscores the extensive research that has led to a better understanding of the mechanisms involved in the generation of seizures and to the development of several highly effective anticonvulsant drugs for the management of seizures in man. Attempts have been made to find out the mechanism of action of anticonvulsants, but the precise mechanism of action of several of them is still not known. Advancement in neurosciences has revealed several cellular targets for interaction of anticonvulsant agents viz. sites on EAA receptor, benzodiazepine receptors, neuronal voltage-dependent sodium, potassium and calcium T type channels. These targets need to be further explored by new and promising anticonvulsant agents. Several QSAR and molecular modelling based models also need to be explored. The application of quantum pharmacology and computer-aided rational drug design (CARDD) leading to the modelling of voltage-regulated sodium ion channel protein, model of the NMDA antagonist sites, and design of anticonvulsant cyclic peptide has provided a new direction to the design of more specific anticonvulsants.

Acknowledgement

We are thankful to Dr. S. Bhattacharji and Mr. A.S. Kushwaha for their invaluable help in the preparation of this manuscript.

References

1   A. Spinks, W.S. Waring: in Progress in Medicinal Chemistry Vol. III (G.P. Ellis and G.B. West. Eds.), Butterworths, Washington, D.C., 1963 pp. 161.
2   A.V. Delgaelo-Escueto, A.A.Jr. Ward, D.M. Woodbury and R.J. Porter: Adv. Neurol. 44, 1 (1986).
3   Collaborative group for the study of Epilepsy: Epilepsia 33, 45 (1992).
4   R.D.C. Elwes, A.L. Johnson, S.D. Shorvon, E.H. Reynolds: New England Journal of Medicine 311, 944 (1984).
5   D.B. Smith, R.H. Mattson, J.A. Cramer, J.F. Collins, R.A. Novelly et al.: Epilepsia 28, S50 (1987).
6   T. Keränen and P. Reikkinen: Acta Neurologica Scandinavica 78, 7 (1988).
7   T.A. Pedley: Epilepsia 28, S1 (1987).
8   M.A. Rogawski and R.J. Porter: Pharmacol. Rev. 42, 223 (1990).

9   R.J. Porter: In New anticonvulsant drugs (B.S. Meldrum and R.J. Porter eds.). John Libby, London 1986 pp. 3.

10   B.S. Meldrum: In New anticonvulsant drugs (B.S. Meldrum and R.J. Porter eds.). John Libby, London 1986 pp. 17.

11   H. Kohn and J.D. Conley: Chem. Br. *24*, 231 (1988).

12   E. Benassi: Curr. Probl. Epilepsy *5*, 33 (1988).

13   M. Dragunow: Prog. Neurobiol. *31*, 85 (1988).

14   M.A. Mikati and T.R. Browne: Clin. Neuropharmacol. *11*, 130 (1988).

15   G. Avanzini and M. De Curtis: Curr. Probl. Epilepsy *5*, 3 (1988).

16   R. Kälviäinen, T. Keränen and P.J. Reikkinen Sr: Drugs *46*, 1009 (1993).

17   R.J. Porter and S. Sato: in Advances in epileptology: XIII epilepsy international symposium (Eds. H. Akimoto, H. Kazamatsuri, M. Seino and A.A. Ward Jr.) Raven Press, New York 1982, pp. 47.

18   J.K. Penry, R.J. Porter and F.E. Dreifuss: Brain *98*, 427 (1975).

19   H. Gastaut and R. Broughton: in Epileptic seizures: Clinical and electrographic features, diagnosis and treatment (Eds. C.C. Thomas). Springfield 1972.

20   M.H. Charleton: in Myoclonic seizures. Excerpta Medica, Amsterdam 1975.

21   C.D. Marsden, M. Hallet and S. Fahn: in Neurology 2: movement disorders (C.D. Marsden and S. Fahn eds.) Butterworths, London 1982 pp. 196.

22   W.A. Hauser, J.F. Annegers and V.E. Anderson: in Epilepsy (A.A. Ward Jr., J.K. Penry and D. Purpura eds.), Research Publications, Association for Research in Nervous and Mental Diseases 61, Raven Press, New York 1983 pp.267.

23   W.J. Close and M.A. Spielman: in Medicinal Chemistry, Vol. V (eds. W.H. Hartung) Wiley, New York 1961 pp. 1.

24   H.H. Jasper, A.A. Ward and A. Pope (eds.): in Basic mechanisms of the epilepsies. Little Brown, Boston 1969.

25   D.B. Tower: in Neurochemistry of Epilepsy (C.C. Thomas eds.). Springfield, III, 1960.

26   A. Lajtha: in International Review of Neurobiology (C.C. Pfeifer and J.R. Symthies Eds.). Vol VI Academic Press New York, 1964 pp. 1.

27   A. Kreindler: in Progress in Brain Research. Vol. XIX, Elsevier Publisher, New York, 1965 pp. 168.

28   R.D. Traub and R.K.S. Wong: Neurol. *33*, 257 (1983).

29   R.D. Traub and R.K.S. Wong: J. Neurophysiol. *49*, 459 (1983).

30   P.A. Schwartzkroin and H.V. Wheal: in Electrophysiology of Epilepsy. Academic Press London, 1984 pp. 420.

31   W. Penfield and H.H. Jasper: in Epilepsy and the functional anatomy of the human brain. Little Brown, Boston, 1954.

32   A.R. Wyler and A.A. Ward: in Epilepsy – a window to brain mechanisms (J.S. Rockard and A.A. Ward eds.) Raven Press, New York 1980 pp. 51.

33   P. Singh and J. Huot: in Anticonvulsant Drugs, Vol 2, I.E.P.T. Pergamon, New York, 1973 pp. 427.

34   A.A. Ward Jr: in International review of neurobiology, Vol. III (C.C. Pfeifer and J.R. Symthies eds.). Academic Press, New York, 1961 pp. 137.

35   G.B. Koelle: in The Pharmacological Basis of Therapeutics, 3rd edition. (L.S. Goodman and A. Gilman eds.), Macmillan, New York 1955 pp. 428.

36   O.P. Ottersen and J. Storm-Mathisen: in Handbook of chemical neuroanatomy. Vol.3:

Classical transmitters and transmitter receptors in the CNS. Part II. (eds. A. Bjorklund, T. Hokfelt and M.J. Kuhar. Elsevier Science Publisher, Amsterdam 1984 pp. 141.

37   B.S. Meldrum: in Handbook of experimental pharmacology. Antiepileptic drugs (M.M. Frey and D. Hanz eds.). Springer-Verlag, Berlin 1985 pp.153.

38   B.S. Meldrum and B. Braestrup: in Actions and interactions of GABA and ben-zodiazepines. (N.G. Bowery ed.), Raven Press, New York 1984 pp. 133.

39   H.A. Harper: in Review of physiological chemistry. Lange, Los Altos, California, 1973 pp. 102.

40   A. White, P. Handler and E.L. Smith: in Principles of biochemistry. 6th ed., McGraw-Hill, New York, 1978 pp. 1344.

41   T.A. Pedley, R.W. Horton and B.S. Meldrum: Epilepsia 20, 409 (1979).

42   B.S. Meldrum and R.W. Horton: Eur. J. Pharmacol. 61, 231 (1980).

43   P. Krogsgaard-Larsen: Molec. Cell Biochem. 31, 105 (1980).

44   M.J. Chroucher, B.S. Meldrum and P. Krogsgaard-Larsen: Eur. J. Pharmacol. 89, 217 (1983).

45   R.W. Horton, J.F. Collins, G.M. Anlezark and B.S. Meldrum: Eur. J. Pharmacol. 59, 75 (1979).

46   B.S. Meldrum: Epilepsia 25, S140 (1984).

47   D.R. Curtis and J.C. Watkins: in Inhibition in the Nervous System and g-Aminobutyric Acid. (Ed. E. Roberts). Pergamon, Oxford 1960. pp. 424.

48   D.R. Curtis: Pharmacol. Rev. 15, 333 (1963).

49   D.W. Esplin and B. Zablocka: in The Pharmacological Basis of Therapeutics, 3rd edition. (Eds. L.S. Goodman and A. Gilman). Macmillan, New York 1965. pp. 349.

50   R.H. Travis and G. Sayers: in The Pharmacological Basis of Therapeutics, 3rd edition. Eds. L.S. Goodman and A. Gilman. Macmillan, New York 1965. pp. 1627.

51   A. Sytinskii and T.N. Priyatkina: Biochem. Pharmacol. 15, 49 (1966).

52   N.M. van Gelder: Biochem. Pharmacol. 15, 533 (1966).

53   R. Tapia, H. Pasantes, M. Perez de la Mora, B.G. Ortega and G.H. Massieu: Biochem. Pharmacol. 16, 483 (1967).

54   T. Hayashi: Jap. J. Physiol. 3, 46 (1952).

55   S.H. Chung and M.S. Johnson: Proc. Roy. Soc. B 221, 145 (1984)

56   A. Baba, S. Okumura, H. Mizuo and H. Iwata: J. Neurochem. 40, 280 (1983).

57   S.J. Potashner: J. Neurochem. 32, 103 (1979).

58   A.C. Dolphin and E.R. Archer: Neurosci. Lett. 43, 49 (1983).

59   J.C. Watkins and R.H. Evans: Ann. Rev. Pharmacol. Toxicao. 21, 165 (1981).

60   M.L. Mayer and G.L. Westbrook: J. Physiol. 354, 29 (1984).

61   G.H. Glaser, J.K. Penry and D.M. Woodbury: in Antiepileptic drugs: Mechanisms of action. Raven Press, New York 1980. pp. 1.

62   R.L. Macdonald, M.J. Mclean and J.H. Skerritt: Fed. Proc. 44, 2643 (1985).

63   C. Locock (discussion of) E.H. Sieveking: Lancet 1, 327 (1857).

64   A. Hauptmann: Münch. Med. Wochenscher 59, 1907 (1912).

65   E. Blum: Dtsch. Med. Wochenscher 58, 696 (1932).

66   H. Weese: Dtsch. Med. Wochenschr. 58, 696 (1932).

67   L.G.M. Page: Br. Med. J. 1, 531 (1936)

68   C.G. Millman: J. Ment. Sci. 85, 971 (1939).

69   P. Albertoni: Arch. Exp. Pathol Pharmacol. 15, 248 (1982).

70   F. Hildebrandt: Naunyn Schmiedebergs Arch Exp. Pathol. Pharmakol. 116, 100 (1926).

71   W.E. Stone: in Experimental models of epilepsy – A manual for the laboratory worker (D.P. Purpura, J.K. Penry, D.B. Tower, D.M. Woodbury and R.D. Walter Eds.) Raven Press, New York 1972, pp. 407.
72   H.H. Merritt, T.J. Putnam: Arch. Neurol. Psychiatry *39*, 1003 (1938).
73   H.H. Merritt, T.J. Putnam: JAMA *111*, 1068 (1938).
74   Federal Food and Drugs Act of 1906. Public Law 384, 59th Congress.
75   R.K. Richards, G.M. Everett: Fed. Proc. *3*, 39 (1944).
76   H. Spielman and C. Landis: J. Am. Chem. Soc. *66*, 1244 (1944).
77   L.S. Goodman, M.S. Grewal, W.C. Brown, E.A. Swinyard: J. Pharmacol. Exp. Ther. *108*, 168 (1953).
78   J.E.P. Toman, E.A. Swinyard and L.S. Goodman: J. Neurophysiol. *9*, 231 (1946).
79   L.S. Goodman, E.A. Swinyard and J.E.P. Toman: Proc. Am. Fed. Clin. Res. *2*, 100 (1945).
80   L.B. Kalinowsky and F. Kennedy: J. Nerv. Ment. Dis. *98*, 56 (1943).
81   H. Strauss and C. Landis: Proc. Soc. Exp. Biol. Med. *38*, 369 (1938).
82   W.G. Lennox: JAMA *129*, 1069 (1945).
83   J.P. Davis and W.G. Lennox: Res. Publ. Assoc. Res. Nerv. Ment. Dis. *26*, 423 (1947).
84   W.G. Lennox: JAMA *134*, 138 (1947).
85   E.A. Swinyard: J. Am. Pharm. Assoc. *38*, 201 (1949).
86   G. Chen, R. Portman, C.R. Ensor, A.C. Jr. Bratton: J. Pharmacol Exp. Ther. *103*, 54 (1951).
87   F.T. Zimmerman and B.B. Burgemeister: Neurology *8*, 769 (1958).
88   R.J. Porter, J.K. Penry, J.R. Lacy, M.E. Newmark and H.J. Kuferberg: Neurology *27*, 375 (1977).
89   G. Chen, J.K. Weston and A.C. Jr. Bratton: Epilepsia *4*, 66 (1963).
90   D.M. Woodbury, J.K. Penry and R.P. Schmidt (Eds.): in Antiepileptic Drugs. Raven Press, New York 1972, pp. 536.
91   C.V. Pryles, J.M. Burnett and S. Livingston: JAMA *148*, 536 (1952).
92   R.L. Krall, J.K. Penry, H.J. Kufferberg and E.A. Swinyard: Epilepsia *19*, 393 (1978).
93   Federal Register 31: 8380, June 15, 1966.
94   Federal Register 31: 2786, February 16, 1966.
95   Drug Amendments Act of 1962. Public Law 87-781, 21 USC 355.
96   J.J. Cereghino and J.K. Penry: in Antiepileptic Drugs. D.M. Woodbury, J.K. Penry and R.P. Schmidt (Eds.), Raven Press, New York, 1972 pp. 63.
97   Public Health Service Advisory Committee on the Epilepsies. Minutes of meeting, February 9, 1967. Md. Bethesda: National Institutes of Health, 1967.
98   J.J. Coatsworth: in Studies on the Clinical Efficacy of Marketed Antiepileptic Drugs. NINDS Monograph No. 12, DHEW Publication No. (NIH) 73-51, U.S. Govt. Printing Office, Washington, D.C. 1971.
99   H. Gastaut: Epilepsia *11*, 102 (1970).
100 S.W. Rose, L.D. Smith and J.K. Penry: Blood level determinations of antiepileptic drugs – Clinical value and methods. National Institutes of Health, Bethesda 1971.
101 H.J. Kupferberg: J. Pharm. Sci. *61*, 284 (1972).
102 H. Kutt and J.K. Penry: Arch. Neurol. *31*, 283 (1974).
103 H.J. Kupferberg and J.K. Penry: in Clinical Pharmacology of Antiepileptic Drugs (Eds. H. Schneider, D. Janz, C. Gardner-Thorpe, H. Meinardi and A.L. Sherwin). Springer-Verlag, Berlin 1975, pp. 304.

104   C.E. Pippenger, J.K. Penry, B.G. White, D.D. Daly and R. Buddington: Arch. Neurol. *33*, 351 (1976).

105   C.E. Pippenger, J.K. Penry and H. Kutt: in Antiepileptic Drugs: Quantitative Analysis and Interpretation. Raven Press, New York, 1978 pp. 367.

106   W.C. Brown, D.O. Schiffman, E.A. Swinyard and L.S. Goodman: J. Pharmacol. Exp. Ther. *107*, 273 (1953).

107   J.G. Millichap: in Anticonvulsant Drugs. Vol. 1, I.E.P.T., Pergamon, New York, 1973, pp. 189.

108   S.G. Pirreda, J.H. Woodhead and E.A. Swinyard: J. Pharmacol. Exp. Ther. *222*, 741 (1985).

109   R.L. Krall, J.K. Penry, B.G. White, H.J. Kupferberg and E.A. Swinyard: Epilepsia *19*, 409 (1978).

110   E.A. Swinyard and H.J. Kupferberg: Fed. Proc. *44*, 2629 (1985).

111   J.F. Reinhard and J.F. Jr. Reinhard: in Anticonvulsants (ed. J. AAvida), Academic Press, New York 1977, pp. 57.

112   R.J. Porter, J.J. Cereghino, G.D. Gladding, B.J. Hessie, H.J. Kupferberg, B. Scoville and B.G. White: Cleveland Clin. Q. *51*, 293 (1984).

113   B.S. Meldrum: in New Anticonvulsant Drugs (eds. B.S. Meldrum and R.J. Porter). John Libbey, London 1986, pp. 31.

114   P.C. Jobe and H.E. Laird II: Neurotransmitters and Epilepsy. Humana Press, Clifton, NJ 1987.

115   E.W. Lothman, R.A. Salerno, J.B. Perlin and D.L. Kaiser: Epilepsy Res. *2*, 367 (1988).

116   H.J. Kupferberg: Epilepsia *30* (suppl.1), S51 (1989).

117   R.S. Fisher: Brain Res. Rev. *14*, 245 (1989).

118   W. Löscher and D. Schmidt: Epilepsy Res. *456*, 139 (1988).

119   R. Mutani, F. Monaco and S. Gentile: Curr. Probl. Epilepsy *5*, 15 (1988).

120   D.E. Woolley, P.S. Timiras, M.R. Rosenzweig, D. Krech and E.L. Bennett: Nature *190*, 515 (1961).

121   M.L. Torchiana and C.A. Stone: Proc. Soc. Exp. Biol. Med. *100*, 290 (1959).

122   E.A. Swinyard, J.H. Woodhead, H.S. White and M.R. Franklin: in Antiepileptic Drugs, 3rd edition (eds. R. Levy, R. Mattson, B. Meldrum, J.K. Penry and F.E. Dreifuss). Raven Press Ltd., New York 1989, pp. 85.

123   V.D. Davenport and H.W. Davenport: J. Nutr. *36*, 139 (1948).

124   T.J. Putman and H.H. Merritt: Science *85*, 525 (1937).

125   L.A. Woodbury and V.D. Davenport: Arch. Int. Pharmacodyn. Ther. *92*, 97 (1952).

126   R.L. Krall, J.K. Penry, B.G. White, H.J. Kupferberg and E.A. Swinyard: Epilepsia *19*, 404 (1978).

127   S.J. Enna and S.H. Synder: Mol. Pharmacol. *13*, 442 (1977).

128   C. Braestrup and R.F. Squires: Proc. Nat. Acad. Sci. U.S.A. *74* (9), 3805 (1977).

129   S.R. Zukin, A.B. Young and S.H. Synder: Proc. Natl. Acad. Sci. U.S.A. *71* (12), 4802 (1974).

130   J.W. Phillis, P.H. Wu and A.S. Bender: General Pharmacol. *12*, 67 (1981).

131   C.W. Cotman: Methods in Enzymology *31A*, 445 (1974).

132   C.L. Faingold: Gen. Pharmacol. *19*, 331 (1988).

133   W. Löscher and H.H. Frey: Eur. J. Pharmacol. *143*, 335 (1987).

134   D.D. Johnson, R. Wilcox, J.M. Tuchek and R.D. Crawford: Epilepsia *26*, 466 (1985).

135 J.L. Noebels: in Electrophysiology of epilepsy (eds. P.A. Schwartzkroin and H.V. Wheal). Academic Press, London 1984, pp. 201.

136 T.N. Seyfried and G.H. Glaser: Epilepsia 26, 143 (1985).

137 A. Lehmann: Life Sci. 20, 2047 (1977).

138 A.G. Chapman, M.J. Croucher and B.S. Meldrum: Arzneimittel-Forsch. 34, 1261 (1984).

139 A.G. Chapman and B.S. Meldrum: in Neurotransmitters and epilepsy (eds. P.C. Jobe and H.E. Laird). Humana Press, Clifton 1986.

140 H.E. Laird and P.C. Jobe: in Neurotransmitters and epilepsy (eds. P.C. Jobe and H.E. Laird). Humana Press, Clifton 1986.

141 R. Naquet and B.S. Meldrum: in Experimental models of epilepsy (eds. D. Purpura et al.,). Raven Press, New York 1972, pp. 373.

142 R. Naquet and B.S. Meldrum: in Advances in neurology, Vol. 43, Myoclonus (eds. F. Fahn, C.D. Marsden and M. van Woert). Raven Press, New York 1985, pp. 579.

143 B.S. Meldrum, R.W. Horton and P.A. Toseland: Arch. Neurol. 32, 289 (1975).

144 B.S. Meldrum, G. Anlezark, E. Balzano, R.W. Horton and M. Trimble: in Advances in neurology (eds. B.S. Meldrum and C.D. Marsden) Vol. 10. Raven Press, New York 1975, pp. 119.

145 B.S. Meldrum: in Contemporary clinical neurophysiology suppl. No. 34, Electroenceph. clin. neurophysiol. (eds. W.A. Cobb and H. van Duijn). Elsevier Scientific Publishing Co., Amsterdam 1978, pp. 317.

146 B.S. Meldrum and R.W. Horton: Psychopharmacol. 60, 277 (1979).

147 D.C. Piper, B. S. Meldrum and C. R. Gardner: Drug Development Res. 1, 77 (1981).

148 B.S. Meldrum, M.J. Croucher, G. Badman and J.F. Collins: Neurosci. Lett. 39, 101 (1983).

149 J.S. Lockard, R.H. Levy, L.L. DuCharme and W.C. Congdon: Epilepsia 20, 339 (1979).

150 J.S. Lockard: in Epilepsy, a window to brain mechanisms (eds. J.S. Lockard and A.A. Ward). Raven Press, New York 1980, pp. 11.

151 J.S. Lockard, R.H. Levy, P.H. Rhodes and D.F. Moore: Epilepsia (in press) 1986.

152 J.A. Wada: Kindling, Raven Press, New York 1976, pp. 260.

153 J.A. Wada: Kindling 2, Raven Press, New York 1081, pp. 361.

154 R.J. Racine and W.M. Burnham: in Electrophysiology of epilepsy (eds. P.A. Schwartzkroin and H.V. Wheal). Academic Press, London 1984, pp. 153.

155 M. Schmutz: Prog. Neuropsychopharmacol. Biol. Psychiat. 11, 505 (1987).

156 A. Vezzani, H.Q. Wu, E. Moneta and R. Samanin: Neurosci. Lett. 87, 63 (1988).

157 I. Mody, P.K. Stanton and U. Heinemann: J. Neurophysiol. 59, 1033 (1988).

158 J.O. McNamara, R.D. Russell, L. Rigskee and D.W. Bonhans: Neuropharmacol. 27, 653 (1988).

159 M.J. Croucher, H.F. Bradford, D.C. Sunter and J.C. Watkins: Eur. J. Pharmacol. 152, 29 (1988).

160 J.D. Leander, R.C. Rathbun and D.M. Zimmerman: Brain Res. 454, 368 (1988).

161 A.C. Chapman, B. Engelsen and B.S. Meldrum: J. Neurochem. 49, 121 (1987).

162 I.E. Leppik, K. Marienan, N.M. Graves and C.A. Rark: Neurology 35, 405 (1988).

163 N.W. Dunham and T.A. Miya: J. Amer. Pharm. Ass. Sci. Ed. 46, 208 (1957).

164 E.A. Swinyard: Epilepsia 10, 107 (1969).

165. S. Irwin: Psychopharmacologia (Berl.) 13, 222 (1968).

166 G.G. Somjen and M. Gill: J. Pharmacol. Exp. Ther. 140, 19 (1963).

167   L.S. Goodman and A. Gillman: in The pharmacological basis of therapeutics. Macmillan, New York 1975, pp. 102–113 and 209–211.

168   H. Downes, R.S. Perry, R.E. Ostlund and R. Karler: J. Pharmacol. Exp. Ther. *175*, 692 (1970).

169   J.H. Skerritt and R.L. Macdonald: J. Pharmacol Exp. Ther. *230*, 82 (1984).

170   E.A. Swinyard, W.C. Brown and L.S. Goodman: J. Pharmacol. Exp. Ther. *106*, 47 (1952).

171   C.R. Craig and F.E. Shideman: J. Pharmacol. Exp. Ther. *176*, 35 (1971).

172   E.K. Killam: Fed. Proc. *35*, 2264 (1976).

173   D.A. Callaghan and W.S. Schwark: Neuropharmacology *19*, 1131 (1980).

174   B.B. Gallagher: in Epileptic drugs, 3rd edition (eds. R. Levy, R. Mattson, B. Meldrum, J.K. Penry and F.E. Dreifuss). Raven Press, New York 1989, pp. 103.

175   M.J. Painter: in Epileptic drugs, 3rd edition (eds. R. Levy, R. Mattson, B. Meldrum, J.K. Penry and F.E. Dreifuss). Raven Press, New York 1989, pp. 329.

176   E.P.G. Vining. E.D. Mellitis, M.M. Dorsen, M.F. Cataldo, S.A. Quaskey, S.P. Spielberg and J.M. Freeman: Pediatrics *80*, 165 (1987).

177   D.A. Brent, P.K. Crumrine, R.E. Varma, M. Allan and C. Allman: Pediatrics *80*, 909 (1987).

178   W.G. Mitchell and J.M. Chavez: Epilepsia 28, 56 (1987).

179   J.R. Farwell, Y.J. Lee, D.G. Hirtz, S.I. Sulzbacher, J.H. Ellenberg and K.B. Nelson: N. Engl. J. Med. *322*, 364 (1990).

180   C.M. Regan, A.M.C. Gorman, O.M. Larson, C. Maguire, M.L. Martin, A. Schousboe' and D.C. Williams: International J. Developmental Neuroscience 8, 143 (1990).

181   C.M. Regan, O.M. Larson, M.L. Martin, A. Schousboe and D.C. Williams: Toxic in vitro *5*, 77 (1991).

182   M.J. Eadie: in Epileptic drugs, 3rd edition (eds. R. Levy, R. Mattson, B. Meldrum, J.K. Penry and F.E. Dreifuss). Raven Press, New York 1989, pp. 357.

183   T.W. Rall and L.S. Schleifer: in Goodman and Gilman's the Pharmacological Basis of Therapeutics, 6th edition (eds. A.G. Gilman, L.S. Goodman and A. Gilman). Macmillan publishing Co., New York 1980, pp. 448.

184   C.M. Samour, J.F. Reinhard and J.A. Vida: J. Med. Chem. *14*, 187 (1971).

185   G. Gobbi, E.P. Maglietta, P. Stanzani, M.G. Costanzo, P. Folegani, M. Santucci and P.G. Rossi: in Book of abstracts, 18th International epilepsy congress, New Delhi, India 1989, pp. 79.

186   D.B. Smith, S.G. Goldstein and A. Roomet: Epilepsia *27*, 149 (1986).

187   B.D. Bernardina, E. Fontana, V. Sgro, R. Cellino and M. Simeoni: in Book of abstracts, 18th International epilepsy congress, New Delhi, India 1989, pp. 156.

188   J.A. Vida, W.R. Wilber and J.F. Reinhard: J. Med. Chem. *14*, 191 (1971).

189   J.A. Vida, M.L. Hooker and J.F. Reinhard: J. Med. Chem. *16*, 602 (1973).

190   J.A. Vida, M.L. Hooker and C.M. Samour: J. Med. Chem. *16*, 1378 (1973).

191   F.F. Blicke and R.H. Cox: in Medicinal chemistry. Vol. IV, Wiley-Interscience, New York 1959.

192   P.R. Andrews, G.P. Jones and D. Lodge: Eur. J. Pharmacol. *55*, 115 (1979).

193   P.R. Andrews, G.P. Jones and D. Lodge: Eur. J. Pharmc *61* (1982).

194   J.A. Vida, C.M. Samour, M.H. O'Dea, T.S. Wang and W.R. Wilber: J. Med. Chem. *17*, 32 (1974).

195   J.K. Barker, D.O. Rauls and R.F. Borma: J. Med. Chem. *22*, 1301 (1979).

196 J. Knabe, W. Rummel, H.P. Bluch and N. Franz: Arzneim. Forsch. *28*, 1048 (1978).

197 H.P. Bluch, F. Schneider-Affeld and W. Rummel: Naunyn Schmiedepers Arch. Pharmacol. *27*, 191 (1973).

198 G.P. Jones and P.R. Andrews: J. Med. Chem. *23*, 244 (1980).

199 P.R. Andrews and G.P. Jones: Eur. J. Med. Chem. *16*, 139 (1980).

200 B. Pullman, J.L. Coubeils and P. Courriere: J. Theor. Biol. *35*, 375 (1972).

201 P.R. Andrews, A.J. Jones, G.P. Jones, A. Marker and E.A. Owen: Eur. J. Med. Chem. *16*, 145 (1980).

202 F.I. Carrol, A.H. Lewin, E.E. Williams, J.A. Berdasco and C.G. Moreland: J. Med. Chem. *27*, 1191 (1984).

203 J.P. Bideau, L. Marly and J. Housty: Compt. Rend. Acad. Sci. *269*, 549 (1969).

204 S.H. Kim and A. Rich: Proc. Natl. Acad. Sci. USA *60*, 402 (1968).

205 P.P. Williams: Acta Crystallogr. *B29*, 1572 (1973).

206 P.R. Andrews, L.C. Mark, D.A. Winkler and G.P. Jones: J. Med. Chem. *26*, 1223 (1983).

207 F.F. Blicke and M.F. Zienty: J. Am. Chem. Soc. *63*, 2991 (1941).

208 L. Velluz, J. Mathieu and R. Jequier: Ann. Pharm. Fr. *9*, 271 (1951).

209 P.K. Knoefel: Exp. Ther. *84*, 26 (1945).

210 A.M. Allan and R.A. Harris: J. Pharmacol. Exp. Ther. *238*, 763 (1986).

211 R.W. Olsen: Int. Anesthesiol. Clin. *26*, 254 (1988).

212 E.S. Levitan, L.A.C. Blair, V.E. Dionne and E.A. Barnard: Neuron *1*, 773 (1988).

213 D.W. Schulz and R.L. Macdonald: Brain Res. *209*, 177 (1981).

214 H. Kalant and W. Grose: J. Pharmacol. Exp. Ther. *158*, 386 (1967).

215 J.A. Richter and M.B. Waller: Biochem. Pharmacol. *26*, 609 (1977).

216 D. Coleman-Riese and R.W.P. Cutler: Neurochem. Res. *3*, 423 (1978).

217 R.A. Nicoll and E.T. Ewamoto: J. Neurophysiol. *41*, 977 (1978).

218 S.J. Potashner, N. Lake, E.A. Langlois, L. Plouffe and D. Lecavalier: Brain Res. Bull. *5*, 659 (1980).

219 M.P. Blaustein and A.C. Ector: Mol. Pharmacol. *11*, 369 (1975).

220 M.G. Ondrusek, J.K. Belknap and S.W. Leslie: Mol. Pharmacol. *15*, 386 (1979).

221 S.W. Leslie, M.B. Friedman, R.E. Wilcox and S.V. Elrod: Brain Res. *185*, 409 (1980).

222 J.W. Haycock, W.B. Levy and C.W. Cotman: Biochem. Pharmacol. *26*, 159 (1977).

223 M.C. Nowycky, A.P. Fox and R.W. Tsien: Nature (lond.) *316*, 440 (1985).

224 R.J. Miller: Science (Wash. DC) *235*, 46 (1987).

225 J.R. Huguenard and W.A. Wilson: J. Pharmacol. Exp. Ther. *234*, 821 (1985).

226 D.M.T. Politi, S. Suzuki and M.A. Rogawski: Eur. J. Pharmacol. *168*, 7 (1989).

227 R.A. Gross and R.L. Macdoald: Neurology *38*, 443 (1988).

228 M.A. Rogawski, N. Hershkowitz, D.M. Politi, S. Suzuki, A. Thürkauf and S. Yamaguchi: in Current and future trends in anticonvulsant, anxiety and stroke therapy (Princeton drug research symposium vol.1) (eds. B.S. Meldrum and M. Williams). Wiley-Liss, New York 1990, pp. 91.

229 C. Zona, V. Tancredi, E. Palma, G.C. Pirrone and M. Avoli: Can. J. Physiol. Pharmacol. *68*, 545 (1990).

230 M.A. Simmonds and A.L. Horne: in Excitatory amino acids in health and disease (ed. D. Lodge). John Wiley and Sons, Chichester 1988, pp. 219.

231 L. Sivilotti and A. Nistri: Neuropharmacology *28*, 1107 (1989).

232 S.K. Kulkarni and M.K. Ticku: Life Sci. *44*, 1317 (1989).

233   P.W. Gage, D. McKinnon and B. Robertson: in Molecular and cellular mechanisms of anesthetics (eds. S.H. Roth and K.W. Miller). Plenum, New York 1986, pp. 139.

234   L.B. Kier and L.H. Hall: Pharm. Res. 7, 801 (1990).

235   G. Bursot and J.L. Bursot: Ann. Pharm. Fr. 47, 361 (1989).

236   S.C. Basak, D.K. Harriss and V.R. Masnuson: J. Pharm. Sci. 73, 429 (1984).

237   S.C. Basak, L.J. Monsrud, M.E. Rosen, C.M. Frane and V.R. Masnuson: Acta Pharm. Jugosl. 36, 81 (1986).

238   D. Henry, J.H. Block, J.L. Anderson and G.R. Carlson: J. Med. Chem. 19, 619 (1976).

239   J.S. Millership and A.D. Woolfson: J. Pharm. Pharmacol. 30, 483 (1978).

240   D.A. Brent, J.J. Sabatka, D.J. Minick and D.W. Henry: J. Med. Chem. 26, 1014 (1983).

241   E.J. Lien and X.C. Ou: Acta Pharm. Jugosl. 34, 123 (1984).

242   N. Watari, Y. Susiyama, N. Kaneniwa and M. Hiura: J. Pharmacokinet. Biopharm. 16, 279 (1988).

243   G.L. Tons and E.J. Lien: J. Pharm. Sci. 65, 1651 (1976).

244   S. Toon and M. Rowland: J. Pharmacol. Exp. Ther. 225, 752 (1983).

245   J.M. Plia-Delfina, J. Moreno, J. Duran and A. Pozo: J. Pharmacokinet. Biopharm 3, 115(1975).

246   A. Lopate, F. Darvas, A. Stadler-Szoke and J. Szejtli: J. Pharm. Sci. 74, 211 (1985).

247   W.J. Murray, L.B. Kier and L.H. Hall: J. Med. Chem. 19, 573 (1976).

248   G. Klopman and C. Raychaudhury: J. Chem. Inf. Comput. Sci. 30, 12 (1990).

249   B.F.D. Bourgeois: in Antiepileptic Drugs 3rd edition (eds. R. Levy, R. Mattson, B. Meldrum, J.K. Penry and F.E. Dreifuss). Raven Press, New York 1989, pp. 401.

250   H.H. Frey: in Antiepileptic Drugs (eds. H.H. Frey and D. Janz). Handbook of experimental pharmacology, Vol. 74. Springer-Verlag, Berlin 1985, pp. 283.

251   K.W. Leal, R.L. Rapport, A.J. Wilensky and P.N. Friel: Ann. Neurol. 5, 470 (1979).

252   B.F.D. Bourgeois, W.E. Dodson and J.A. Ferrendelli: Neurology 33, 283 (1983).

253   G.L. Jones and G.H. Wimbish: in Antiepileptic Drugs (eds. H.H. Frey and D. Janz). Handbook of experimental pharmacology. Vol 74, Springer-Verlag, Berlin 1985, pp. 351.

254   M.J. Eadie and J.H. Tryer: in Pharmacological basis and practice, 3rd edition. Churchill Livingstone, Edinburgh 1989.

255   J. Majkowski, A. Sobieszek, B. Bilinska-Nigot and A. Karlinski: Epilepsia 17, 257 (1976).

256   J.O. McNamara, L.C. Rigsbee, L.S. Butler and C. Shin: Ann. Neurol. 26, 675 (1989).

257   M.E. Selzer, E.M. Edler, G. David and Y. Yaari: in Mechanisms of epileptogenesis: The transition to seizure (ed. M.A. Dichter). Plenum Press, New York 1988, pp. 221.

258   R.J. De Lorenzo: in Antiepileptic Drugs 3rd edition (eds. R. Levy, R. Mattson, B. Meldrum, J.K. Penry and F.E. Dreifuss). Raven Press, New York 1989, pp. 143.

259   Y. Yaari, M.E. Selzer and J.H. Pincus: Ann. Neurol. 20, 171 (1986).

260   M.J. McLean and R.L. Macdonald: J. Pharmacol. Exp. Ther. 227, 779 (1983).

261   T. Naraheshi: in Calculations Drugs in Action (ed. P.F. Baker). Handbook of experimental Pharmacology, Vol. 83. Springer-Verlag, Berlin 1988, pp. 255.

262   S. Kaneko, T. Hirano, T. Kondo, K. Otani, Y. Fukushima, R. Hishida and M. Matsunga: Jpn. J. Psychiatry Neurol. 42, 643 (1988).

263   M.P. Earnest, J.A. Marx and L.R. Drury: JAMA 249, 762 (1983).

264   H. Masur, C.E. Elger, A.C. Ludolph and M. Galanski: Neurology 39, 432 (1989).

265   H.J. Kupferberg: in Antiepileptic Drugs 3rd edition (eds. R. Levy, R. Mattson, B. Meldrum, J.K. Penry and F.E. Dreifuss). Raven Press, New York 1989, pp. 257.

266   A.S. Troupin, L.M. Ojemann and C.B. Dodrill: Epilepsia *17*, 414 (1976).

267   M.M. Robins: Am. J. Dis. Child. *104*, 614 (1962).

268   R.J. Porter: in Epilepsy: in One hundred elementary principles, 2nd edition. W.B. Saunders Co., London 1989.

269   E. Campaigne and H.L. Thomas: J. Am. Chem. Soc. *77*, 5365 (1955).

270   J. Klosa: Arch. Pharm. *289*, 223 (1956).

271   J.A. Vida, W.R. Wilber and J.F. Reinhard: J. Med. Chem. *14*, 190 (1971).

272   D.K. Yung, T.P. Forrest, M.L. Gilroy and M.M. Vohra: I. Pharm. Sci. *62*, 1764 (1973).

273   J.A. Vida, M.H. O'Dea, C.M. Samour and J.F. Reinhard: J. Med. Chem. *18*, 383 (1975).

274   A. Blade Font, J.N. Torres Estaban: Span. Pat. *389*, 999 (1975) [Chem. Abstr. *83*, 179062k (1975)].

275   W. Oldfield and C.H. Cashin: J. Med. Chem. *8*, 239 (1965).

276   A. Spinks and W.S. Waring: in Progress in Medicinal Chemistry Vol. III (eds. G.P. Ellis and G.B. West). Butterworths, Washington, D.C., 1963, pp. 261.

277   M.A. Davis, S.O. Winthrop, R.A. Thomas, F. Herr, M.P. Charest and R. Gaudry: J. Med. Chem. *7*, 439 (1964).

278   C.H. Carter: Clin. Med. *78*, 33 (1971).

279   L. Musial, M.J. Korohoda, A. Szadowski and H. Szmigielska: Acta Pol. Pharm. *29*, 573 (1972).

280   C.H. Kwon, M.T. Iqbal and J.N Wulpel: J. Med. Chem. *34*, 1845 (1991).

281   J.H. Poupaert, D. Vaderuorst, P. Guiot, M.M.M. Morestata and P. Dument: J. Med. Chem. *27*, 76 (1984).

282   F.A. Gibbs, G.M. Everett and R.K. Richards: Dis. Nerv. Syst. *10*, 47 (1949).

283   S.B. Coker, E.W. Holmes and R.T. Egal: Neurology *37*, 1861 (1987).

284   D.M. Woodbury and E. Fingl: in The pharmacological basis of therapeutics, 5th ed. (L.S. Goodman and A. Gilman Eds.). MacMillan, New York 1975 pp. 201.

285   A.G. Pechenkin, L.G. Thgnibidina, A. Pigilev, V.K. Gorshkova and V.M. Kurilenko: Khim. Farm. Zh. *7*, 16 (1973).

286   M.S. Dhar: Arch. Int. Pharmacodyn. Ther. *219*, 103 (1976).

287   M.R. Pavia, S.J. Lobbestael, C.P. Taylov, F.M. Hershenson and D.L. Miskell: J. Med. Chem. *33*, 854 (1990).

288   M. Khalil and D.F. Weaver: J. Pharm. Pharmacol. *42*, 349 (1990).

289   G.L. Jones, R.J. Amato, G.H. Wimbish and G.A. Peyton: J. Pharm. Sci. *70*, 618 (1981).

290   P.W. Codding, T.A. Lee and J.F. Richardson: J. Med. Chem. *27*, 649 (1984).

291   H. Kutt: in Antiepileptic Drugs 3rd ed. (R. Levy, R. Mattson, B. Meldrum, J.K. Penry and F. E. Dreifuss). Raven Press, New York 1989, pp. 457.

292   J.A. Wada: Arch. Neurol. *34*, 389 (1977).

293   R.M. Julien and R.P. Hollister: Adv. Neurol. *11*, 263 (1975).

294   J. David and R.S. Grewal: Epilepsia *17*, 415 (1976).

295   M. Schmutz: in Antiepileptic Drugs (H.H. Frey and D. Janz Eds.). Handbook of Experimental Pharmacology, Vol. 74. Springer-Verlag, Berlin 1985, pp. 479.

296   B.M. Kerr and R.H. Levy: in Antiepileptic Drugs 3rd (Eds. R. Levy, R. Mattson, B. Meldrum, J.K. Penry and F.E. Dreifuss). Raven Press, Ney York 1989, pp. 505.

297   P.S. Albright and J. Bruni: Neurology *34*, 1383 (1984).

298   B.F.D. Bourgeois and N. Wad: J. Pharmacol. Exp. Ther. *231*, 411 (1984).

299   I. Altafulla, D. Talwar, R. Loewenson, K. Olson and L.A. Lockman: Epilepsy Res. 4, 72 (1989).

300   P.L. Morselli, G. Bartholini and K.G. Lloyd: in New Anticonvulsant Drugs (B.S. Meldrum and R.J. Porter Eds.). John Libbey, London 1986, pp. 237.

301   R.H. Mattson, J.A. Cramer, J.F. Collins, D.B. Smith, A.V. Delgadoescueta, T.R. Browne, P.D. Williamson, D.M. Treiman, J.O. McNamara, C.B. McCutchen, R.W. Homan, W.E. Crill, M.F. Lubozynski, N.P. Rosenthal and A. Mayersdorf: N. Engl. J. Med. 313, 145 (1985).

302   K.J. Meador, D.W. Loring, K. Huh, B.B. Gallager and D.W. King: Neurology 40, 391 (1990).

303   K.J. Jones, R.Y. Lacro, K.A. Johnson and J. Adams: N. Engl. J. Med. 320, 1661 (1989).

304   T.R. Browne, G.K. Szabo, J.E. Evans, B.A. Evans, D.J. Greenblatt and M.A. Mikati: Neurology 38, 1146 (1988).

305   B.F.D. Bourgeois and N. Wad: Epilepsia 29, 482 (1988).

306   M. Willow, T. Gonoi and W.A. Catterall: Mol. Pharmacol. 27, 549 (1985).

307   M.J. Mclean and R.L. Macdonald: J. Pharmacol. Exp. Ther. 238, 727 (1986).

308   J.R. Schwarz and G. Grigat: Epilepsia 30, 286 (1989).

309   P.F. Worley and J.M. Baraban: Proc. Natl. Acad. Sci. USA 84, 3051 (1987).

310   M. Willow and W.A. Catterall: Mol. Pharmacol. 22, 627 (1982).

311   H.-R. Olpe, M. Baudry and R.S.G. Jones: Eur. J. Pharmacol. 110, 71 (1985).

312   E.T. MacNeal, G.A. Lewandowski, J.W. Daly and C.R. Creveling: J. Med. Chem. 28, 381 (1985).

313   P.J. Marangos, P. Montgomery, S.R.B. Wess, J. Patel and R.M. Post: Clin. Neuropharmacol. 10, 443 (1987).

314   R.L. Weir, S.M. Anderson and J.W. Daly: Epilepsia, 31, 503 (1990).

315   P.J. Marangos, R.M. Post, J. Patel, K. Zander, A. Parma and S. Weiss: Eur. J. Pharmacol. 93, 175 (1983).

316   S.R.B. Weiss, R.M. Post, J. Patel and P.J. Marangos: Lif. Sci. 36, 2413 (1985).

317   H. Schtz, K.F. Feldmann, J.W. Faigle, H.-P. Kriemler and T. Winkler: Xenobiotica 16, 769 (1986).

318   V. Baltzer and M. Schmutz: Advances in Epileptology, 295–299 (1977).

319   J. Wagner and K. Schmidt: Xenobiotica 17, 951 (1987).

320   P.N. Patsalos, T.J. Stephenson, S. Krishna, A.A. Elyas, P.T. Lascelles and C.M. Wiles: Lancet 2, 496 (1985).

321   M. Dam, R. Ekberg, Y. Löyning, O. Waltimo and K.A. Jakobsen: Epilepsy Res. 3, 70 (1989).

322   M.L. Friis, O. Kristensen, J. Boas, M. Dalby, S.H. Deth et al.: Acta Neurologica Scandinavica 87, 224 (1993).

323   S.M. Grant and D. Faulds: Drugs 43, 873 (1991).

324   B.J. Steinhoff, K.-D. Stoll, S.R.G. Stodieck and W. Paulus: Epilepsy Res. 11, 67 (1992).

325   M. Sillanpää: in The treatment of epilepsy: principles and practice (Wyllie, Ed.). Lea and Febiger, Philadelphia 1993, pp. 867.

326   G. Krämer, B. Tettenborn, J.P. Klosterskov, G.P. Menge and K.D. Stoll: Epilepsia 33, 1145 (1992).

327   T.C. Butler, W.J. Waddell and D.T. Poole: Biochem. Pharmacol. 14, 937 (1965).

328   3H.H. Frey and B.H. Kretschmer: Arch. Int. Pharmacodyn. Ther. 193, 181 (1971).

329 H.E. Booker: in Antiepileptic Drugs 3rd ed. (R. Levy, R. Mattson, B. Meldrum, J.K. Penry and F.E. Dreifuss). Raven Press, Ney York 1989, pp. 715.

330 D.A. Coulter, J.R. Huguenard and D.A. Prince: Neurosci. Lett. 98, 74 (1989).

331 P. Emig, J. Engel, B. Nickel, I. Szelenyi and U. Werner: Drugs Future 15, 223 (1990).

332 G. Chen, J.K. Weston and A.C. Jr. Bratton: Epilepsia 4, 66 (1963).

333 T.R. Browne, R.H. Mattson, J.K. Penry, D.B. Smith, D.M. Treiman, B.J. Wilder, E. Ben-Menachem, R.M. Miketta, K.M. Sherry and G.K. Szabo: Br. J. Pharmacol. 27 (suppl. 1), 95S (1989).

334 R.V. Andrews, F.J. Ritter and J. Mims: Epilepsia 30, 736 (1989).

335 A.H. Heller, M.A. Dichter and R.L. Sidman: Epilepsia 25, 25 (1983).

336 C. Marescaux, G. Micheletti, M. Vergnes, A. Depaulis, L. Rumbach and J.M. Warter: Epilepsia 25, 326 (1984).

337 M. Sasa, Y. Ohno, H. Ujihara, Y. Fujita, M. Yoshimura, S. Takaori, T. Serikawa and J. Yamada: Epilepsy 29, 505 (1988).

338 J. Veliskova, L. Velisek, P. Mases, R. Rokyta and D. Micianikova: Pharmacol. Biochem. Behav. 44, 975 (1993).

339 T.R. Browne, F.E. Dreifuss, P.R. Dyken, D.J. Goode, J.K. Penry, R.J. Porter, B.G. White and P.T. White: Neurology 25, 515 (1975).

340 A.L. Sherwin, J.P. Robb and M. Lechter: Arch. Neurol. 28, 178 (1973).

341 M.J. McLean and R.L. Macdonald: J. Pharmacol. Exp. Ther. 237, 1001 (1986).

342 D.M. Barnes and M.A. Dichter: Neurology 34, 620 (1984).

343 P.P. De Deyn and R.L. Macdonald: Epilepsia 30, 17 (1989).

344 D.A. Coulter, J.R. Huguenard and D.A. Prince: Epilepsia 30, 734 (1989).

345 D.A. Coulter, J.R. Huguenard and D.A. Prince: J. Physiol. (Lond.) 414, 587 (1989). 734 (1989).

346 D.A. Coulter, J.R. Huguenard and D.A. Prince: Ann. Neurol. 25, 582 (1989).

347 D.A. Coulter, J.R. Huguenard and D.A. Prince: Br. J. Pharmacol. 100, 800 (1990).

348 N.E. Akopyan and D.A. Gerasimyan: Biol. Zh. Arm. 24, (1971).

349 N.E. Akopyan and D.A. Gerasimyan and Dzh.A. Melkonyan: Biol. Zh. Arm. 27, 52 (1974).

350 Z. Alfud, O. Jolanta and J. Izabela: Acta Pol. Pharm. 48, 39 (1991).

351 W. Kwiatkowski, J. Karolak-Wojciechowska, J. Obniska and A. Zejc: Acta Crystallogr. C46, 108 (1990).

352 J. Lange, W. Kazmierski and J. Daroszewski: Pol. J. Pharmacol. Pharm. 43, 71 (1991).

353 H.Y. Aboul-Enein, C.W. Schauber, A.R. Hansen and L.J. Fisher: J. Med. Chem. 18, 736 (1975).

354 D.T. Witiak, S.K. Seth, E.R. Baizman, S.L. Weibel and H.H. Wolf: J. Med. Chem. 15, 1117 (1972).

355 D.T. Witiak, W.L. Cook, T.K. Gupta and M.C. Gerald: J. Med. Chem. 19, 1419 (1976).

356 Y. Tateoka, T. Kimura, H. Kamiyama, K. Watanabe, I. Yamamoto and I.K. Ho: Res. Commun. Chem. Pathol. Pharmacol. 61, 315 (1988).

357 R.R. Goehring, T.D. Greenwood, G.C. Nwokogu, J.S. Pisipati, T.G. Rogers and J.F. Wolfe: J. Med. Chem. 33, 926 (1990).

358 H.H. Frey and W. Loescher: Arzneim-Forsch. 26, 299 (1976).

359 A. Chapman, P.E. Keane, B.S. Meldrum, J. Simiand Vernières: Prog. Neurobiol. 19, 315 (1982).

360 W. Löscher and D. Schmidt: Epilepsy Res. 2, 145 (1988).

361 G.D. Bartoszyk, Dooley, E. Fritschi and G. Satzinger: in New anticonvulsant drugs (eds. B.S. Meldrum and R.J. Porter). John Libbey, London 1986, pp. 309.

362 W. Löscher: in Antiepileptic drugs (eds. H.H. Frey and D. Janz). Hand book of Experimental Pharmacology, Vol. 74. Springer-Verlag, Berlin 1985, pp. 507.

363 J.A. Ferrendelli, K.D. Holland, A.C. McKeon and D.F. Covey: Epilepsia 30, 617 (1989).

364 N.Y. Walton and D.M. Treiman: Epilepsy Res. 12, 199 (1992).

365 R.H. Levy and D.D. Shen: in Antiepileptic Drugs 3rd ed. (R. Levy, R. Mattson, B. Meldrum, J.K. Penry and F.E. Dreifuss). Raven Press, Ney York 1989, pp. 583.

366 T.A. Baillie and A.W. Rettenmeier: in Antiepileptic Drugs 3rd ed. (R. Levy, R. Mattson, B. Meldrum, J.K. Penry and F.E. Dreifuss). Raven Press, Ney York 1989, pp. 601.

367 S. Sato, B.G. White, J.K. Penry, F.E. Dreifuss and H.J. Kupferberg: Neurology 32, 157 (1982).

368 J.C. Dean and J.K. Penry: Epilepsia 29, 140 (1988).

369 D. Chadwick: Am. J. Med. 84, 3 (1988).

370 W. Löscher: Arch. Int. Pharmacodyn. Ther. 276, 263 (1985).

371 D. Cotariu and J.L. Zaidman: Life Sci. 48, 1341 (1991).

372 H. Nau, R.S. Hauck and K. Ehlers: Pharmacol. Toxicol. 69, 310 (1991).

373 R.S. Hauck, M.M. Elmazar, C. Plum and H. Nau: Toxicol. Lett. 60, 145 (1992).

374 H. Nau and W.J. Scott: Arch. Toxicol. Suppl. 11, 128 (1987).

375 H. Nau: Acta Pharm. Jugosl. 40, 291 (1990).

376 R.L. Macdonald: J. Neural Transm. 72, 173 (1988).

377 H.J. Kupferberg, W.G. Lust and J.K. Penry: Fed. Proc. 34, 283 (1975).

378 H. Nau and W. Löscher: J. Pharmacol. Exp. Ther. 220, 654 (1982).

379 A.G. Chapman, B.S. Meldrum and E. Mendes: Life Sci. 32, 2023 (1983).

380 M. Willow, E.A. Kuenzel and W.A. Catterall: Mol. Pharmacol. 25, 228 (1984).

381 G. Carraz: Agressoligie 8, 13 (1967).

382 G. Taillandier, J.L. Benoît-Guyod, A. Boucherle, M. Broll and P. Eymard: Eur. J. Med. Chem.-Chim. Ther. 10, 453 (1975).

383 S. Hadad, T.B. Vree, K.E. Vander and M. Bialer: J. Pharm. Sci. 81, 1047 (1992).

384 M. Morre, P.E. Keane, J.C. Verières, J. Simiand and R. Roncucci: Epilepsia 25, S5 (1984).

385 W. Löscher and H. Nau: Neuropharmacol. 24, 427 (1985).

386 F.S. Abbott and A.A. Acheampong: Neuropharmacol. 27, 287 (1988).

387 S.N. Calderon, A.H. Newman and F.C. Tortella: J. Med. Chem. 34, 3159 (1991).

388 R. Dingledine, C.J. McBain and J.O. McNamara: TIPS 11, 334 (1990).

389 J.O. McNamara, R.D. Russell, L. Rigsbee and D.W. Bonhaus: Neuropharmacol. 27, 563 (1988).

390 S.C.J. Pedder, R. Wilcox, J.M. Tuchek, D.D. Johnson and R.D. Crawford: Neuropharmacol. 28, 753 (1989).

391 M.J. Croucher, J.F. Collins and B.S. Meldrum: Science (Wash. DC) 216, 899 (1982).

392 S. Patel, S.G. Chapman, M.H. Millan and B.S. Meldrum: in Excitatory amino acids in Health and disease (ed. D. Lodge). John Wiley and Sons, Chichester 1988, pp. 353.

393 S.J. Czuczwar and B.S. Meldrum: Eur. J. Pharmacol. 83, 335 (1982).

394 G. De Sarro, B.S. Meldrum and C. Reavill: Eur. J. Pharmacol. 106, 175 (1984).

395 J.A. Aram, D. Martin, M. Tomczyk, S. Zeman, J. Millar, G. Pohler and D. Lodge: J. Pharmacol. Exp. Ther. 248, 320 (1989).

396   G.E. Fagg, H.-R. Olpe, M.F. Pozza, J. Baud, M. Steinmann, M. Schmutz, C. Portet, P. Baumann, K. Thedinga, H. Bittiger, H. Allgeier, R. Heckendorn, C. Angst, D. Brundish and J.G. Dingwall: Br. J. Pharmacol. *99*, 791 (1990).

397   M. Schmutz, Ch. Portet, A. Jeker, K. Klebs, A. Vassout, H. Allgeeier, R. Heckendorn, G.E. Fagg, H.-R. Olpe and H. van Riezen: Nauyn-Schmiedeberg's Arch. Pharmacol. *101*, 456 (1990).

398   P.L. Herrling, B. Aebischer, P. Frey,- H.J. Oliverman and J.C. Watkins: Soc. Neurosci. Abst. *15*, 327 (1989).

399   S. Patel, A.G. Chapman, J.L. Graham, B.S. Meldrum and P. Frey: Epilepsy Res. *7*, 3 (1990).

400   J.W. Ferkany, D.J. Kyle, J. Willets, W.J. Rzeszotarski, M.E. Guzewska, S.R. Ellenberger, S.M. Jones, A.I. Sacaan, L.D. Snell, S. Borosky, B.E. Jones, K.M. Johnson, R.L. Balster, K. Burchett, K. Kawasaki, D.B. Hoch and R. Dingledine: J. Pharmacol. Exp. Ther. *250*, 100 (1989).

401   J. Davies, R.H. Evans, P.L. Herrling, A.W. Jones, H.J. Oliverman, P. Pook and J.C. Watkins: Brain Res. *382*, 169 (1986).

402   A.G. Chapman, B.S. Meldrum, N. Nanji and J.C. Watkins: Eur. J. Pharmacol. *139*, 91 (1987).

403   J. Lehmann, A.J. Hutchison, S.E. McPherson, C. Mondadori, M. Schmutz, C.M. Sinton, C. Tsai, D.E. Murphy, D.J. Steel, M. Williams, D.L. Cheney and P.L. Wood: J. Pharmacol. Exp. Ther. *246*, 65 (1988).

404   K. Anayama, N. Miyagi, S. Nakajima, H. Kawawaki, R. Namata and S. Natsura: Jpn. J. Psychiatry Neurol. *46*, 521 (1992).

405   A.J. Hutchison, M. Williams, C. Angst, R. de Jesus, L. Blanchard, R.H. Jackson, E.J. Wilusz, D.E. Murphy, P.S. Bernard, J. Schneider et al.: J. Med. Chem. *32*, 2171 (1989).

406   R.G.M. Morris, S. Davis and S.P. Butcher: in The NMDA, (eds. J.C. Watkins and G.L. Collingridge). IRL Press Oxford 1989, pp. 137.

407   M.D. Tricklebank, L. Singh, R.J. Oles, C. Preston and S.D. Iversen: Eur. J. Pharmacol. *167*, 127 (1989).

408   R. Zand and I. Izquierdo: Neurochem. Res. *5*, 1 (1980).

409   U. Erez, H. Frenk, O. Goldberg, A. Cohen and V.I. Teichberg: Eur. J. Pharmacol. *110*, 31 (1985).

410   P.L. Oinstein, M.B. Arnold, N.K. Angenstein, D. Lodge, J.D. Leander and D.D. Schoepp: J. Med. Chem. *36*, 2046 (1993).

411   M.L. Vazquez: US Pat. US 5,216,003, 01 Jun. 1993 [C.A. 119, 181017e (1993)].

412   M. Rowley, P. Leeson, G. Stevenson, A. Moseley, I. Stansfield, I. Sanderson, L. Robinson, R. Baker and J. Kemp: J. Med. Chem. *36*, 3386 (1993).

413   S.L. Peterson: Epilepsy Res. *13*, 73 (1992).

414   K.W. Moore, P.D. Leeson, R. Carling, M.D. Tricklebank and L. Singh: Bioorg. Med. Chem. Lett. *3*, 61 (1993).

415   K.G. Lloyd, S. Arbilla, K. Beaumont, M. Briley, G. De Montis, B. Scatton, S.Z. Langer and G. Bartholini: J. Pharmacol. Exp. Ther. *220*, 672 (1982).

416   N.G. Bowery, D.R. Hill and A.L. Hudson: Neuropharmacology *21*, 391 (1982).

417   P.J. Schechter, Y. Tranier, M.J. Jung and P. Böhlen: Eur. J. Pharmacol. *45*, 319 (1977).

418   E. Ben-Menachem, L.I. Persson, P.J. Schechter, K.D. Haegele, N. Huebert, J. Hardenberg, L. Dahlgren and J.P. Mumford: Epilepsy Res. *2*, 96 (1988).

419 P.J. Riekkinen, A. Pitkanen, A. Ylinen, J. Sivenius and T. Halonen: Epilepsia *30*, S18 (1989).

420 A. Pitkanen, R. Matilainen, T. Ruutiainen, M. Lehtinen and P. Riekkinen: J. Neural Neurosurg. Psychiatry *51*, 1395 (1988).

421 C. Shin, L.C. Rigsbee and J.O. McNamara: Brain Res. *398*, 370 (1986).

422 R. Bernasconi, M. Klein, P. Martin, P. Christen, T. Hafner, C. Portet and M. Schnutz: in J. Neural Trans. *72*, 213 (1988).

423 A.M.A. Ylinen, R. Miettinen, A. Pitkanen, A.I. Gulyas, T. Freund et al.: in Proceedings of the National Academy of Sciences of the United States of America, Vol. 88, 1991, pp. 7650.

424 B.S. Meldrum and K. Murugaiah: Eur. J. Pharmacol. *89*, 149 (1983).

425 S.M. Grant and R.C. Heel: Drugs *41*, 889 (1991).

426 A. Ylinen, J. Sivenius, A. Pitanen, T. Halonen, J. Partanen et al.: Epilepsia *33*, 917 (1992).

427 A. Tartara, R. Manni, C.A. Galimberti, R. Morini, J.P. Mumford et al.: Acta Neurologica Scandinavica *86*, 247 (1992).

428 R. Matilainen, A. Pitkanen, T. Ruutiainen, E. Mervaala, H. Sarlund et al.: Neurology *38*, 743 (1988).

429 C. Chiran, O. Dulac, D. Beaumont, L. Palacios, N. Pajot et al.: J. Child Neurology *6*, 52 (1991).

430 A.M. McGuire, J.S. Duncan and M.R. Trimble: Epilepsia *33*, 128 (1992).

431 C.B. Dodrill, J. Arnett, K. Sommerville, N. Sussman: Neurology *43*, 306 (1993).

432 R. Kalviainen, M. Aikia, P.J. Riekkinen: Epilepsia *33*, 118 (1992).

433 J.P. Gibson, J.T. Yarrington, D.E. Loudy, C.G. Gerbig, G.H. Hurst et al.: Toxicologic Pathology *18*, 225 (1990).

434 J. Sivenius, L. Paljarvi, M. Vapalahti, U. Nousiainen and P.J. Riekkinen: Epilepsia *34*, 196 (1993).

435 O.M. Larsson, E. Flach, P. Krogsgaard-Larsen and A. Schousboe: J. Neurochem. *50*, 818 (1988).

436 M.C. Heit and W.S. Schwark: Neuropharmacol. *27*, 367 (1988).

437 C. Braestrup, E.B. Nielsen, K.H. Wolffbrandt, K.E. Andersen, L.J.S. Knutsen and U. Sonnewald: Int. Cong. Ser. Excerpta Med. *750*, 125 (1987).

438 C.P. Taylor, M.G. Vartanian, R.D. Schwarz, D.M. Rock, M.J. Callahan and M.D. Davis: Drug Dev. Res. 21, 151 (1990).

439 A.J. Sedman, G.P. Gilmet, A.J. Sayed and E.L. Posvar: Drug Dev. Res. 21, 235 (1990).

440 E. Ben-Menachem, T. Hedner, R.I. Persson and B. Söderfeldt: Neurology *40*, 158 (1990).

441 K.L. Goa and E.M. Sorkin: Drugs *46*, 409 (1993).

442 G.D. Bartoszyk, N. Meyerson, W. Reimann, G. Satzinger and A. von·Hodenberg: in Current problems in epilepsy (Eds. Meldrum and Porter), Vol. 4. John Libbey, London 1986, pp. 147.

443 W. Loscher, D. Honack and C.P. Taylor: Neuroscience Letters *128*, 150 (1991).

444 D.R. Hill, N. Suman Chauhan and G.N. Woodruff: British J. Clinical Pharmacol. *104*, 72 (1991).

445 D.K. Naritoku, M.T. Stryker, L.B. Mecozzi, C.A. Copley and C.L. Faingold: Epilepsia *29*, 693 (1988).

446 B. Abou-Khalil, M.K. Shellenberger and H. Anhut: Epilepsia *33*, 77 (1992).

447 G. Bauer, D. Bechinger, M. Castell, E. Deisenhammer, M. Egli et al.: Advances in Epileptology *17*, 219 (1989).

448 J. Bruni, M. Saunders, H. Anhut and W. Sauermann: Neurology *41*, 330 (1991).

449 R.E. Ramsay, J. Wallace, K. Shellenberger, A. Arbor: Neurology *41*, 330 (1991).

450 T.R. Browne: Neurology *43*, 307 (1993).

451 A.J. Wilensky, N.R. Temkin, L.M. Ojeman, B. Riscker, A. Holubkov et al.: Epilepsia *33*, 77 (1992).

452 C.B. Dodrill, A.J. Wilensky, L. Ojeman, N. Temkin, K. Shellenberger et al.: Epilepsia *33*, 117 (1992).

453 H.F. Schwartz and R.F. Doerge: J. Am. Pharm. Assoc. Sci. Ed. *44*, 80 (1955).

454 H.F. Schwartz, L.F. Worrell and J.N. Delgado: J. Pharm. Sci. *56*, 80 (1967).

455 A.M.A. Department of Drugs, Americal Medical Association, A.M.A. Drug Evaluations, 3rd ed., Publishing Sciences Group, Inc. Littleton, Mass, 1977, pp. 452.

456 A. Haj-Yehia: Pharmaceutical Res. *6*, 683 (1989).

457 A. Balsamo, P.L. Barili, P. Crotti, B. Macchia, F. Macchia, A. Pecchia, A. Cuttica and N. Passerini: J. Med. Chem. *18*, 842 (1975).

458 A. Balsamo, P.L. Barili, P. Crotti, B. Macchia, F. Macchia, A. Cuttica and N. Passerini: J. Med. Chem. *20*, 48 (1977).

459 A. Balsamo, P. Crotti, A. Lapucci, B. Macchia, F. Macchia, A. Cuttica and N. Passerini: J. Med. Chem. *24*, 525 (1981).

460 G.H. Wimbish, G.L. Jones, R.J. Amato and G. A. Peyton: Proc. West. Pharmacol. Soc. *23*, 75 (1980).

461 W. Koek and F.C. Colpaert: J. Pharmacol. Exp. Ther. *252*, 349 (1990).

462 A.A. Cordi and C.L. Gillet: U.S. Pat. US 5,141,960 (1992).

463 C.R. Clark, M.J.M. Wells, R.T. Sansom, G.N. Norris, R.C. Dockens and W.R. Ravis: J. Med. Chem. *27*, 779 (1984).

464 C.R. Clark, R.T. Sansom, C.M. Lin and G.M. Norris: J. Med. Chem. *28*, 1259 (1985).

465 C.R. Clark, C.M. Lin and R.T. Sansom: J. Med. Chem. *29*, 1534 (1986).

466 C.R. Clark and T.W. Davenport: J. Med. Chem. *30*, 1214 (1987).

467 D.W. Robertson, J.D. Leander, R. Lawson, E.E. Beedle, C.R. Clark, B.D. Potts and C.J. Parli: J. Med. Chem. *30*, 1742 (1987).

468 J.D. Leander, D.W. Robertson, C.R. Clark, R.R. Lawson and R.C. Rathbun: Epilepsia *29*, 83 (1988).

469 33W. Lubisch, S. Schult, R. Binder, M. Raschack, R. Reinhordt and D. Seemann: Eur. Pat. appl. EP,534,246 (1993).

470 C.R. Clark: Epilepsia *29*, 198 (1988).

471 J.D. Leander, R.R. Lawson and D.W. Robertson: Neuropharmacology *27*, 623 (1988).

472 C.J. Parli, E. Evenson, B.D. Potts, E. Beedle, R. Lawson, D.W. Robertson and J.D. Leander: Drug Metab. Dispos. *16*, 707 (1988).

473 D.W. Robertson, E.E. Beedle, J.H. Krushinski, R.R. Lawson, C.J. Parli, B. Potts and J.D. Leander: J. Med. Chem. *34*, 1253 (1991).

474 C.R. Clark and C.L. McMillian: J. Pharm. Sci. *79*, 220 (1990).

475 N.E. Duke and P.W. Codding: J. Med. Chem. *35*, 1806 (1992).

476 P.F. VonVoigtlander, E.D. Hall, M.C. Ochoa, R.A. Lewis and H.J. Triezenberg: J. Pharmacol. Exp. Ther. *243*, 542 (1987).

477 P.F. VonVoigtlander, J.S. Althaus, R.A. Lewis and D.S. Green: Drug Dev. Res. *18*, 205 (1989).

478   Y. Zhu, W.B. Im, R.A. Lewis, J.S. Althans, A.R. Cazers, J.W. Nielsen, J.R. Palmer and P.F. Vonvoigtlander: Brain Res. *606*, 50 (1993).

479   D.N. Johnson, C.R. Taylor, B.E. Tomczuk and E.A. Swinyard: Epilepsia *29*, 694 (1988).

480   M.A. Osman, L.K. Cheng, D.N. Johnson and G.J. Wright: Epilepsia *29*, 694 (1988).

481   W. von Dorsser, D. Barris, A. Cordi and J. Roba: Arch. Int. Pharmacodyn. Ther. *266*, 239 (1983).

482   H. Kohn, K.N. Sawhney, P. LeGall, J.D. Conley, D.W. Robertson and J.D. Leander: J. Med. Chem. *33*, 919 (1990).

483   H. Kohn, K.N. Sawhney, P. LeGall, D.W. Robertson and J.D. Leander: J. Med. Chem. *34*, 2444 (1991).

484   H.L. Koln and D. Watson: U.S. Pat. (appl.) US 710,610 (1991) [C.A. 119, 8508t (1994)].

485   A.J. Bower, M. Noyer, R. Verloes, J. Gobut and E. Wulfert: Eur. J. Pharmacol. *222*, 193 (1992).

486   R.W. Carling, P.D. Leeson, A.M. Moseley, M. Smith, R. George, A.C. Foster, S. Grimwood: Bioorg. Med. Chem. Lett. *3*, 65 (1993).

487   P. George, D. DePeretti, F.J. Gilbert, M. Mangane and O. LeGalloudec: Eur. Pat. EP 524,055 (1993) [C.A. 119, 8810k (1994)].

488   P. Janssens de Varebeke, R. Cavalier, M. David-Remacle and M.B.H. Youdim: J. Neurochem. *50*, 1011 (1988).

489   P. Janssens de Varebeke, G. Pauwels, C. Buyse, M. David-Remacle, J. De Mey, J. Roba and M.B.H. Youdim: J. Neurochem. *53*, 1109 (1989).

490   D.D. Truong, B. Diamond, G. Pezzoli, M.A. Mena and S. Fahn: Life Sci. *44*, 1059 (1989).

491   A.G. Chapman and G.P. Hart: J. Neural. Transm. *72*, 201 (1988).

492   L.C. Norton, K.D. Laxer, D. Schomer and P. Osborn: Epilepsia *27*, 648 (1986).

493   M.A. Houtkooper, C.A.E.H. van Oorschot, T.W. Rentmeester, P.J.E.A. Hoppener and C. Onkelinx: Epilepsia *27*, 255 (1986).

494   L.M. Donune, M.I. Gaunlov, S.N. Shurov and M.E. Konshin: Khim Geberotsikl Soedin *11*, 1506 (1992).

495   R.A. Akhundov, S.A. Dzhafarova and A.N. Aliev: Eksp. Kline. Farmakol. *55*, 27 (1992).

496   W.J. Jr. Welsheed and S. LoYoung: US Pat. US 5,183,903 (1993) [C.A. 119, 28000z (1994)].

497   G. Singh, N. Siddiqui and S.N. Pandeya: Arch Pharmacol. Res. *15*, 272 (1992).

498   R.W. Carling, P.D. Leeson, K.W. Moore, J.D. Smith, C.R. Moyes, I.M. Mawer, S. Thomas, T. Chan, R. Baker et al.: J. Med. Chem. *36*, 3397 (1993).

499   P. Albaugh: US Pat. US 5,182,290 (1993) [C.A. 119, 49380p (1994)].

500   D. Ashton, E. DePrins, R. Willems, H. VanBelle and A. Wauquire: Epilepsy Res. *2*, 65 (1988).

501   Z.S. Quan, R.L. Li and Y.Z. Ling: Yaoxue Xuebao *27*, 711 (1992) [C.A. 119, 195097t (1994)].

502   P. Xu, S. Wang and W. Liu: J. Clin. Pharm. Sci. *1*, 27 (1992).

503   I.Y. Belavin, N.F. Krokhina, Y.I. Bankov and T.A. Zharkovskaya: Khim-Farm. Zh. *26*, 74 (1992).

504   T. Isobe: Jpn. Pat. JP 0559,064 (1993) [C.A. 119, 139281m (1994)].

505   G.D. Bartoszyk and M. Hamer: Pharmacol. Res. Commun. *19*, 429 (1987).

506   B. Wagner, G. Strumpf and G.D. Bartoszyk: Pharmacol. Res. Commun. *19*, 591 (1987).

507   H. Tanimukai, M. Inui, S. Hariguchi and Z. Kaneko: Biochem. Pharmacol. *14*, 961 (1965).

508   W.D. Grey, T.H. Maren, B.M. Sisson and F.H. Smith: J. Pharmacol. Exp. Ther. *121*, 160 (1957).

509   R.E. Anderson, R.A. Howard and D.M. Woodbury: Epilepsia *27*, 504 (1986).

510   D.M. Woodbury and J.W. Kemp: in Antiepileptic Drugs 3rd ed. (R. Levy, R. Mattson, B. Meldrum, J.K. Penry and F.E. Dreifuss). Raven Press, New York 1989, pp. 855.

511   F.L. Engstrom, H.S. White, J.W. Kemp and D. M. Woodbury: Epilepsia *27*, 19 (1986).

512   C.T. Supuran, G. Mande, A. Dinculescu, A. Schiketunz, M.D. Gheorghiu, I. Puscas and A.T. Balaban: J. Pharm. Sci. *81*, 716 (1992).

513   G.H. Hamore and B.L. Reavlin: J. Pharm. Sci. *56*, 134 (1967).

514   Y. Masuda, T. Karasawa, Y. Shiraishi, M. Hori, K. Yoshima and M. Shimizu: Arzneim. Forsch. Drug Res. *30*, 477 (1980).

515   C. Kamei, M. Oka, Y. Masuda, K. Yoshida and M. Shimizu: Arch. Int. Pharmacodyn. Ther. *249*, 164 (1981).

516   T. Ito, M. Hori, Y. Masuda, K. Yoshida and M. Shimizu: Arzneim. Forsch. Drug Res. *30*, 603 (1980).

517   T. Ito, M. Hori and T. Kadokawa: Epilepsia *27*, 367 (1986).

518   C.L. Schauf: Brain Res. *413*, 185 (1987).

519   D.M. Rock, R.L. Macdonald and C.P. Taylor: Epilepsy Res. *3*, 138 (1989).

520   T. Mimaki, Y. Suzuki, T. Tagawa, J. Tanaka, N. Itoh and H. Yabuuchi: Jpn. J. Psychiatry Neurol. *42*, 640 (1988).

521   G.H. Fromm, T. Shibuya and C.F. Terrence: Epilepsia *28*, 673 (1987).

522   K.S. Okada, T. Hirano, M. Ishida, T. Kondo, K. Otani and Y. Fukushima: Epilepsy Res. *13*, 113 (1992).

523   A.J. Wilensky, P.N. Friel, L.M. Ojemann, C.B. Dodrill, K.B. McCormick and R.H. Levy: Epilepsia *26*, 212 (1985).

524   J.C. Sachellares, P.D. Donofrio, J.G. Wagner, B. Abou-Khalil, S. Berent and K. Aasved-Hoyt: Epilepsia *26*, 206 (1985).

525   T.R. Henry, I.E. Leppik, R.J. Gumnit and M. Jacobs: Neurology *38*, 928 (1988).

526   A. Takeda, J. Inaguma and A. Shimizu: Jpn. Pharmacol. Ther. *15*, 397 (1987).

527   A. Shimizu, J. Yamamoto, Y. Yamada, M. Tanaka and T. Kawasaki: Curr. Ther. Res. *42*, 147 (1987).

528   H. Oguni, T. Hayakawa and Y. Fukayama: J. Jpn. Epilepsy Soc. *7*, 43 (1989).

529   K. Iinuma, I. Handa, N. Fueki, K. Yamamoto, A. Kojima and K. Haginoya: Curr. Ther. Res. Clin. Exp. *43*, 281 (1988).

530   H. Shuto, T. Sugimoto, A. Yasuhara, T. Hatanaka, M. Woo, K. Murakami, A. Áraki and Y. Kobayashi: Curr. Ther. Res. Clin. Exp. *45*, 1031 (1989).

531   B.E. Maryanoff, S.O. Nortey, J.F. Gardocki, R.P. Shank and S.P. Dodgson: J. Med. Chem. *30*, 880 (1987).

532   A.J. Wilensky, L.M. Ojemann, T. Chmelir, B.L. Margul and D.R. Doose: Epilepsia *30*, 645 (1989).

533   K.L. Floren, N.M. Graves, I.E. Leppik, R.P. Remmel, B.L. Morgul and D.R. Doose: Epilepsia *30*, 646 (1989).

534   P. Kontro and S.S. Oja: Neuropharmacology *26*, 19 (1987).

535 K. Nakagawa and R.J. Huxtable: Neurochem. Int. 7, 819 (1985).

536 P. Kontro and S.S. Oja: Neuroscience 23, 567 (1987).

537 O. Malminen and P. Kontro: Neuropharmacology 28, 907 (1989).

538 M. Iivanainen, O. Waltimo, O. Tokola, J. Parantainen, H. Allonen and P.J. Neuvonen: in Book of abstracts, 18th International epilepsy congress. New Delhi, India, 1989, pp. 29.

539 E.M. Airaksinen, K. Koivisto, T. Keranen, A. Pitkanen, P.J. Riekkinen, S.S. Oja, K.-M. Marnela, J.V. Partanen, O. Tokola, G. Gothoni, P.J. Neuvonen and M.M. Airaksinen: Epilepsy Res. 1, 308 (1987).

540 D.J. Watjen and L.H. Jensen: Eur. Pat. EP 522,494 (1993) [C.A. 118, 254746h (1993)].

541 D. Schmidt: in Antiepileptic Drugs 3rd ed. (R. Levy, R. Mattson, B. Meldrum, J.K. Penry and F.E. Dreifuss). Raven Press, Ney York 1989, pp. 735.

542. L.O. Randall, W. Schallek, L.H. Sternbach and R.Y. Ning: in Psychopharmacological agents (M. Gordon, Ed.) Vol. III. Academic Press, New York 1974, pp. 175.

543 R.W. Homan and D.H. Unwin: in Antiepileptic Drugs 3rd ed. (R. Levy, R. Mattson, B. Meldrum, J.K. Penry and F.E. Dreifuss). Raven Press, New York 1989, pp. 841.

544 R.W. Homan and J.E. Walker: Adv. Neurol. 34, 493 (1983).

545 P.S. Albright and W.M. Burnham: Epilepsia 21, 681 (1980).

546 S. Sato: in Antiepileptic Drugs 3rd ed. (R. Levy, R. Mattson, B. Meldrum, J.K. Penry and F.E. Dreifuss). Raven Press, Ney York 1989, pp. 765.

547 F. Barzaghi, R. Fournex and P. Mantegazza: Arzneim. Forsch. 23, 683 (1973).

548 M.R. Trimble and M.M. Robertson: in New anticonvulsant drugs (B.S. Meldrum and R.J. Porter, Eds.). John Libbey, London 1986, pp. 65.

549 A.G. Chapman, R.W. Horton and B.S. Meldrum: Epilepsia 19, 293 (1978).

550 Y. Ichimaru, Y. Gomita and M. Moriyama: J. Pharmacobiodyn. 10, 189 (1987).

551 H.C. Rosenberg, E.I. Tietz and T.H. Chiu: Epilepsia 30, 276 (1989).

552 E.I. Tietz, H.C. Rosenberg and T.H. Chiu: Epilepsy Res. 3, 31 (1989).

553 B. Hentschel: in Clobazam in the treatment in epilepsy. Hoechst Aktiengesellschaft, Frankfurt, Germany 1987.

554 S.D. Shorvon: in Antiepileptic Drugs 3rd ed. (R. Levy, R. Mattson, B. Meldrum, J.K. Penry and F.E. Dreifuss). Raven Press, Ney York 1989, pp. 821.

555 L. Steru, R. Chermat, B. Millet, J.A. Mico and P. Simon: Epilepsia 27 (suppl. 1), S14 (1986).

556 I. Hindmarch: Br. J. Clin. Pharmacol. 7 (suppl. 1), 77S (1979).

557 J.R. Haigh, T. Pullar, J.P. Gent, C. Dailley and M. Feely: Br. J. Clin. Pharmacol. 23, 213 (1987).

558 J.P. Gent, J.R.M. Haigh, A. Mehta and M. Feely: Drugs Exp. Clin. Res. 10, 867 (1984).

559 N.A. Young, S.J. Lewis, Q.l. Harris, B. Jarrott and F.J. Vajda: J. Pharm. Pharmacol. 40, 365 (1988).

560 A.J. Heller, H.A. Ring and E.H. Reynolds: Epilepsy Res. 2, 276 (1988).

561 R.E. Study and J.L. Barker: Proc. Natl. Acad. Sci. (USA) 78, 7180 (1981).

562 R.E. Twyman, C.J. Rogers and R.L. Macdonald: Ann. Neurol. 25, 213 (1989).

563 H. Mohler and T. Okada: Science (Wash. DC) 198, 849 (1977).

564 S.M. Paul, P.J. Syapin, B.A. Paugh, V. Moncada and P. Skolnick: Nature (Lond.) 281, 688 (1979).

565 R. Young and R.A. Glennon: Psychopharmacol. 93, 529 (1987).

566 D.J. Nutt, P.J. Cowen and H.J. Little: Nature (Lond.) 295, 426 (1982).

567 S.C.J. Pedder, R. Wilcox, J.M. Tuchek, R.D. Crawford and D.D. Johnson: Brain Res. *424*, 139 (1987).

568 A. Doble and I.L. Martin: Trends in Pharm. Sci. *13*, 76 (1992).

569 D.B. Pritchett, H. Luddens and P.H. Seeburg: Science (Wash. DC) *242*, 1306 (1988).

570 P.A. Borea, G. Gilli, V. Bertolasi and V. Ferretti: Mol. Pharmacol. *31*, 334 (1987).

571 P.A. Borea and G. Gilli: Arzneim. Forsch. *34*, 649 (1984).

572 G. Wong and P. Skolnick: Eur. J. Pharmacol. *225*, 63 (1992).

573 J.K. Wang, T. Taniguchi and S. Spector: Mol. Pharmacol. *25*, 349 (1984).

574 H.O. Villar, E.T. Uyeno, L. Toll, W. Polgar, M.F. Davies and G.H. Loew: Mol. Pharmacol. *36*, 589 (1989).

575 G.H. Loew, J.R. Nienow and M. Poulsen: Mol. Pharmacol. *26*, 19 (1984).

576 P.A. Borea: Arzneim. Forsch. *33*, 1086 (1983).

577 A.K. Ghose and G.M. Crippen: Mol. Pharmacol. *37*, 725 (1990).

578 S.P. Hollinshead, M.L. Trudell, P. Skolnick and J.M. Cook: J. Med. Chem. *33*, 1062 (1990).

579 B. Brandau, J.-J. Bourguignon and C.G. Wermuth: J. Med. Chem. 34, 1754 (1991).

580 H. Diaz-Arauzo, G.E. Evoniuk, P. Skolnick and J.M. Cook: Life Sci. 49, 207 (1991).

581 H. Diaz-Arauzo, K.F. Koehler, T.J. Hagen and J.M. Cook: Quant. Struct.-Act. Relat. *11*, 102 (1992).

582 R.W. Lucek, W.A. Garland and W. Dairman: Fed. Proc. *38*, 541 (1979).

583 T. Blair and G.A. Webb: J. Med. Chem. *20*, 1206 (1977).

584 E.J. Lien: J. Med. Chem. *13*, 1189 (1970).

585 E.J. Lien, R.C.H. Liao and H.G. Shinouda: J. Pharm. Sci. *68*, 463 (1979).

586 E.J. Lien, G.L. Tong, J.T. Chou and J. Lien: J. Pharm. Sci. *62*, 246 (1973).

587 P.A. Borea: Boll. Soc. Ital. Biol. Sper. *57*, 628 (1981).

588 A. Camerman and N. Camerman: J. Am. Chem. Soc. *94*, 268 (1972).

589 A. Camerman and N. Camerman: Acta Crystallogr. *B37*, 1677 (1981).

590 G.L. Jones and D.M. Woodbury: in Antiepileptic drugs (D.M. Woodbury, J.K. Penry and C.E. Pippenger, Eds.). Raven Press, New York 1982, pp. 83.

591 G. Klopman and R. Contreras: Mol. Pharmacol. *27*, 86 (1984).

592 D. Nardi, A. Tajana, A. Leonardi, R. Pennini, F. Portioli, M.J. Magistretti and A. Subissi: J. Med. Chem. *24*, 727 (1981).

593 G. Graziani, F. Tirone, E. Barbadoro and R. Testa: Arzeim. Forsch. Drug Res. *33*, 1155 (1983).

594 K.A. Walker, M.B. Wallach and D.R. Hirschfeld: J. Med. Chem. *24*, 67 (1981).

595 W.C. Jr. Buhles, M.B. Wallach, M.D. Chaplin and D.M. Treiman: in New anticonvulsant drugs (B.S. Meldrum and R.J. Porter, Eds.). John Libbey, London 1986, pp. 203.

596 G.B. De Sarro, V. Libri, C. Ascioti, R. Testa and G. Nistico: Neuropharmacology *26*, 1425 (1987).

597 R. Testa and D. Bertin: in New anticonvulsant drugs (B.S. Meldrum and R.J. Porter, Eds.). John Libbey, London 1986, pp. 85.

598 E. Benassi, G. Besio, G.P. Bo, L. Cocito, M. Maffini, P. Mainardi, P.L. Morselli and C. Loeb: Int. J. Clin. Pharmacol. Res. *8*, 353 (1988).

599 T.E. Albertson and W.F. Walby: Epilepsy Res. *2*, 20 (1988).

600 D.M. Treiman, A.J. Wilensky, E. Ben-Menachem, L. Ojemann, M. Yerby, K.O. Barber, K.B. McCormick, J.J. Cereghino, B.G. White and K. Swisher: Epilepsia *26*, 607 (1985).

601   D.W. Robertson, J.H. Krushinski, E.E. Beedle, J.D. Leander, D.T. Wong and R.C. Rathbun: J. Med. Chem. *29*, 1577 (1986).

602   A. Chiminri, A. De Sarro, G. De Sarro, S. Grasso, G.R. Trimarchi and M. Zappal: J. Med. Chem. *32*, 93 (1989).

603   P. Bernard, W. Brown, M. Williams, J. Lehmann, J. Kapeghian, J. Liebman and R. Robson: in Abstracts of the first princeton drug research symposium (Ed. M. Williams), 1989, pp. 42.

604   P.K. Kadaba: J. Med. Chem. *31*, 196 (1988).

605   C.L. Zhang and U. Heinemann: N-S. Arch. Pharmacol. *346*, 581 (1992).

606   N. Ates, E.L.J.M. Van Luijtelaar, W.H.I.M. Drinkenburg, J.M.H. Vossen and A.M.L. Coenen: Epilepsy Res. *13*, 43 (1992).

607   T.R. Deshmukh and P.K. Kadaba: Med. Chem. Res. *3*, 223 (1993).

608   J.M. Kane, B.M. Baron, M.W. Dudley, S.M. Sorensen, M.A. Staeger and F.P. Miller: J. Med. Chem. *33*, 2772 (1990).

609   J.M. Kane, M.A. Staeger, C.R. Dalton, F.P. Miller, M.W. Dudley, A.M.L. Ogden, J.H. Kehne, H.J. Ketteler, T.C. McCloskey, Y.S.P.A. Chmielewski and J.A. Miller: J. Med. Chem. *37*, 125 (1994).

610   A. Chapman and B.S. Meldrum: Eur. J. Pharmacol. *166*, 201 (1989).

611   G.C. Ormandy, R.C. Jope and O.C. Snead 3rd: Exp. Neurol *106*, 172 (1989).

612   A.C. Foster and E.H.F. Wong: Br. J. Pharmacol. *91*, 403 (1987).

613   R.F. Halliwell, J.A. Peters and J.J. Lambert: Br. J. Pharmacol. *96*, 480 (1989).

614   P.D. Leeson, K. James, R.W. Carling, E.H. Wong and R. Baker: Prog. Clin. Biol. Res.' *361*, 513 (1990).

615   P.D. Leeson, R.W. Carling, K. James, J.D. Smith, K.W. Moore, E.H. Wong and R. Baker: J. Med. Chem. 33, 1296 (1990).

616   T.A. Lyle, C.A. Magill, S.F. Britcher, G.H. Denny, W.J. Thompson, J.S. Murphy, A.R. Knight, J.A. Kemp, G.R. Marshall, D.N. Middlemiss et al.: J. Med. Chem. *33*, 1047 (1990).

617   A.S. Troupin, J.R. Mendius, F. Cheng and M.W. Risinger: in New anticonvulsant drugs (eds. B.S. Meldrum and R.J. Porter). John-Libbey, London, 1986, pp. 191.

618   Y. Wata, H. Hasegawa, M. Nakamura and N. Yamaguchi: Pharmacol. Biochem. Behav. *43*, 1269 (1992).

619   C.E. Stafstarm, G.L. Holmes and J. Thompson: Epilepsy Res. *14*, 41 (1993).

620   L. Velisek and P. Mares: in Ligands mech. neuromodulation neuroprot. (Eds. J.-M. Kamenka and E.F. Domino). US Semin, CNRS-NSF, 1992, pp. 779.

621   W.J. Thompson, P.S. Anderson, S.F. Britcher, T.A. Lyle, J.E. Thies, C.A. Magill, S.L. Varga, J.E. Schwering, P.A. Lyle, M.E. Christy et al.: J. Med. Chem. *33*, 789 (1990).

622   K.M. Johnson and S.M. Jones: Annu. Rev. Pharmacol. Ther. Toxicol. *30*, 707 (1990).

623   G. Chen and B. Bohner: Proc. Soc. Exp. Biol. Med. *106*, 632 (1961).

624   A.P. Leccese, K.L. Marquis, A. Mattia and J.E. Moreton: Brain Res. *19*, 163 (1986).

625   M.A. Rogawski, A. Thürkauf, S. Yamaguchi, K.C. Rice, A.E. Jacobson and M.V. Mattson: J. Pharmacol. Exp. Ther. *249*, 708 (1989).

626   E.B. Geller, L.H. Adler, C. Wojno and M.W. Adler: Psychopharmacology *74*, 97 (1981).

627   D.A. Bennett, P.S. Bernard and C.I. Amrick: Life Sci. *42*, 447 (1988).

628   F.G. Freeman, M.F. Jarvis and P.M. Duncan: Pharmacol. Biochem. Behav. *16*, 1009 (1982).

629   M.E. Gilbert: Brain Res. *463*, 90 (1988).

630   B.A. Hayes and R.L. Blaster: Eur. J. Pharmacol. *117*, 121 (1985).

631   D. Lodge, M. Jones and E. Fletcher: in The NMDA receptor (eds. J.C. Watkins and G.L. Collingridge). IRL press, Oxford, 1989, pp. 37.

632   S.N. Davies, D. Martin, J.D. Millar, J. Church and D. Lodge: Eur. J. Pharmacol. *145*, 141 (1988).

633   J.F. MacDonald and L.M. Nowak: Trends Neurosci. *11*, 167 (1990).

634   A. Thürkauf, B. DeCosta, S. Yamaguchi, M.V. Mattson, A.E. Jacobson, K.C. Rice and M.A. Rogawski: J. Med. Chem. *33*, 1452 (1990).

635   F.C. Tortella, J.M. Witkin and J.M. Musacchio: Eur. J. Pharmacol. *155*, 69 (1988).

636   H.R. Feeser, J.L. Kadis and D.A. Prince: Neurosci. Lett. *86*, 340 (1988).

637   T. Kuko and J.A. Wada: Epilepsia *30*, 669 (1989).

638   F.C. Tortella, J.W. Ferkany and M.J. Pontecorvo: Life Sci. *42*, 2509 (1988).

639   A.E. Cole, C.U. Eccles, J.J. Aryanpur and R.S. Fisher: Neuropharmacology *28*, 249 (1989).

640   R.S. Fisher, B.J. Cysyk, R.P. Lesser, M.J. Pontecorvo, J.T. Ferkany, P.R. Schwerdt, J. Hart and B. Gordon: Neurology *40*, 547 (1990).

641   J.L. Perhach, I. Weliky, J.J. Newton, R.D. Sofia, M.W. Romanyshyn and W.F.Jr. Arndt: in Antiepileptic Drugs (B.S. Meldrum and R.J. Porter). John Libbey, London, 1986, pp. 117.

642   R.D. Sofia, R. Gordon, M. Gels and W. Diamantis: Res. Commun. Chem. Pathol. Pharmacol. *79*, 335 (1993).

643   I.E. Leppik and N.M. Grave: in Antiepileptic Drugs 3rd ed. (R. Levy, R. Mattson, B. Meldrum, J.K. Penry and F.E. Dreifuss). Raven Press, Ney York 1989, pp. 983.

644   E. Faught, R.C. Sachdeo, M.P. Remler, S. Chayasirisobhon, V.J. Iragui-Mandoz et al.: Neurology *43*, 688 (1993).

645   R.C. Sachdeo and S.K. Sachdeo: Abstract Neurology *43*, 308 (1993).

646   R.C. Sachdeo, J.V. Murphy and M. Kamin: Abstract Epilepsia *33*, 118 (1992).

647   I.E. Leppik, F.E. Dreifuss, G.W. Pledger, N.M. Graves, N. Santilli, I. Drury, J.Y. Tsay, M.P. Jacobs, E. Bertram, J.J. Cereghino, G. Cooper, P. Sheridan and M. Ashworth: Epilepsia *30*, 661 (1989).

648   M. Poisson, F. Huguet, A. Savattier, F. Bakri-Logeais and G. Narcisse: Arzneim. Forsch. Drug Res. *34*, 199 (1984).

649   J.C. Vincent: in New Anticonvulsant Drugs (Eds. B.S. Meldrum and R.J. Porter). John Libbey, London, 1986, pp. 255.

650   R. Wegmann, A. Ilies and M. Aurousseau: Cell Mol. Biol. *23*, 455 (1978).

651   J.R. Farwell, R.H. Levy and G. Anderson: in Book of abstracts, 18th International Epilepsy Congress. New Delhi, India, 1989, pp. 109.

652   P. Loiseau and B. Duche: in Antiepileptic Drugs 3rd ed. (R. Levy, R. Mattson, B. Meldrum, J.K. Penry and F.E. Dreifuss). Raven Press, Ney York 1989, pp. 955.

653   A.A. Miller, P. Wheatley, D.A. Sawyer, M.G. Baxter and B. Roth: Epilepsia *27*, 483 (1986).

654   P.L. Wheatley and A.A. Miller: Epilepsia *30*, 34 (1989).

655. K.H. Stankova and P. Mares: Epilepsy Res. *13*, 17 (1992).

656   H. Cheung, D. Kamp and E. Harris: Epilepsy Res. *13*, 107 (1992).

657   K.L. Goa, S.R. Ross and P. Chrisp: Drugs *46*, 152 (1993).

658   M.J. Leach, C.M. Marden and A.A. Miller: Epilepsia *27*, 490 (1986).

659   C. Binnie: International Practice Series, No. 2, 1992, pp. 31.

660   L. Oller, A. Russi and D.L. Oller: Abstract Epilepsia *32*, 58 (1991).

661   E. Schlumberger, F. Chavez, L. Palacios, O. Dulac, S. Kouzan et al.: Abstract Epilepsia *32*, 58 (1991).

662   A.W.C. Yuen and J.E.W. Rafter: Epilepsia *33*, 82 (1992).

663   T. Betts, G. Goodwin, R.M. Withers and A.W.C. Yuen: Epilepsia *32*, 17 (1991).

664   J. Tytgat, J. Vereecke and E. Carmeliet: Arch. Pharmacol. *337*, 690 (1988).

665   L.K. Desmedt, C.J. Niemegeers and P.A. Janssen: Arzneim. Forsch. Drug Res. *25*, 1408 (1975).

666   A. Wauquier, D. Ashton, G. Clincke, J. Fransen, J.M. Gillardin and P.A.J. Janssen: Drug. Dev. Res. *7*, 49 (1986).

667   G.B. De Sarro, G. Nistico and B.S. Meldrum: Neuropharmacology *25*, 695 (1986).

668   D. Ashton and A. Wauquier: Psychopharmacology *65*, 7 (1979).

669   A. Vezzani, H.-Q. Wu, M.A. Stasi, P. Angelico and R. Samanin: Neuropharmacology *27*, 451 (1988).

670   A. Wauquier, D. Ashton and W. Melis: Exp. Neurol. *64*, 579 (1979).

671   G.B. De Sarro, B. S. Meldrum and G. Nistico: Br. J. Pharmacol. *93*, 247 (1988).

672   F.B. Meyer, R.E. Anderson and T.M. Sundt Jr.: Epilepsia *31*, 68 (1990).

673   A. Popoli, A. Pezzola and A. Scotti De Carolis: Arch. Int. Pharmacodyn. Ther. *292*, 58 (1988).

674   W.-S. Wong and R.G. Rahwan: Gen. Pharmacol. *20*, 309 (1989).

675   M.J. McLean: Pol. J. Pharmacol. Pharm. *39*, 513 (1987).

676   W. Frosher, P. Bulau, W. Burr, H. Penin, M.L. Rao and F. De Beukelaar: Clin. Neuropharmacol. *3*, 232 (1988).

677   C.D. Binnie: in Antiepileptic Drugs 3rd ed. (R. Levy, R. Mattson, B. Meldrum, J.K. Penry and F.E. Dreifuss). Raven Press, New York 1989, pp. 971.

678   O.L. Vizyunova, Yu.V. Kozhevnikov, L.M. Obvintseva and V.S. Zalesov: Khim. Farm. Zh. *20*, 1047 (1986).

679   S. Buyuktimkin: Arch. Pharm. *319*, 933 (1986).

680   M.J. Kornet: Eur. J. Med. Chem. Chim. Ther. *21*, 529 (1986).

681   C. Dwivedi and G.W. Omodt: PCT Int. 9213,535 (1992) [C.A. 117, 234037d (1992)].

682   M. Shrimalli, R. Kalsi, K.S. Dixit and J.P. Barthwal: Arzneim. Forsch. *41*, 514 (1991).

683   M.A. Khalil and M.M.M. El-Din: Alexandria J. Pharm. Sci. *3*, 190 (1989).

684   N. Despande, Y.V. Rao, R.P. Kandlikar, A.D. Rao and V.M. Reddy: Ind. J. Pharmacol. *18*, 127 (1987).

685   S. Buyuktimkin: Arch. Pharm. *319*, 933 (1986).

686   M.J. Kornet, T. Varia and W. Beaven: J. Heterocycl. Chem. *21*, 1709 (1984).

687   M. Hori, R. Iemura, H. Hara, A. Ozaki, T. Sukamoto and H. Ohtaka: Chem. Pharm. Bull. *38*, 1286 (1990).

688   K.D. Holland, A.C. McKeon, D.F. Covey and J.A. Ferrendelli: J. Pharmacol. Exp. Ther. *254*, 578 (1990).

689   D.J. Canney, K.D. Holland, J.A. Levine, A.C. McKeon, J.A. Ferrendelli and D.F. Covey: J. Med. Chem. *34*, 1460 (1991).

690   A.R. Martin, P. Consroe, V.V. Kane, V. Shah, V. Singh, N. Lander, R. Mechoulam and M. Srebnik: NIDA Res. Monogr. *79*, 48 (1987).

691   P. Consroe and R. Mechoulam: NIDA Res. Monogr. *79*, 59 (1987).

692   K.D. Holland, D.K. Naritoku, A.C. McKeon, J.A. Ferrendelli and D.F. Covey: Mol. Pharmacol. *37*, 98 (1990).

693   A. Chimirri, S. Grasso, A.M. Monforte, M. Zappala, A. De Sarro and G.B. De Sarro: Pharmacology *46*, 935 (1991).

694   A. Arnoldi, A. Bonsignori, P. Melloni, L. Merlini, M.L. Quadri, A.C. Rossi and M. Valsecchi: J. Med. Chem. *33*, 2865 (1990).

695   M.R. Stillings, A.P. Welbourn and D.S. Walter: J. Med. Chem. *29*, 2280 (1986).

696   C.B. Chapleo, M. Myers, P.L. Myers, J.F. Saville, A.C. Smith, M.R. Stillings, I.F. Tulloch, D.S. Walter and A.P. Welbourn: J. Med. Chem. *29*, 2273 (1986).

697   S.N. Pandeya and A.A. Khan: Ind. J. Physiol. Pharmacol. *32*, 164 (1988).

698   W.J. Brouillette, G.B. Brown, T.M. DeLorey, S.S. Shirali and G.L. Grunewald: J. Med. Chem. *31*, 2218 (1988).

699   K.A. Gupta, A.K. Saxena, P.C. Jain, R.C. Srimal, K. Kar and N. Anand: Ind. J. Chem. *22B*, 384 (1983).

700   K.A. Gupta, A.K. Saxena and P.C. Jain: Ind. J. Chem. *21B*, 228 (1982).

701   K.A. Gupta, A.K. Saxena, P.C. Jain, P.R. Dua, C.R. Prasad and N. Anand: Ind. J. Chem. *22B*, 789 (1983).

702   M. Bruce, G.K. Wellman, L.N.T. Yun, B. Delia, M. Syed, P.R. Hyde and T.S. Hasan: U.S. Pat. WO 745,216 (applied) (1993) [C.A. 119, 49738m (1994)].

703   R.C. Griffith, R.J. Murray and R.J. Schmiesing: Eur. Pat. EP 540,318 (1993) [C.A. 119, 160120u (1994)].

704   A.K. Saxena, V.A. Murthy, G.K. Patnaik, P.C. Jain and N. Anand: Ind. J. Chem. *19B*, 873 (1980).

705   E.K. Moltzen and J.K. Perregaard: Eur. Pat. EP 518,805 (appl.) (1992) [C.A. 119, 117118m (1994)].

706   P. Martine and G. Umberto: Eur. Pat. EP 535,626 (1993) [C.A. 119, 20513y (1994)].

707   P. Lardenois, J. Frost, M.C. Renones and C. Roussella: Fr. Demande FR 2,681,319 (1993) [C.A. 119, 160122v (1994).

708   M. Veda, T. Gemba, M. Eigyo and I. Adachi: Eur. Pat. EP 519,602 (appl.) (1992) [C.A. 118, 94335t (1993)].

709   G. Singh, N. Siddique and S.N. Pandeya: Arch. Pharm. Res. *15*, 272 (1992).

710   J.R. Dimmock, K.K. Sidhu, R.S. Thayer, P. Mack, M.J. Duffy, R.S. Reid, J.W. Quarl, V. Pugazhenthi, A. Ong et al.: J. Med. Chem. *36*, 2243 (1993).

711   H.S. White, J. Hunt, H.H. Wolf, E. Swinyard, E. Falch, P. Krogsgaard-Larsen and A. Schousboe: Eur. J. Pharmacol. *236*, 147 (1993).

712   S. Selleri, F. Bruni, A. Costanzo, G. Guerrini, A. Malmberg, G. Lavarone and C. Martini: Eur. J. Med. Chem. *27*, 985 (1992).

713   K. Srivastava and S.N. Pandeya: Boll. Chim. Farm. *131*, 313 (1992).

714   J.L. Kelley: U.S. Pat. US 5,166,209 (1992) [C.A. 118, 234066h (1993)].

715   V.S. Lebedev, T.I. Kostenko, N.V. Lukoyanov, G.I. Vankin, B.K. Beznosko, L.V. Zhuravleva and O.A. Raevskij: U.S.S.R. SU 1,410,476 (1992) [C.A. 119, 188561m (1994)].

716   D.F. Weaver, K.E. Edgecombe, H. Smith and M.N. Anderson: Chemical Design Automation News *6* (12), 1 (1991).

717   D.F. Weaver, K.E. Edgecombe, H. Smith and M.N. Anderson: Chemical Design Automation News *7* (1), 11 (1992).

Index Vol.44

The references of the Subject Index are given in the language of the respective contribution
Die Stichworte des Sachregisters sind in der jeweiligen Sprache der einzelnen Beiträge aufgeführt.
Les termes repris dans la Table des Matières sont donnés selon la langue dans laquelle l'ouvrage est écrit.

Index of titles
Verzeichnis der Titel
Index des titres
Vol. 1–44 (1959–1995)

Author and paper index
Autoren- und Artikelindex
Index des auteurs et des articles
Vol. 1–44 (1959–1995)

Recent advances in electrophysiology of antiarrhythmic drugs *17*, 33 (1973)	A. L. Bassett A. L. Wit
Chirality and future drug design *41*, 191 (1993)	Sanjay Batra Manju Seth A. P. Bhaduri
Drugs for treatment of patients with high cholesterol blood levels and other dyslipidemias 43, 9 (1994)	Harold E. Bays Carlos A. Dujovne
Stereochemical factors in biological activity *1*, 455 (1959)	A. H. Beckett
Molecular modelling and quantitative structure-activity analysis of antibacterial sulfanilamides and sulfones *36*, 361 (1991)	P. G. De Benedetti
Industrial research in the quest for new medicines *20*, 143 (1976) The experimental biologist and the medical scientist in the pharmaceutical industry *24*, 38 (1980)	B. Berde
Newer diuretics *2*, 9 (1960)	K. H. Beyer, Jr. J. E. Baer
Recent developments in 8-aminoquinoline antimalarials *28*, 197 (1984)	A. P. Bhaduri B. K. Bhat M. Seth
Studies on diphtheria in Bombay *19*, 241 (1975)	M. Bhaindarkar Y. S. Nimbkar
Bitoscanate in children with hookworm disease *19*, 6 (1975)	B. Bhandari L. N. Shrimali
Recent studies on genetic recombination in *Vibriocholerae* *19*, 460 (1975)	K. Bhaskaran
Interbiotype conversion of cholera vibrios by action of mutagens *19*, 466 (1975)	P. Bhattacharya S. Ray
Experience with bitoscanate in hookworm disease and trichuriasis in Mexico *19*, 23 (1975)	F. Biagi

Contributions of medicinal chemistry to medicine – from 1935 *12*, 11 (1968) Changing influences on goals and incentives in drug research and development *20*, 159 (1976) Quaternary ammonium salts – advances in chemistry and pharmacology since 1960 *24*, 267 (1980)	C. J. Cavallito
Über Vorkommen und Bedeutung der Indolstruktur in der Medizin und Biologie *2*, 227 (1960)	A. Cerletti
The new generation of monoamine oxidase inhibitors *38*, 171 (1992)	Andrea M. Cesura Alfred Pletscher
Cholesterol and its relation to atherosclerosis *1*, 127 (1959)	K. K. Chen Tsung-Min Lin
Effect of hookworm disease on the structure and function of small bowel *19*, 44 (1975)	H. K. Chuttani R. C. Misra
The psychomimetic agents *15*, 68 (1971)	S. Cohen
Implementation of disease control in Asia and Africa *18*, 43 (1974)	M. J. Colbourne
Structure-activity relationships in certain anthelmintics *3*, 75 (1961)	J. C. Craig M. E. Tate
Contribution of Haffkine to the concept and practice of controlled field trials of vaccines *19*, 481 (1975)	B. Cvjetanovic
Antifungal agents *22*, 93 (1978)	P. F. D'Arcy E. M. Scott
Carcinogenecity, mutagenecity and cancer preventing activities of flavanoids: A structure-system-activity relationship (SSAR) analysis *42*, 133 (1994)	A. Das J. H. Wang E. J. Lien
Some neuropathologic and cellular aspects of leprosy *18*, 53 (1974)	D. K. Dastur Y. Ramamohan A. S. Dabholkar

Mechanism of action of anxiolytic drugs *31*, 315 (1987)	T. Mennini S. Caccia S. Garattini
Pathogenesis of amebic disease *18*, 225 (1974) Protozoan and helminth parasites – a review of current treatment *20*, 433 (1976)	M. J. Miller
Medicinal agents incorporating the 1,2-diamine functionality *33*, 135 (1989)	Erik T. Michalson Jacob Szmuszkovicz
Fluorinated quinolones-new quinolone antimicrobials *38*, 9 (1992)	S. Mitsuhashi (Editor) T. Kojima, N. Nakanishi, T. Fujimoto, S. Goto, S. Miyusaki, T. Uematsu, M. Nakashima, Y. Asahina, T. Ishisaki, S. Susue, K. Hirai, K. Sato, K. Hoshino, J. Shimada, S. Hori
Synopsis der Rheumatherapie *12*, 165 (1968)	W. Moll
On the chemotherapy of cancer *8*, 431 (1965) The relationship of the metabolism of anticancer agents to their activity *17*, 320 (1973) The current status of cancer chemotherapy *20*, 465 (1976)	J. A. Montgomery
Present status of Leishmaniasis *34*, 447 (1990)	Anita Mukherjee Manju Seth A. P. Bhaduri
The significance of DNA technology in medicine *33*, 397 (1989)	Hansjakob Müller
Der Einfluß der Formgebung auf die Wirkung eines Arzneimittels *10*, 204 (1966) Galenische Formgebung und Arzneimittelwirkung. Neue Erkenntnisse und Feststellungen *14*, 269 (1970)	K. Münzel
A field trial with bitoscanate in India *19*, 81 (1975)	G. S. Mutalik R. B. Gulati A. K. Iqbal

Problems of malaria eradication in India *18*, 245 (1974)	V. N. Rao
Pharmacology of migraine *34*, 209 (1990)	Neil H. Raskin
The photochemistry of drugs and related substances *11*, 48 (1968)	S. T. Reid
Orale Antikoagulantien *11*, 226 (1968)	E. Renk W. G. Stoll
Mechanism-based inhibitors of monoamine oxidase *30*, 205 (1986)	Lauren E. Richards Alfred Burger
The hopanoids, bacterial triterpenoids, and the biosynthesis of isoprenic units in prokaryote *37*, 271 (1991)	Michael Rohner Philippe Bisseret Bertrand Sutter
Tetrahydroisoquinolines and β-carbolines: Putative natural substances in plants and animals *29*, 415 (1985)	H. Rommelspacher R. Susilo
Functional significance of the various components of the influenza virus *18*, 253 (1974)	R. Rott
Drug receptors and control of the cardiovascular system: Recent advances *36*, 117 (1991)	Robert R. Ruffolo Jr J. Paul Hieble David P. Brooks Giora Z. Feuerstein Andrew J. Nichols
Behavioral correlates of presynaptic events in the cholinergic neurotransmitter system *32*, 43 (1988)	Roger W. Russell
Epidemiology of pertussis *19*, 257 (1975)	J. A. Sa
Surgical amoebiasis *18*, 77 (1974)	A. E. de Sa
Role of beta-adrenergic blocking drug propranolol in severe tetanus *19*, 361 (1975)	G. S. Sainani K. L. Jain V. R. D. Deshpande A. B. Balsara S. A. Iyer

Studies on *Vibrio parahaemolyticus* in Bombay *19*, 586 (1975)	F. L. Saldanha A. K. Patil M. V. Sant
Leukotriene antagonists and inhibitors of leukotriene biosynthesis as potential therapeutic agents *37*, 9 (1991)	John A. Salmon Lawrence G. Garland
Pharmacology and toxicology of axoplasmic transport *28*, 53 (1984)	Fred Samson Ralph L. Smith J. Alejandro Donoso
Clinical experience with bitoscanate *19*, 96 (1975)	M. R. Samuel
Tetanus: Situational clinical trials and therapeutics *19*, 367 (1975)	R. K. M. Sanders M. L. Peacock B. Martyn B. D. Shende
Epidemiological studies on cholera in non-endemic regions with special reference to the problem of carrier state during epidemic and non-epidemic period *19*, 594 (1975)	M. V. Sant W. N. Gatlewar S. K. Bhindey
Epidemiological and biochemical studies in filariasis in four villages near Bombay *18*, 269 (1974)	M. V. Sant W. N. Gatlewar T. U. K. Menon
Hookworm anaemia and intestinal malabsorption associated with hookworm infestation *19*, 108 (1975)	A. K. Saraya B. N. Tandon
The effects of structural alteration on the anti-inflammatory properties of hydrocortisone *5*, 11 (1963)	L. H. Sarett A. A. Patchett S. Steelman
The impact of natural product research on drug discovery *23*, 51 (1979)	L. H. Sarett
Aldose reductase inhibitors: Recent developments *40*, 99 (1993)	Reinhard Sarges Peter J. Oates
Anti-filariasis campaign: Its history and future prospects *18*, 259 (1974)	M. Sasa

Pharmacological Sciences:
Perspectives for Research and Therapy in the Late 1990s

Edited by
A.C. Cuello and **B. Collier**
McGill University, Montreal, Quebec, Canada

1995. Approx. 460 pages. Hardcover.
ISBN 3-7643-5072-5

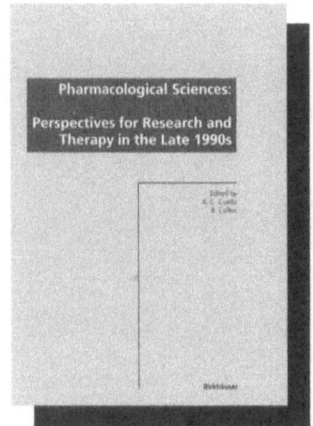

Containing fifty-one outstanding, reviewed chapters, this volume presents a comprehensive picture of the research challenges and novel therapies emerging as we approach the year 2000.

Highly distinguished scientists, all at the very forefront of their fields, were invited to condense into succinct surveys their plenary lectures and symposia from the *XIIth International Congress of Pharmacology*, Montreal, 1994. Highlighting the current developments and future directions in the pharmacological sciences, the chapters span the entire scope from molecular mechanisms to clinical use. They enable the reader to acquire, very rapidly, a panorama of the numerous fields of research. These include drug receptors; signal transduction; ion channels; drug metabolism; neuropharmacology; purines; cardiovascular, endocrine and pulmonary pharmacology; nitric oxide; immunopharmacology; the pharmacology of gene expression; chemotherapy; toxicology; regulatory requirements for drug registration, and pharmacological and instructional methods.

All researchers, teachers, clinicians and graduate students in basic and clinical pharmacology as well as related areas in biochemistry, physiology and pharmacy will find this highly authoritative volume an inspiring and invaluable reference.

Birkhäuser

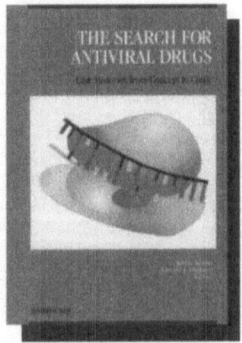

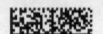